# On trial

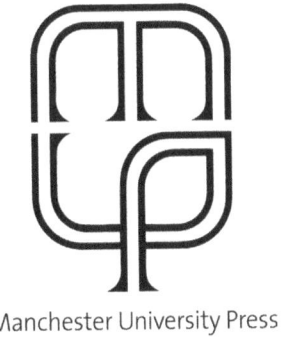

# SOCIAL HISTORIES OF MEDICINE

Series Editors
David Cantor, Anne Hanley and Elaine Leong

Editorial Board
Diego Armus, Swarthmore College, PA, USA
Rana Hogarth, University of Illinois, Urbana-Champaign, USA
Angela Ki Che Leung, University of Hong Kong, China
Ian Miller, Ulster University, Northern Ireland

*Social Histories of Medicine* is concerned with all aspects of health, illness and medicine, from prehistory to the present, in every part of the world. The series covers the circumstances that promote health or illness, the ways in which people experience and explain such conditions, and what, practically, they do about them. Practitioners of all approaches to health and healing come within its scope, as do their ideas, beliefs, and practices, and the social, economic and cultural contexts in which they operate. Methodologically, the series welcomes relevant studies in social, economic, cultural, and intellectual history, as well as approaches derived from other disciplines in the arts, sciences, social sciences and humanities. The series is a collaboration between Manchester University Press and the Society for the Social History of Medicine.

To buy or to find out more about the books currently available in this series, please go to: https://manchesteruniversitypress.co.uk/series/social-histories-of-medicine/

# On trial

## Testing new drugs in psychiatry, 1940–1980

Marietta Meier,
Mario König, and Magaly Tornay

with the collaboration of Ursina Klauser
and translated by Bernard Heise

MANCHESTER UNIVERSITY PRESS

Copyright © Marietta Meier, Mario König, and Magaly Tornay 2024

The right of Marietta Meier, Mario König, and Magaly Tornay to be identified as the authors of this work has been asserted in accordance with the Copyright, Designs and Patents Act 1988.

Published by Manchester University Press
Oxford Road, Manchester, M13 9PL

www.manchesteruniversitypress.co.uk

British Library Cataloguing-in-Publication Data
A catalogue record for this book is available from the British Library

ISBN 978 1 5261 6980 8 hardback
ISBN 978 1 5261 9482 4 paperback

First published 2024
Paperback published 2026

The publisher has no responsibility for the persistence or accuracy of URLs for any external or third-party internet websites referred to in this book, and does not guarantee that any content on such websites is, or will remain, accurate or appropriate.

EU authorised representative for GPSR:
Easy Access System Europe – Mustamäe tee 50,
10621 Tallinn, Estonia
gpsr.requests@easproject.com

Typeset by Newgen Publishing UK

# Contents

| | |
|---|---|
| *List of figures* | *page* vi |
| *Preface* | vii |
| *Acknowledgements* | ix |
| *List of abbreviations* | xii |
| Introduction | 1 |
| 1 The 1940s: The ball gets rolling | 18 |
| 2 The 1950s: Testing frenzy with Geigy | 48 |
| 3 Test patients | 92 |
| 4 The 1960s: A flood of substances and new dimensions of testing | 117 |
| 5 Substance logistics, information streams, and money flows | 168 |
| 6 The 1970s: Between doldrums and success | 195 |
| 7 Fatal incidents | 229 |
| 8 The 1980s: A long, restless finale | 249 |
| Conclusion | 280 |
| *Chronology* | 302 |
| *List of test substances* | 307 |
| *Bibliography* | 317 |
| *Index* | 337 |

# Figures

1.1 Clinic with lakeshore and fence, around 1950 (StATG, 9'40, 11.7/0) *page* 19
1.2 Roland and Verena Kuhn at a congress in Rome, 1958 (StATG, 9'40, 8.0/311, 312, 6) 34
2.1 Advertising brochure for Tofranil, 1969 (CA Novartis) 55
3.1 Drawing test by Franz Traber, 1965 (StATG, ZA KAs 18405) 93
3.2 'Not eye to eye', trainee nurses scrubbing the floor, 1960 (photo album of a former trainee nurse) 102
4.1 Roland Kuhn ('Daddy-Long-Legs') with staff, 1961 (photo album of Marlies Verhofnik) 155
5.1 Metal boxes with three different test substances, late 1960s (StATG, 9'40, 15.2/0; 9'40, 15.2/1; 9'40, 15.2/10) 173
5.2 Test substances with at least 25,000 delivered units, 1946–1980 (calculations based on StATG, 9'10 and 9'40, especially 9'40, 5) 174
6.1 Ludio and Mili, Carnival 1979 (StATG, 9'10, 1.7.0.1/5) 196
7.1 Corridor of a ward for chronically ill and disabled women, 1980 (StATG, 9'10, 1.7.0/3) 232
8.1 Roland Kuhn's desk drawer, 2013 (StATG, office archive) 250

# Preface

It was a brisk spring day in 2016 as five historians boarded a train to meet Roland Kuhn, the famous 'father' of the first antidepressant – or, more precisely, his vestiges. Waiting for us in the Thurgau State Archives in Frauenfeld, Switzerland was a newly accessible treasure trove of immense historical value: the private archive of Kuhn and his wife Verena. A few years earlier, the media had shone a scandalous spotlight on the drug trials that Kuhn had conducted at the Münsterlingen Psychiatric Clinic and criticised his approach as unethical. It was now our job to look into these testing practices.[1]

At the Thurgau State Archives, we were led to the first basement level, where the aforementioned private archive is stored. It makes an imposing sight. The files are packed into 457 cartons, which together run to 45 linear metres. We pulled a few cartons off the shelf. They contained massive amounts of paper, sheets in A4 format, along with numerous carbon copies, letters, notes of various sizes, daily calendar sheets filled with entries, used letter envelopes, and deposit slips. A few notes with red writing immediately caught the eye. As soon as we had deciphered the first one it became clear that Kuhn was talking to us: 'The files per se are worthless, but are of substantial scientific-historical interest and therefore should be preserved!'

As we would quickly notice, Roland Kuhn had used a ruler to mark important concepts and passages, sometimes with red ink; the combination of red, double-underlining, and exclamation marks was thus an especially urgent signal. The note signed by 'Prof. R. Kuhn' had been written exactly twelve years ago – a day on which the 92-year-old had evidently gone through his documents again, rearranging them, writing messages for posterity, and thereby preparing for his own historicisation. In so doing, he probably had a different goal in mind than the one we were tackling that spring day. Concerned about his fame, he had been hoping for due recognition of his achievements in psychopharmacology. But in the meantime, there had been a sea change in societal thought, which challenged medical authority, raised ethical questions, and placed greater priority on patient rights. His clinical trials, which we were now poised to investigate, appeared in a different, more ambivalent light.

### Note

1 The team initially consisted of Marietta Meier (project management), Mario König, Magaly Tornay, and two junior researchers, Ursina Klauser and Francesco Spöring, who subsequently pursued their own projects. Ursina Klauser remained closely affiliated with the book project and gave it substantial support.

# Acknowledgements

*On trial* grew out of a research project that was supported by many people and institutions, and we would like to thank them here. The translation is a slightly shortened and updated version of *Testfall Münsterlingen: Klinische Versuche in der Psychiatrie, 1940–1980* (Zurich, Chronos: 2019).

To begin with, we would like to express our gratitude to the team at the Thurgau State Archives. Our project was only possible because the state archivist André Salathé campaigned to have the private archive of Roland and Verena Kuhn brought to Frauenfeld and to secure funding for a historical research project. The archive employees, who through years of careful work organised and indexed the private archive, created the preconditions that enabled our historical research in the first place. Knowledgeable and keen, Kim de Solda, Beat Oswald, André Salathé, Urban Stäheli, and Erich Trösch consistently stood by us during our source work and research. During the final phase, Nathalie Kolb helped to edit the manuscript and Martin Polt took over the photography and the processing of the illustrations. At the historical archive of Novartis we were graciously supported by Carole Billod, Walter Dettwiler, Philipp Gafner, and Florence Wicker; at the company's clinical and research archives, Felix Brugger, Maha Khaled, Matthias Leuenberger, and Robert Sieber did the same. We were advised by Alexander Bieri at the Roche archive, and by Andreas Altorfer at the archive of the Psychiatry Museum in Bern. Swissmedic, the Münsterlingen Psychiatric Clinic, and *Der Schweizerische Beobachter* all gave us access to specific holdings. We also extend our immense gratitude to the many contemporary witnesses who came forward and shared their memories with us; their interviews gave us invaluable information and perspectives on the Münsterlingen trial site.

Our project was aided by an advisory group of representatives and experts from various disciplines, and we would like to thank them for their support, feedback, and specialised assistance: Rainer Andenmatten (pharmacology), Monika Dommann (history), Thomas Geiser (law), Daniel Hell (psychiatry), Andreas Keller (general secretary of the Department for Internal and Economic Affairs of the Canton of Thurgau), Stephan Krähenbühl (pharmacology), Martha Monstein (head of the Cultural Office of the Canton of Thurgau), André Salathé (advisory group president at the Thurgau State Archives), and Urban Stäheli (advisory group secretary at the Thurgau State Archives). The chemist Daniela Hoegger, the legal expert Margot Michel, and the historian of medicine Maike Rotzoll stood at our beck and call with their expertise. We discussed our initial results and research questions with a group of historians – Cornelius Borck, Cornelia Brink, Monika Dommann, Maike Rotzoll, Carola Sachse, and Jakob Tanner – as part of a workshop. Francesco Spöring collaborated on the project during the first year and contributed substantially to the groundwork; Niklaus Müller conducted research for us and read the manuscript during the final phase. Joanna Haupt and Florian Müller took care of the economic-historical calculations, and we thank Stefan Klauser and Gerold Ritter for their IT assistance. We discussed specific issues and larger interconnections with a range of other people, particularly Beat Bächi, Thomas Bein, Anna Joss, Oliver König, Luzia Meier, and Felix Waldmeier, with whom we exchanged ideas about material traces and sources, medical questions, and daseinsanalysis. Bernard Heise translated this book skilfully and the lottery fund of the Canton of Thurgau generously financed the translation, and Meredith Carroll and David Cantor carefully oversaw its publication with Manchester University Press.

This book is the result of a close, fruitful collaboration. In this respect, we would especially like to thank Ursina Klauser and Mario König. Ursina Klauser initially worked in the project as a junior academic. After she had subsequently accepted her dissertation fellowship, she nonetheless remained closely linked with us, read all of the chapters, and demonstrated great circumspection and knowledge of her field. When Mario König fell ill, she came to our aid as soon as we needed help. It is in large part thanks to her that our book was completed more or less on time. We are sad that Mario König never managed to hold the published book in his hands. He was a wonderful, spirited colleague, and over the last few years he also became our friend. We thank him for all that we lived through together and deeply appreciate that he ultimately entrusted us with our collective book.

# Abbreviations

| | |
|---|---|
| ARM | annual report, Münsterlingen Psychiatric Clinic |
| CA | company archive |
| FDA | Food and Drug Administration |
| FMH | Foederatio Medicorum Helveticorum (Swiss Medical Association) |
| HAR | Roche Historical Collection and Archive |
| HLS | *Historisches Lexikon der Schweiz* |
| IKS | Interkantonale Kontrollstelle für Heilmittel (Intercantonal Office for the Control of Medicines; now Swissmedic) |
| KA | medical file |
| KAa | outpatient medical file |
| KAs | inpatient medical file |
| PKM | Psychiatrische Klinik Münsterlingen (Münsterlingen Psychiatric Clinic) |
| SAMS | Swiss Academy of Medical Sciences |
| StATG | Staatsarchiv des Kantons Thurgau (Thurgau State Archives) |
| WHO | World Health Organization |
| ZA | Zwischenarchiv (transitional archive) |

# Introduction

Medications are everywhere today. Before a drug comes onto the market, it must be tested – not only on healthy subjects, but also on patients with symptoms or diseases against which the relevant substance is supposed to be used, for a chemical substance does not reveal its effectiveness on its own. It is only turned into a medication if its effects can be identified, evaluated, and established. Thus the course of substance testing includes deliberations, negotiations, and rejections. The path from the laboratory to potential market readiness is long, and, in the case of psychotropic drugs, it passes through psychiatric clinics. That is the subject of this book. Based on the Münsterlingen Psychiatric Clinic in eastern Switzerland, where a large number of substances were tested over decades, this is the first detailed account of how clinical trials were conducted in psychiatry.

Apart from chemical substances, many further actors are involved in the multilayered process of making sense of drugs.[1] Hence, clinical research, especially in psychiatry, takes place in a field of tensions – between economic, scientific, ethical, and therapeutic interests; between the individual and society; between law, guidelines, and the need for safety and the understanding that clinical studies always entail residual risk. In other words: clinical trials are ambivalent and also raise ethical questions, which recede to the background, however, as soon as chemical substances are turned into approved products. This ambivalence has also shaped the image of the internationally renowned psychiatrist Roland Kuhn. Hailed by many as the 'discoverer' of the first antidepressant Tofranil (imipramine), Kuhn was the driving force behind the Münsterlingen trials. But in Switzerland after his death in 2005, his reputation as a researcher began to tarnish as journalists and concerned individuals spoke out, criticising him for conducting experiments under ethically questionable, scientifically dubious conditions. In the end, his experiments became the subject of a heated public debate. Roland Kuhn left behind a private archive that for the first time offers the opportunity to examine the practices of clinical trials up close. These holdings are the most important source material for our book, almost every page of which mentions his name. Even so, in our view Kuhn should be understood as only a part of the 'trial operation', as a node in a network of actors and substances. *On trial* therefore goes beyond a biographical perspective. The focus is on how knowledge about the possible psychoactive effects of substances was produced at the Münsterlingen trial site, which practices were applied in the process, and what changes can be identified for the three decades after the Second World War. How were effects determined and objectivised, and which actors were involved in the process? In what ways did trial practices in the clinic and on the part of the pharmaceutical industry change, and how were these modification processes related?

The trials at the Münsterlingen Psychiatric Clinic in eastern Switzerland will therefore be historically situated. Clinical research and the pharmaceutical industry have changed considerably since the end of the Second World War, but so too have medicine, psychiatry, pharmaceutics, and society. New research methods have been developed, norms and regulations set in place. Therefore, it is important not to assess clinical trials against seemingly self-evident, immutable criteria but rather to historicise the latter just like the trials themselves. Only then can we evaluate and contextualise Kuhn's research.

In terms of methodology and theory, this study locates itself in the history of knowledge, which is closely linked to the history of science and science and technology studies. An important result of historical research into science and technology over recent decades has been the widening and pluralisation of the understanding of knowledge. Knowledge has since come to be understood as everything that historical actors defined or accepted as knowledge. This has fundamentally shifted research interests and perspectives. The focus is no longer on the history of scientific discoveries and theories but rather on the practical dimensions of the production and circulation of knowledge. Locations, infrastructures, instruments, and recording and classification systems come into view in the same manner as the interactions and negotiation processes between varying groups of actors. The goal is to investigate the generation of knowledge as a temporally, spatially, and culturally specific process that is closely linked to political, social, and economic factors.[2] Proceeding with such an approach, *On trial* combines a micro-historical analysis of the way in which knowledge about the effects of psychoactive substances was produced in a specific clinic with an investigation into the local, regional, national, and international conditions under which these practices were applied.

## State of research

Our study interweaves the local, situated history of a clinic in eastern Switzerland with the international development of clinical trials of psychotropic drugs. Münsterlingen, a completely 'normal' psychiatric clinic with a regional service mission, intersects with globally aligned pharmaceutical companies based in Basel. One of the central developments of the second half of the twentieth century – the rise of psychotropic drugs – was advanced not just by the laboratories and marketing divisions of the pharmaceutical industry but also in clinics like Münsterlingen. Thus the book examines local practices as part of a decentralised but clearly Western-dominated history of broader dimensions.[3] Which patients stood at the start of the long chain of people who have received a dose of a psychoactive substance such as Tofranil and still take it today? How exactly was its effect determined? And what substances were tested – perhaps on a large scale – but were then forgotten because they were deemed a failure?

Studies on clinical testing in psychiatry are a desideratum of research. Admittedly, such trials have started to come under public scrutiny in recent years in the German-speaking world, which has resulted in a series of studies on individual clinics or regions that have provided the historical groundwork. From a praxeological or epistemological perspective, however, the history of clinical trials in psychiatry remains largely unwritten.[4] *On trial* helps close this gap.

At the same time, however, it builds on studies from other research fields that extend from the history of pharmacology and psychiatry to the history of the pharmaceutical industry and human experiments. Historical scholarship on modern psychotropic drugs started in the 1990s. As is often the case, the first publications came from historians of medicine or people who personally worked in this field, and they often adopted an industry-focused perspective. Noteworthy are Edward Shorter's history of psychiatry, which tends to argue in terms of historical progress,[5] and the publications of David Healy. The latter are mostly based on interviews with contemporary witnesses of the development of psychotropic drugs, which were published in three volumes. Appearing in 1997 was *The Antidepressant Era*, in which Healy shows how depression developed into one of the most frequently diagnosed mental disorders and antidepressants became a booming business. This was followed in 2002 by the study *The Creation of Psychopharmacology*, which focused on the development of antipsychotic substances and their consequences.[6] Additional materials and commentary – including from Roland Kuhn – appeared in four anthologies.[7]

There is an abundance of literature on mental disorders, especially on depression, which was Kuhn's main bailiwick. Conceptually challenging contributions on the social contouring of the depression diagnosis – *The Weariness of the Self* by Alain Ehrenberg, for example – and on the cultural stabilisation of antidepressants have come from France.[8] At the heart of these studies is the question of whether more and more people actually suffer from depressive disorders or if it is only the willingness to diagnose depressions that has grown. Joanna Moncrieff, Martin Dornes, and Jonathan Sadowksy have also dealt with the sociopolitical backgrounds of such illnesses and their medication.[9]

Viola Balz, Sabine Braunschweig, and Benoît Majerus have dealt with the testing of the first neuroleptic drugs in psychiatric clinics and shown how the psychopharmacological turn changed the routines of everyday nursing. They relied on medical files and interviews for this purpose.[10] Marietta Meier's book on the history of psychosurgery after the Second World War provides a look into the operating principle of psychiatric clinics and clinical research that is based on an in-depth examination of case and clinical files.[11]

For her study on psychotropic drugs, Magaly Tornay used, among other things, sources from the pharmaceutical industry and the Münsterlingen clinic, and in the process also dealt with Roland Kuhn's experiments.[12]

Also central for *On trial* were works on the history of the pharmaceutical industry. Whereas various investigations have focused more on specific substances than on the history of the industry, Mario König has provided a comprehensive survey on the development of the chemical industry in Basel.[13] Internal company sources on marketing strategy were analysed for the first time in an anthology on scientific marketing.[14] Jeremy A. Greene has comprehensively dealt with the sales and branding strategies of pharmaceutical companies in the United States, while David Herzberg has investigated the interplay between various social connotations of narcotics and medications.[15] Jean-Paul Gaudillière, Volker Hess, and Arthur Daemmrich have provided groundwork on the history of regulation.[16]

An entire series of works, some by investigative journalists, has examined the history of human experiments, the testing on particularly vulnerable population groups, and the associated ethical questions.[17] With *The Progress of Experiment*, Harry M. Marks produced a standard work on the experimentalisation of medicine.[18] Erika Dyck and Emmanuel Delille have recently published an overview on human experimentation in psychiatry, while around a decade earlier Edward Shorter provided an illuminating outline on the role of placebos in clinical trials.[19]

## Sources and source criticism

There is no direct access to the past that we are tracking down in this book, only traces – texts, objects, pictures, and recountable memories – that can be analysed and pieced together into a history. Such traces form the basis of every historical study; the view of the past is therefore also shaped by the sources. A multitude of archives, holdings, and types of sources were consulted for *On trial* – apart from Kuhn's private archive, also medical records and other files of the Münsterlingen Psychiatric Clinic; archives of the pharmaceutical industry and the Intercantonal Office for the Control of

Medicines (now Swissmedic); conversations with contemporary witnesses; and specialised publications and media reports.

The mainstay of the project was the extensive private archive of Roland and Verena Kuhn, which was placed in the Thurgau State Archives in 2012/2013. It includes a section entitled *Fonds zur Psychopharmakologie* (psychopharmacological holdings), which documents the clinical trials and consists of twenty-four archive boxes. These holdings contain the test reports to the pharmaceutical companies, the accompanying correspondence, and a wide range of other documents created during the trials, including numerous handwritten notes and lists with the names of patients who were given test substances. In addition, the private archive contains large inventories of correspondence, medical files, manuscripts for publications and lectures, files from Kuhn's teaching activities, and documents relating to his time as clinical director. Verena Kuhn's papers are comparatively modest; her activities are far more poorly documented in these holdings than those of her spouse.

Also playing an important role is the archive of the Münsterlingen Psychiatric Clinic, which contains files from the period 1840–1980. The extensive inventory of medical files, which consists of approximately 15,000 inpatient and 15,000 outpatient dossiers, is extremely valuable.[20] Many of these files contain nursing reports and tables that provide information about the administration of pharmacological substances that are not noted in the actual medical histories. The preservation of such sources was by no means standard practice; they are often missing from the medical files of other clinics.

Apart from the medical files, the clinic archive also contains directorate and administrative files, which provide an insight into clinic operations and the collaboration with other institutions; the bookkeeping records are missing, however. The clinic comes into view from another perspective in the archives of the cantonal health office and medical services department. Located here, for example, are documents of the supervisory commission for the hospitals, but there are also additional documents that show how communications occurred through and with the Münsterlingen clinic.

The excellent sources in the Canton of Thurgau contrast with the records of the pharmaceutical companies Kuhn worked with – primarily the predecessor companies of Novartis: Geigy,

Ciba, Ciba-Geigy, Sandoz, and Wander, which gradually merged starting in the late 1960s.[21] Notwithstanding the support of Novartis, the sources proved to be fragmentary and heterogeneous, which was due in part to the many mergers, something that evidently had a negative impact on the written record.[22]

The holdings of the Novartis historical archive document the committees at the middle or higher level of the corporate hierarchy. The closer to the executive level, the greater the focus is on marketing and country reports; psychopharmaceutical products are rarely discussed. The research and the clinical trials are hardly documented, while the name of an investigator only emerges every now and then. Often an interesting series of annual reports or committee minutes will break off after a short time without it being clear whether this was due to organisational reforms or disruptions of the written record. But despite the fragmentary transmission, the documents we found are very important, for they fill significant gaps that Kuhn's private archive leaves unresolved.

It was long unclear whether, apart from its historical archive, Novartis had any other archival holdings. It turned out that the company has clinical and research archives as well, but with almost no records predating the 1970s. The few exceptions we caught sight of were evidently fragments that had survived by chance. Along with plenty of insignificant material, a few relevant documents emerged here too, for example, documents from Wander in which company employees discuss Kuhn with unusual candour.

Despite these gaps and complications, working with the sources at Novartis offered an important, complementary perspective, especially with regard to marketing strategies and the development of psychopharmaceuticals. Thanks to the holdings in Basel, we could clearly reconstruct how the pharmaceutical industry reacted to increasing international regulation and how this process affected the status of Kuhn's trials. The survival of a dossier with payments transferred to Kuhn by Geigy and Ciba-Geigy is owed to chance; it supplements the information available in his private archive.

Less fruitful, on the other hand, was the source research at Swissmedic, formerly the Intercantonal Office for the Control of Medicines, which today is responsible for the approval and monitoring of medicines in Switzerland. Once Novartis declared its agreement to having Swissmedic allow us access to the granted approval applications for substances that its predecessor companies had tested in Münsterlingen, we were able to examine the records in the approval dossiers. These records contain documents that the pharmaceutical companies wanted to use to substantiate the effectiveness and harmlessness of the tested products.[23] However, we were not permitted to view the associated correspondence because it might include patent-protected information on drugs for which file access was not approved. Documents such as patient information leaflets were copied for us. More extensive information, pertaining, for example, to approval applications that were denied, could not be gained because a close inspection of the archive was impossible. We were also prevented from viewing the private accounting records and social insurance information of Roland and Verena Kuhn, which might hold further information on remunerations from the pharmaceutical industry.

Along with working with written sources, we also conducted discussions with contemporary witnesses, which showed the Kuhns as a married couple and the Münsterlingen clinic from yet another perspective. We spoke with twenty-four people in personal meetings and conducted twenty-nine telephone interviews. It was important for us to speak with the broadest possible spectrum of contemporary witnesses – former patients, nurses, assistant physicians, pharmaceutical industry employees, and politicians, as well as fellow specialists who likewise had conducted clinical trials.[24]

The memories reported by our interlocutors deviated greatly at times. This is unsurprising, given that the role of an outpatient differs substantially from that of a senior nurse or of a physician employed in a pharmaceutical company's research division. Moreover, memories are always subjective in nature. But if one surveys the various discussions from a distance, two general points stand out. First, the interviews show the great ambivalence with which Roland Kuhn is remembered. Apparently, he was a very polarising figure. Second, it becomes clear that the everyday – often oppressive – experiences people had in the clinic etched themselves more deeply into their memory than did the tests. Hardly anything could be learned from the interviews about testing practices and the concrete circumstances in which trial preparations were discussed, administered, and evaluated.

## Introduction

What conclusions can we draw in light of all of these holdings? On the one hand, we are dealing with an undoubtedly unique body of sources. We looked at a massive quantity of files; the sources are extremely diverse, rich, fruitful, and by no means fully explored. This abundance makes it possible to uncover contradictions; what Kuhn wrote was often inconsistent with what he did. His private archive is invaluable, for it contains – along with many other items – reports and correspondence on successful and less successful trials, as well as plenty of information on how the effectiveness of psychoactive substances was established. In addition, it provides an insight into Kuhn's extensive network of contacts and a plethora of patient names, which open the path to numerous medical files. There, one can find much more information on the trials, which also leads beyond Kuhn's private archive and Münsterlingen.[25]

On the other hand, it must be noted that the available holdings also have gaps. Thanks to the abundance of sources, gaps emerged that would otherwise not have been detectable. Thus we soon noticed that certain incidents were not systematically recorded. In patient dossiers, for example, we came upon test preparations without finding the names of the corresponding persons in the trial-related material of Kuhn's private archive; conversely, however, we also saw medical files of test patients[26] in which no test substances are documented. Thus the aspiration for quantitative completeness could not be achieved because of the nature of the sources.

In other words, we could not precisely determine how many patients were involved in the trials and how many test substances made their way to Münsterlingen. For some trials, one will never be able to say exactly when they began and when they ended. The plan to register all patients who received test preparations also could not be realised. We registered all of the test patients who could be found and identified in the psychopharmacological holdings of Kuhn's private archive, but we know that this group by far does not include all of the persons who were administered test substances.[27] Thus the question about the dimensions of the trials can only be answered approximately. Nonetheless, the surviving sources provide for an abundance of findings: on the course of the testing, on the transformation of clinical trials, on the role of the patients, and on the microcosm of the clinic.

## Approach and method

If one wants to take account of the interdependency of clinic, research, and industry, one must analyse how these specifically interacted. *On trial* reconstructs this interaction by looking at a variety of types of sources. Because the groups of sources were all created in different contexts and therefore also pursued different goals and logics, we assign an important role to filtering and translation processes. For example, we investigate how information from nursing records found its way into reports or published research results, which have a very different degree of practical relevance, formalisation, and scientification. To shine light on Kuhn's trials from different perspectives, we look at various actors, their statements, and their conduct while varying the level of analysis. This should clearly show – as per our goal – the multifaceted process of testing chemical substances and 'making' new drugs.

But how was this plan implemented? In a first step, we worked through the psychopharmacological holdings of Kuhn's private archive. All test substances and persons that, according to the inspected sources, received test preparations were registered in a database. Because the Thurgau State Archives and the Münsterlingen Psychiatric Clinic contain thousands of inpatient and outpatient medical files, we decided on a database in which information on substances could be linked with that on test patients, and we defined criteria so as to compile a sample of test patients that, qualitatively, is as representative as possible. If, apart from a legible name, further information was available (for example, a detailed case description or indications of severe side-effects), we registered this as well. If enough information was already available to assess the relevance of a case, we assigned it one of three priorities. This determined the order in which to process the medical files.[28]

In a second step, we went through all of the cases assigned one of the three priorities and compiled a sample of patients who were administered test substances. The goal was to process all first-priority cases as well as a selection of second- and third-priority cases. If we encountered indications that a person had died during or soon after the administration of test substances or suffered from severe side-effects, this person was included as a first-priority case. To achieve maximum heterogeneity, we supplemented the cases of first priority with those of second and third priority – and ultimately also with non-priority cases. The selection was based on factors such as diagnosis, social origin, and the number or nature of the administered test substances. In the end, we processed the medical files of approximately 150 people. This is around one eighth of the cases that are registered in Kuhn's private archive, a fraction of the patients who were administered test substances, and an even smaller fraction of the persons who were treated at Münsterlingen between 1945 and 1980.

At least sixty-seven substances were tested in Münsterlingen. If one counts substances that were retested or ones for which it is unclear whether testing occurred after a pharmaceutical company made an inquiry or delivery, then the number is almost 120. The period of the testing extended from the second half of the 1940s until into the 1980s; Kuhn therefore also conducted tests during his tenure as clinical director and after his retirement from the clinic. Although he primarily worked with Basel chemical companies, he also trialled test preparations of other companies. The trials varied widely; on one end of the spectrum were rapid tests on individual inpatients; on the other, there were multiyear, large-scale studies involving hundreds of inpatients and outpatients.

Thus well over 1,000 patients were involved in the tests. At certain times, more than half of the clinic's residents must have been receiving test preparations. The spectrum of affected persons is broad, reaching from severely ill inpatients, to outpatients stemming from all segments of Thurgau's population, to private patients from abroad. Many people were involved in multiple tests. Some received various test substances simultaneously; more frequently, however, test preparations were combined with registered substances. Certain preparations were used for years on end without anyone keeping trial-appropriate records of them. Certain remedies were still being delivered to Kuhn even after the company had stopped testing them. In other words, clinical testing and therapy flowed seamlessly from one to the other.

Many findings presented in this book reveal practices and ideas that stand diametrically opposed to those that prevail today, whether these are ideas about clinical trial procedures, the role of supervisory authorities, or the appropriate handling of patients. The closer something is to people – thematically, temporally, geographically – the more they tend to take it for granted and to believe that it has always existed everywhere. This study scrutinises such assumptions (for example, the idea of cross-temporal and cross-cultural norms) and shows that they are made, historically evolved, and thus also mutable. It places Kuhn's tests as far as possible into a larger context, which does not mean, however, that everything can be reduced to a so-called *Zeitgeist*. *On trial* seeks neither to valorise nor to demonise, but rather to work out differentiated subtleties. In the testing at the Münsterlingen clinic, medical, scientific, social, ethical, legal, and other fields intersect, all of which changed in the course of the long investigation period. If one looks closely, it becomes apparent that ostensibly clear boundaries (for instance, between research and therapy or between scientific and financial interests) could shift or dissolve or only came to exist in the course of time.

The longtime fluidity of the boundaries between the therapeutic and experimental application of substances can also be seen from the terminology that was used. In Münsterlingen, new medications were first referred to as *Präparate* (preparations); therapies and experiments were called *Kuren* (cures). Hence, we speak in the book about substances, or preparations that were either approved – then they were described as *Medikamente* (medications) or *Arzneimittel* (medicinal products) – or not. If terms like test, trial, experiment, or test substance are used, we do not rule out that the administration occurred for therapeutic purposes. If a case seems unequivocal, we point this out. The transitions between therapy and research and between test preparation and medication are sometimes fluid – as is shown simply by the fact that previously approved substances were also tested for new indications.

History is not a court of law; historians evaluate, but they do not judge. This book illustrates the perspectives of various historical actors and compares them with each other. Our goal is to reconstruct, analyse, and interpret statements, practices, events, processes, and structures, and to shape the results of our research into a story that stimulates reflection and discussion. We strive for as much precision and clarity as possible, but present our actors in terms of their different facets, illuminating one or the other depending on the context. In this way we try to create a reflective distance that facilitates the historical analysis and critical scrutiny

# Introduction

of the oft-invoked assumption of progress – for example, in clinical research or state supervision. In short, we assume responsible readers will form their own opinion.

## Structure

*On trial* combines a chronological structure with a thematic one. Apart from the Introduction and Conclusion, the book contains eight chapters. Three extensive main chapters deal with three decades (the 1950s, 1960s, and 1970s), portraying the various stages of clinical research and the trials at the Münsterlingen Psychiatric Clinic. In between are three shorter longitudinal sections dedicated to three key thematic areas. These six chapters are flanked by a prologue on the 1940s and an epilogue on the 1980s, which deal with the beginnings and the end of Kuhn's trials.

Chapter 1 introduces several of the important actors: the Münsterlingen Psychiatric Clinic, its location and institutional context, the patients, and the clinic staff. Key roles are played by Roland and Verena Kuhn, Director Adolf Zolliker, as well as the Basel pharmaceutical industry and its development in the first half of the twentieth century. Parpanit, a substance made by the Geigy company for the alleviation of movement disorders that arrived in Münsterlingen in 1946, ultimately kicks off the roundelay of test substances. The testing of this preparation established the collaboration between Kuhn and Geigy; the trial would be followed by a longer series of additional tests.

Chapter 2 deals with the early stages of psychopharmaceutical research in Münsterlingen, which started in the 1950s. It tells the story of the arrival of the first neuroleptic drug from the perspective of Münsterlingen, rewriting the well-known 'discovery narrative' of the first antidepressant. Using new sources, it also shows how the development of Tofranil turned into a battle over ranking orders and intellectual authorship. The first Geigy substances still evoked great enthusiasm in Münsterlingen. But then, as the serial testing of a second generation of Geigy preparations failed to yield successes, a certain scepticism spread.

Chapter 3 looks at a large, heterogeneous group of actors: the patients of the Münsterlingen Psychiatric Clinic. It reveals the breadth of the range of persons who were treated at the clinic over time, investigates to whom test substances were administered, and works out various patterns in the process. This makes it possible to get a sense of the broad spectrum of test patients and explain why patients perceived and assessed the administration of test preparations very differently.

Chapter 4 deals with the 1960s, a time of intensive, sprawling trials and large numbers of test substances, which followed directly from the 'discoveries' of the 1950s and which in Münsterlingen was characterised by the search for a better, more specific antidepressant. For Kuhn, the development of clinical research in the 1960s had an ambivalent effect: He was still in demand as an investigator. But at the same time, signs were growing that he could not keep up with the increasing standardisation and regulation of clinical research.

Chapter 5 examines three different types of flows that arose through the clinical trials and simultaneously fostered them: flows of material, information, and finances. The pharmaceutical industry provided test preparations and pharmacological and toxicological reports; it transferred money and received orders for substances. Kuhn organised the flow of information and material in the clinic; he administered substances to patients, passed on preparations to their relatives, clinical staff, and other physicians, reported to companies and colleagues on his test results, and read specialised literature. Because the various preparations, items of information, and money went in very different directions, a highly ramified network emerged that extended far beyond the Basel–Münsterlingen line.

Chapter 6 concentrates on the 1970s, a phase of economic and social upheaval that also entailed major changes in the pharmaceutical industry, increased regulation in the area of medicinal products, and the definitive transformation of the clinical trial. Kuhn was now the clinical director, with new responsibilities, and he had to contend with problems internal and external to the clinic. Did the Münsterlingen trials come to an end under these circumstances? Or did testing continue under changed conditions? These are the questions at the heart of this chapter.

Chapter 7 deals with fatal incidents – with patients who received test substances and died during or shortly after the substances' administration. The focus here is not so much on the cause of death itself, but on how Roland Kuhn handled the fatalities, what he attributed them to, and how he provided information about them. His response is then compared with the reactions of other actors – pharmaceutical companies, other physicians, and other clinics. Since the individual cases being analysed are from four different decades, they can also be examined with regard to whether the deaths of test patients were handled differently over time.

Chapter 8 begins with Kuhn's retirement from the clinic in 1980, which at the same time signified his transition into private practice. It deals with Kuhn's last trial and his plans and activities as a pensioner, but also with the scandal surrounding another Thurgau doctor who had administered test preparations to residents of a retirement and nursing home. The idea of writing a history of the development of psychopharmaceuticals first emerged in the 1990s. Kuhn went to great lengths to enter the annals of history with his 'discovery'. At the same time, this nascent historicisation motivated him to deal once more with the reams of paper he had collected during the course of his career.

## Notes

1 Regarding the approach of 'making sense of drugs', see Pignarre, *Psychotrope Kräfte*. On substances as actors, see Van der Geest et al., 'The Anthropology of Pharmaceuticals'.
2 See Burke, *What is the History of Knowledge?*; Lässig, 'The History of Knowledge'; Daston, 'The History of Science'.
3 On the outsourcing of clinical trials to countries with fewer regulations, see Petryna, 'Ethical Variability'; Ehlers, *Europa und die Schlafkrankheit*. On the global perspective, see Petryna et al., *Global Pharmaceuticals*.
4 For Switzerland, see Akermann et al., *Kinder im Klosterheim*; Germann, *Medikamentenprüfungen*; Rietmann et al., ' "Wenn Ihr Medikament" '; Richli, *Bericht über den Umgang mit Arzneimittelversuchen*; Lienhard and Condrau, *Psychopharmakologische Versuche*. For a survey of further studies from the German-speaking world, see Germann, 'Medikamentenversuche'.
5 Shorter, *A History of Psychiatry*.
6 Healy, *The Antidepressant Era*; *The Psychopharmacologists*; *The Creation of Psychopharmacology*.

7 Ban et al., *The Rise of Psychopharmacology*; *The Triumph of Psychopharmacology*; *From Psychopharmacology to Neuropsychopharmacology*; *Reflections*.
8 Pignarre, *Comment la dépression*; *Psychotrope Kräfte*; Ehrenberg, *The Weariness of the Self*.
9 Moncrieff, *The Myth of the Chemical Cure*; Dornes, *Macht der Kapitalismus depressiv?*; Sadowsky, *The Empire of Depression*.
10 Balz, *Zwischen Wirkung und Erfahrung*; Braunschweig, *Zwischen Aufsicht und Betreuung*; Majerus, 'Making Sense of the "Chemical Revolution"'.
11 Meier, *Spannungsherde*.
12 Tornay, *Zugriffe auf das Ich*.
13 König, 'Besichtigung einer Weltindustrie'.
14 Gaudillière and Thoms, *The Development of Scientific Marketing*, therein especially Gerber, 'Marketing Loops'; see also Gerber and Gaudillière, 'Marketing Masked Depression'.
15 Greene, *Prescribing by Numbers*; *Generic*; Herzberg, *Happy Pills*. For a survey regarding Europe, see Rose, 'Psychopharmaceuticals'. On the therapeutic revolution, see Henckes, 'Magic Bullet'.
16 Gaudillière and Hess, 'General Introduction'; Daemmrich, 'A Tale'; *Pharmacopolitics*.
17 See Goliszek, *In the Name of Science*; Hornblum et al., *Against their Will*; Roelcke and Maio, *Twentieth Century Ethics*; Schlich and Troehler, *The Risks of Medical Innovation*; Schmidt and Frewer, *History and Theory*.
18 Marks, *The Progress*. See also Rigal, 'Neo-Clinicians', 511; Valier and Timmermann, 'Clinical Trials'.
19 Dyck and Delille, 'Human Experimentation'; Shorter, 'Brief History of Placebos'. See also Stewart and Dyck, *The Uses of Humans*.
20 The inpatient medical files of the Münsterlingen Psychiatric Clinic are from the period 1840–1960; the outpatient medical files are from the period 1916–1980. Patient files found in the transitional archive are cited with a temporary call number (ZA KA).
21 The Roche archive was also consulted, but Kuhn only conducted a small number of trials with substances from Hoffmann-La Roche.
22 See CA Novartis, Geigy, executive committee GL 27, 14 October 1970, 7.
23 The types of documents that had to be submitted were not regulated until the 1980s. Thus the pharmaceutical companies could themselves decide which documents to submit to the Intercantonal Office for the Control of Medicines (IKS). Until the 1970s, the documentation was limited to publications and lecture manuscripts.

## Introduction

24  Many contemporary witnesses responded to a call put out in the media; some had already established contact with the Thurgau State Archives even before the project began; we approached others directly. Unfortunately, due to a lack of resources we were only able to talk to a portion of the persons who made themselves available for a discussion. Contemporary witnesses who had already spoken to the media were not considered because they already had a certain prominence.

25  The Novartis archives and the focused investigation of psychiatric archives of the cantonal clinic in Marsens (Fribourg) and the Zurich and Bern university clinics suggest that Kuhn's private archive (StATG, 9'40) and the archive of the Münsterlingen Psychiatric Clinic (StATG, 9'10) provide unique documentation that enables a differentiated reconstruction of clinical trials (see Germann, *Medikamentenprüfungen*, 8–9; Rietmann et al., ' "Wenn Ihr Medikament" ', 201–202).

26  We use the term test patient in the following for all patients who were administered test substances. The term implies no disrespect whatsoever.

27  First, not all persons who received test substances are registered in Kuhn's private archive. Second, not all of the registered test patients are clearly identified (illegible, incomplete, or incorrectly spelled names; missing medical files). Third, the administering of test substances is not completely documented in the medical files. Apart from Kuhn's private archive, there are also holdings from the clinic archive that include lists with names of patients. They were also registered.

28  After the completion of the work with StATG, 9'40, 5 (Kuhn's private archive, *Fonds zur Psychopharmakologie*) and 9'10, around 1,200 persons were registered in the database. For the large majority, however, we only had rudimentary information – sometimes not even complete first and last names. We assigned first priority to cases where the information suggested they would be especially relevant (severe side-effects, adverse events, or death, detailed case descriptions, first case of a test or test phase, qualification as a 'model patient', etc.). Cases where we felt that processing might be productive were designated as second-priority cases. Third priority was assigned to cases whose processing we considered negligible within the framework of the available resources.

# 1

# The 1940s: The ball gets rolling

The view of the lake was wonderful, but unfortunately impeded by walls and fences for the compound's slightly fewer than 1,000 residents (Figure 1.1). Not until the start of long-overdue structural renovations of the Münsterlingen Psychiatric Clinic in the 1950s was the architecture of the enclosure reconceptualised as well.

> After we lowered the institution's perimeter fencing opposite the railway by one metre, and thereby found how liberating and aesthetically beneficial this change seemed, did we dare to proceed much more radically along the lakefront. There we completely removed the perimeter fence, which previously was more than two metres high, and this opened the view to a splendid lake landscape for the patients strolling the grounds, for the nursing staff and the visiting relatives.[1]

This was according to the 1957 annual report of the Münsterlingen Sanatorium and Nursing Facility.

Coincidentally, the modification occurred the very same year that the Geigy company's well-known antidepressant Tofranil, associated with the name of Roland Kuhn, was finally ready for approval. However, the clinical testing of previously unknown substances is only briefly mentioned in the annual report. In the next report, one year later, we learn that 'representatives of the Geigy company, Basel', had visited the institution 'repeatedly for inspection'. The reason for these visits is not disclosed. Quite in passing, without making any connections, the report subsequently references the 'increased therapeutic options with the new medications'.[2] This is in fact the first time in decades of close collaboration that the company's name appears in the clinic's public statements of account,

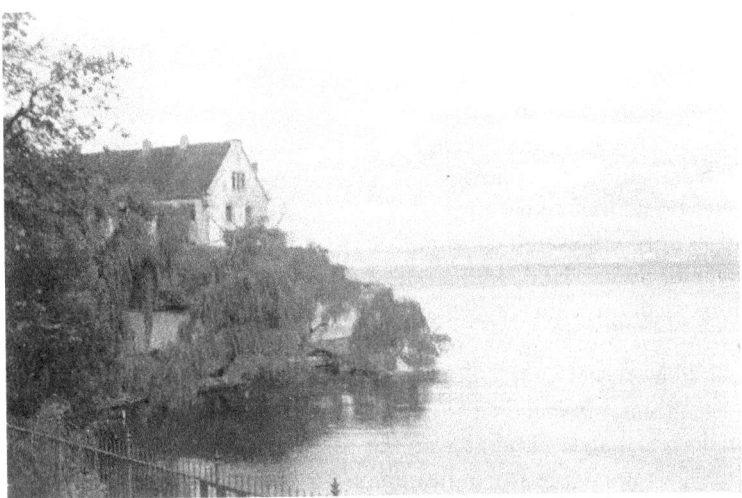

Figure 1.1 Clinic with lakeshore and fence, around 1950

even though the underlying tests constituted an event of completely different dimensions than the removal of a lakeside fence.

The episode of the removal of the fence conveys an initial impression of the institutional setting in which Kuhn's trials took place. For some time now, instead of focusing on the laboratory as the classical locus for experimentation, researchers of the history of knowledge have turned their gaze to those less controllable, socially complex milieus where knowledge is produced, negotiated, and transformed.[3] This approach also seems advantageous in our context; the 'making' of psychoactive substances, namely, occurred not only in the laboratories of pharmaceutical companies – clinics, too, were key sites for the production of knowledge, where the effects and side-effects of substances were stabilized.[4]

## From insane asylum to sanatorium and nursing facility

The Canton of Thurgau in eastern Switzerland founded the institution in Münsterlingen and the neighbouring hospital in 1839/1840 on the shore of Lake Constance, close to the German border.

The seemingly rural canton, which lacked an urban centre, reached a total population of 200,000 people in the 1980s; in 1950, there were only 150,000.[5] The rural appearance concealed an economic structure that was strongly industrial from early on, chiefly characterised by small-scale farmers and proletarians, and politically and culturally controlled by a rural/small-town elite of farmers, entrepreneurs, and educated bourgeoisie. Any socialist opposition only achieved local significance. Just as the canton lay on the edge of Switzerland, Münsterlingen lay on the edge of the canton. Repeatedly a topic of debate, the choice of where to situate the institution was largely decided by the availability of the buildings of an old monastery. Of Switzerland's twenty-one cantonal psychiatric institutions, six emerged from such reutilisations.[6] Münsterlingen's male psychiatric patients were housed in the old buildings of the former monastery on a headland directly on the lakeside; the women were accommodated in the cantonal hospital, inland on a slight rise, in a baroque-style building of the eighteenth century. In 1871, they were cut off from each other by the Romanshorn–Kreuzlingen railway line, which came to run between them. It became the landside border of the psychiatric facility. However, the 'insane asylum' and the 'hospital' were not definitively separated in structural and organisational terms until 1895, when the women, too, were moved to the lakeside.[7]

By the First World War, the number of inmates of the insane asylum had risen to around 400 and henceforth continued to increase. The asylum underwent structural expansion in several phases – in the 1890s, in the second half of the 1920s, and then starting in the second half of the 1950s and accelerating after 1970. With more than 600 patients in 1934, it was the eighth-largest clinic in Switzerland.[8] When Roland Kuhn and Adolf Zolliker began serving, respectively, as Münsterlingen clinic's senior physician and director, the number of patients totalled 635, namely, 311 men and 324 women, while 144 people made up the medical, nursing, and other operational staff. The numbers peaked in 1954, when the institution housed almost 1,000 people: 731 male and female patients plus staff. The patients were categorised and housed according to their behaviour, that is, according to their degree of 'unruliness', and strictly segregated by sex. That year saw the beginning of the intensive testing of the substances that would later be deemed psychopharmaceuticals. A significant decline in the number of occupants only occurred after 1971 as specialised facilities for the chronically ill increasingly relieved the burden of the Münsterlingen clinic.[9]

Reflecting the ratio among the patients, the nursing staff always featured slightly more women than men. The pay was bad, the hours were extremely long, and the overall work and life situation was burdensome. 'Moreover, the female employees also had substantially lower wages than the male staff', noted Kuhn retrospectively in 1990. 'Married staff could only spend the nights before and after the day off and during holidays with the family; for the rest, they had to sleep at the clinic. The directorate, together with the staff association, engaged in a virtual battle for "non-residency" for married staff.'[10] This was only introduced in 1956. At the same time, work time was reduced to sixty hours per week.[11] The VPOD (Union of Public Service Personnel) had continuously called for the ten-hour workday since 1931;[12] but, as Kuhn noted in hindsight,[13] by 1956, one third of all institutions had already reduced their work time to forty-eight hours and another third to fifty-four hours. As of the late 1930s, most of the male nurses were married, whereas the female nurses were single and left when they married. The latters' form of protest against the working conditions was resignation, which led to an extremely high turnover that some years reached 50 per cent. Sometimes female staff actually resigned en masse, such as in 1945/1946, when the directorate secretary, Agathe Christ, spoke of a 'revolutionary mood'.[14] A similar event occurred in 1962; the weekly work time still amounted to fifty-seven hours, and in January ten employees suddenly quit at once.[15] Incidentally, the staff had largely been unionised since the 1930s, with most of them in the VPOD's 'asylum cartel'.[16]

Compared to the constant coming and going among the lower ranks, especially among women, long-term continuity prevailed at the top of the nursing hierarchy. Those entering the clinic had to pass through the iron gate, which from 1904 to 1948 was guarded by the doorman Carl Reutemann. Apart from him, only the physicians had a key. With the new leadership as of 1939, the strict regimen relaxed a little.[17] The head female nurse, Sister Mathilde, had been employed since 1946, until she left prematurely in 1962 as the result of a conflict.[18] Strolling the grounds with her royal poodle, she figured among the establishment's more idiosyncratic characters.[19] Over decades, the activities of the some of the patients permanently living in the clinic's protective confines expanded – Arthur Kreis, for example, whose name can be stated here because Roland Kuhn honoured him by public mention several times.[20] Kreis took care of everything. He was not only an ideal secretary, noted Kuhn as early as 1941; 'he catalogues the library, makes translations of foreign-language works, manages the medical-history archive, in short, asylum life would hardly be conceivable anymore without his energetic help'.[21] Everyone in Münsterlingen knew him back then. He received some pocket money, later a small wage, and thus was privileged. The assistance provided by patients – usually unpaid – was considered a contribution towards the costs they invoked; moreover, it was also seen as part of work therapy.

Starting in 1927, the nursing staff, who were originally trained on the job, could acquire a diploma, part of the effort at professional upgrading. Münsterlingen participated in this program from the start and played a lead role among the larger asylums in the improvement of qualifications. By 1938, 60 per cent of the nursing staff had a diploma, while a further 24 per cent were in training.[22] The senior physician supervised the training operation; apart from that, as personnel manager he was also responsible for hiring the nursing employees.

With regard to the medical staff, as of 1930 the director was assisted by a 'first assistant physician', who acted as deputy and whose title was upgraded to senior physician in 1939. Roland Kuhn was the first to benefit from this; he had previously been a first-class assistant physician at the Waldau clinic in Bern. As of 1934, there were three proper assistant physicians. A second senior physician was added in 1944, followed by a fourth assistant physician position in 1947, filled by Verena Gebhart. For a long time, the medical staff remained at two senior physicians and four assistant physicians. Medical support was then increased again in the 1960s, such that in 1971, when Zolliker retired and Kuhn took over the directorate, the team of doctors had increased to thirteen people, including three women. Verena Gebhart had long been the only woman; she became a 'leading physician' in 1972. As of 1942, the clinic employed one female lab technician, and a second one as of

1956, the costs of which were covered in part by the Geigy company in Basel.

Adolf Zolliker's predecessor as director was Hermann Wille, who had led Münsterlingen since 1912.[23] Under Wille, the name of the institution was changed from *Irrenanstalt* (insane asylum) to *Irrenheilanstalt* (mental sanatorium) in 1929/1930, which underscored the aspired transformation from an asylum to a hospital-like facility. Starting in 1937, the annual reports record new types of therapy, even though the readiness for change waned substantially during the final years of Director Wille's tenure. 'In the 1930s', noted Kuhn retrospectively, 'Dr Wille, probably due to old age, had opposed any even minimal structural change'.[24] The old buildings, in particular, had been in dismal shape.

> The situation was very bad in the wards for unruly sick persons, P and rear building: The staff rooms were distributed across the wards, in part only accessible through sick rooms, mostly in attics and at risk of fire. The sanitation facilities were completely unsatisfactory everywhere. The care of physically frail, above all unclean sick persons, was completely inadequate. The outbreak of war in the beginning of September 1939 substantially delayed any improvement of the conditions.[25]

At the same time, the aforementioned units had the highest occupancy, with around 100 internees. They were much too large for adequate supervision, maintained Roland Kuhn in 1990; but changes did not take place until the early 1970s, when he himself took over the directorate.[26]

It is not unusual for people to portray conditions under their predecessor as gloomy to make their own accomplishments shine all the brighter. But outsiders must certainly have found the Münsterlingen asylum to be oppressive. This was hardly less so in the 1950s than twenty years earlier, for the capital investments briefly envisioned after the Second World War never materialized, frugality being a major priority in the canton. With the restaffing of the directorate and senior physician positions, a certain modernisation set in as of 1939 – thus for example, medical histories were now typewritten, also thanks to the new secretary position. Progress was limited, first due to the frequent absence of the leading physicians because of the war, and then, beyond that, because of the constant lack of finances.

At the same time, the sleep and fever cures started by Wille were continued, and so too the shock therapies with the use of Cardiazol and insulin, which became scarce at times. The artificial triggering of a physical shock reaction had represented the newest standard since the 1930s, with several successes attributed to the method.[27] In 1941, the asylum acquired an electroshock device, a recently available alternative to drug-induced shock therapy. Grave and irreversible were so-called lobotomies, surgical interventions in the brain that after 1945 – and until 1970 – were also performed at Münsterlingen in at least seventy-five cases.[28]

Created under Hermann Wille in 1938/1939, the outpatient department advanced slowly at first; the consulting centre in Frauenfeld was added in 1942 and remained much smaller. Most cases of outpatient consulting and treatment were referred by the cantonal hospital or the various authorities. A few people came on their own initiative. But the big boom only started in 1952/1953, with children and youth quickly gaining importance. Whereas at the beginning, clinicians dealt with no more than a few hundred cases per year, in 1958 the number of consultations reached 1,000 and then 2,000 in 1967, now mostly involving children and adolescents.[29]

The clinic was renamed again in 1939; it was now somewhat awkwardly called the Thurgauische Heil- und Pflegeanstalt Münsterlingen (Thurgau Sanatorium and Care Facility Münsterlingen), thereby officially dispensing with the tainted concept of *Irre* (insane) – yet even at the supervisory commission, people still referred to the *Irrenanstalt*.[30] In common parlance, the term no doubt prevailed for a long time. The final step occurred from 1965 to 1966 – the renaming as the Münsterlingen Psychiatric Clinic, which emphasised the medical aspiration and completed the linguistic convergence with the neighbouring cantonal hospital. Clinical directors from all of Switzerland had thoroughly discussed the issue of names in December 1965. One year later, the Thurgau government council announced the change of name, justifying the move by explaining 'that it is outdated to refer to an asylum. This word is discriminatory. With the new term, one wants to demonstrate that one has completely shifted to modern treatment methods.'[31]

## The institutional framework

An inquiry into the legal framework of Thurgau's postwar healthcare system entails a long search that eventually arrives at the Medical Services Act of 1850, which regulated the canton's healthcare system. Its revision was a long time in coming. A parliamentary motion of 1930 produced no results; not until 1958 was there a draft that reached the consultation process, where it stalled once more. After 1970, the matter was picked up again, with the government council presenting its proposal for a law on the healthcare system in 1981, which was accepted in late 1985.[32]

The supervisory authority of the Thurgau hospitals was the cantonal government, specifically the director of the Department for Medical Services and Education. With regard to Münsterlingen, the reorganisation of the late nineteenth century redefined a number of details. Henceforth, for example, the hospital and asylum kept separate accounts. Even without an updated formulation of the healthcare laws, adjustments were occasionally made at a lower level. Replacing an ordinance of 1898, a stipulation of 1950 on ethical practice stated: 'It is incumbent on the directorate to promote the physical and mental well-being of the sick persons. Their treatment must take place according to the principles of science and humaneness.'[33] Apart from the medical director, the asylum had an economic administrator who also looked after the Münsterlingen state domain, a large neighbouring agricultural estate. The asylum's 'charges' were supposed to be 'used for work on the Münsterlingen state domains', although the instructions of the asylum's directorate took priority over those of the estate's operations.[34] The proximity of the state domain repeatedly proved helpful for provisioning during the war. The tenures of the administrators exceeded even those of the asylum's directors. Upon arriving at Münsterlingen in 1939, Kuhn and Zolliker came across Heinrich Herzog, who had exercised this function since 1903. In 1949, the position devolved to his same-named son, who, apart from looking after his extensive responsibilities as administrator, was also a state council member for the Canton of Thurgau from 1964 to 1979. He remained the administrator until retiring in 1974. Only afterwards were the responsibilities redistributed and the administration of the two clinics separated from the state domain.[35]

A supervisory commission, which functioned as the instrument of cantonal government, existed since the 1890s, initially with five and later as many as nine members. The director of medical services served as president, and members frequently included a second government councillor, along with a district physician or the cantonal physician, and additional parliamentarians and dignitaries. They were all extremely busy men, but the commission's tasks were kept within bounds.[36] It was obliged to show up with all members at each institution at least once per year and primarily had to tend to financial aspects, as well as dealing with building-related issues on a case-by-case basis. The commission only intervened indirectly in the clinical operations insofar as it received and evaluated any complaints against the asylum director submitted to the government.[37]

More active commission members repeatedly spoke out about the inadequacy of their activities. The minutes of September 1954 cited Director of Medical Services Ernst Reiber: 'In a narrower sense, our commission is a very blunt instrument. One cannot give the institutions the desired attention. A better contact with them is absolutely necessary. After all, the current business is limited to only the meetings regarding the budget'.[38] As a stopgap, after 1955 a two-person delegation looked after each health institution – the obligation for all members to visit fell away. However, this alone could not solve the problem. In 1957, the classically liberal businessman and cantonal and national councillor Walter Tuchschmid repeatedly complained that the commission could not adequately do its job.[39] The supervision of the healthcare system's ever-larger and more complex facilities constituted a long-term problem, but the search for a solution seems not to have been especially urgent. Gottlieb Höppli from Wängi, a cantonal councilman and, as a farmer, not a typical commission member, wrote to the department of medical services in 1973: 'I believe that exceedingly few members of the supervisory commission are fighting to get additional tasks, but it seems to me that this institution would need to become substantially energised if it wants to live up to its name.'[40] The key dates cited here – 1954 and 1973 – frame the main period during which substances were clinically tested in Münsterlingen; the testing never shows up the commission's records. Mentioned occasionally is only the amount spent on drugs, which will be addressed in later chapters.[41]

## Roland Kuhn

Roland Kuhn had just turned 27 when he arrived in Münsterlingen in May 1939. The decision to accept the job had been made very quickly. In March, he had come into conflict with Director Jakob Klaesi at Bern University's Waldau clinic, whereupon the aggrieved first-class assistant resigned that same day. They reconciled, but whether immediately or later is unknown.[42] Nonetheless, Kuhn moved quickly when his former Waldau colleague Otto Briner, who first introduced him to psychoanalysis and now worked at the Burghölzli clinic, told him about the job opening. 'I accepted without having seen the new director or the asylum. The head of the Thurgau department of medical services back then, state council member Dr jur. Jakob Müller, ordered me to come to the Federal Palace, where he made it clear to me how beautiful the location of the clinic and how plain and modest the conditions are.'[43]

The quote is from an autobiographical sketch from the 1970s. With a sweeping gesture invoking 'fate' and 'ancestral lines', Roland Kuhn immediately introduces himself in the first sentence as the scion of an old family for whom tradition and origin are not just empty words.

Kuhn was born in March 1912 in Biel at the German–French linguistic border to a Protestant bourgeois family. A sister was born eighteen months later. On his father's side, the family had been part of Bern's urban middle class for generations and thus was of privileged status. His father Ernst Kuhn ran a bookstore and publishing house with locations in Bern and Biel, where his mother came from.

By his own account, Roland Kuhn had disliked school and had performed poorly in languages. In Biel, he grew into French quasi-automatically, but he never properly learned any other foreign languages. His English remained inadequate, which, given the rise of the United States as the pharmacological superpower, would be professionally detrimental in the long term. As with many Swiss intellectuals of his generation, the Anglo-Saxon world remained foreign to him despite later travels. He would later link his early interest in science and medicine to his frequent childhood illnesses, which, among other things, resulted in a stay at a lung clinic. He studied medicine in Bern, with a semester abroad in Paris. His interest in biochemistry was sparked by an organic chemistry lab course; his dissertation set off in a similar direction.[44] The teaching of Jakob

Klaesi, simultaneously a professor, the director of the Waldau clinic, and a pioneer of new forms of therapy, steered him towards psychiatry. And thus, mindful of father's admonishment to heed time and costs, he joined the Waldau clinic immediately after his state exams in June 1937. During the final stages of the world economic crisis, quickly finding a job was a definite plus.[45] Important contacts were made at the new location. Kuhn became friends with the senior physician Jakob Wyrsch, who was twenty years older; Arnold Weber drew his attention to child psychiatry and to the half-artistic/ intuitive diagnostic method known as the Rorschach test; and he followed the teachings of the brain pathologist Ernst Grünthal, who organised scientific presentations as 'lecture evenings', a form and term that Kuhn later adopted as a model.[46] With Grünthal he also shared the fascination with electroencephalography, a new method for visualising brain waves.[47] He became familiar with this technique while still at Waldau, which received its first device in 1938.

Roland Kuhn was a tireless reader, especially during the first ten or fifteen years at Münsterlingen; later, he would not have enough time. He had no family at first; his hometown of Biel was far away; entertainment opportunities at Lake Constance were limited. In such an environment, he noted retrospectively, one has 'only the choice between intellectual impoverishment and the active search and cultivation of relationships and discussions'.[48] An allusion suggests that he played music in his younger years;[49] his predilection for classical concerts and musical interiority were characteristic elements of a traditional cultural conditioning. Artistic and literary modernity remained foreign to him. His willingness to try new things in the field of medical pharmacology stood in obvious contrast to his cultural appreciation of the traditional.

Roland Kuhn was a well-read man, including in areas far beyond the field of medicine, and he shaped himself in accordance with his generation's ideal of the bourgeois intellectual. An important encounter was with the older Ludwig Binswanger in neighbouring Kreuzlingen, who developed so-called daseinsanalysis, an approach located between psychoanalysis and existentialism. Martin Heidegger, whom Kuhn long considered the century's most important philosopher, became a reference point, even though personal contact remained fleeting.[50] In old age he qualified this assessment, speaking now also about the 'very problematic sides of this person' and moving Edmund Husserl to first place.[51]

Kuhn gained his first experiences as a writer with works on the Rorschach test. When Jakob Klaesi and Ernst Grünthal took over the publishing and editing of the prestigious *Monatsschrift für Psychiatrie und Neurologie* in 1938 (the publishing house moved from Berlin to Basel in 1937), Kuhn received the task of preparing a comprehensive literary review of the subject.[52] Further publications in this field followed, which soon earned the young physician a reputation as a specialist and expert on the test and helped establish contacts to prominent figures in Swiss psychiatry. A lecture on 'Mask Interpretations in Rorschach Experiments' led to an extensive treatise published in 1944/1945, which appeared in French translation after the war and became the basis for his postdoctoral qualification at the University of Zurich in 1957.[53] He also made a name for himself with daseinsanalytical deliberations on schizophrenia during the early postwar years. At the time, reflection on that mysterious complex of disorders was considered psychiatry's central intellectual challenge. Although Kuhn emphasised retrospectively that he had already been interested in depression back then, depressive illness was not yet an explicit topic for him.

Kuhn's thought primarily consisted of linguistic and conceptual analysis; social conditions of life interested him less. In a letter of 1964 to the psychoanalyst Gustav Bally, he compared his own viewpoint with that of his older colleague, using the example of an engagement with the texts of Sigmund Freud. 'It seems to me that you give more consideration to sociological and more comprehensive aspects, whereas for me it is more about most appropriately understanding the individual concept, the individual phenomenon, and finally the individual sentence of Freud, and expressing them in the most appropriate language.'[54] Accordingly, the reading and education groups that Kuhn organised for the young assistant physicians at Münsterlingen were focused challengingly on philosophy and textual analysis; this was also true of his lectures at the University of Zurich, which concentrated on examining the literature on daseinsanalysis.[55] When Kuhn nonetheless occasionally invoked the occupational aspect of how people coped with life, it came across as old-fashioned, closer to the ideal of an entrenched order of professions than to the fluid contours of the modern industrialised society and service economy that formed during his lifetime. For him, a successful life was measured by virtue of the 'elation' triggered by the accomplishment of a work.

The artist experiences it in the shaping of a work, the craftsman in the fabrication of a usable object such as a dress, a piece of furniture, a device, a machine. The farmer senses something similar when cultivating the field and when harvesting the fruit, the surgeon with the good conclusion of a difficult operation, the psychiatrist in achieving a free and open discussion with the sick person.[56]

For a long time, the high intellectual aspirations and the externally projected image of the nascent conservative intellectual contrasted starkly with his concrete living conditions. From 1939 to 1944, the war-related cost-of-living allowances increased his annual basic salary at Münsterlingen from almost 6,000 to 7,000 francs a year.[57] This was just slightly higher than the average earnings of a white-collar employee and just under 60 per cent more than blue-collar wages.[58] The inflation allowance was so inadequate that Kuhn – like other canton officials of this salary bracket – had to accept a 25-per-cent loss of purchasing power during the war years.[59] Good comparative data is available for 1944 regarding the earnings of independently practising physicians; they were just shy of three and a half times his basic salary.[60]

In later years, Kuhn liked to point out that his pay was exceedingly modest.[61] However, he always had several sources of additional income whose level we do not exactly know. There were the expert legal opinions and other expert evaluations, then the separate billing for the production of electroencephalograms, but above all his work in the outpatient department, which sharply increased after 1950. More detailed information about the latter is available for the 1970s.[62] In addition to his basic salary, there was also the 'free personal unit' – like all other employees, Kuhn lived on the grounds of the asylum. In principle, he was entitled to a service apartment, but, as per his own description, he only had two modest rooms on a dilapidated property at his disposal, without a bathroom and water supply and almost impossible to heat. He had to share the toilet facilities (which often froze during winter) with employees, patients, and visitors. On some winter days when the icy north wind blew across the lake, even the administrative offices could hardly be used because of the cold.[63] In light of the 'financial weakness of the canton', which was 'repeatedly drawn to [his] attention by higher up', Kuhn wrote with mild sarcasm in 1964, he refrained from filing a complaint regarding the housing situation.[64] In 1939, the director of medical services, Jakob Müller, had announced that the housing situation would be rectified 'as soon as possible', and they would review 'whether perhaps a particular building could be built in which the married senior physicians of the cantonal hospital could live'.[65] After twenty-one years of service, a normally furnished apartment finally became available in January 1961, at which point Kuhn had been married for almost two years.

Kuhn remained in Münsterlingen until his retirement. Looking back, he occasionally said that he never seriously strove for a position at a university clinic,[66] but this was not true. Initially he confidently counted on returning soon to the Waldau clinic. During the war, but also afterwards, he engaged in negotiations with various locations and was also occasionally sought out by external parties.[67] However, in the case of Basel in spring 1942, it turned out that the salary there would have been even less.[68] The motives behind the desire to change locations were more than just financial, as Kuhn explained in 1945 to Jakob Klaesi when looking into a job at the Rosegg Psychiatric Clinic in the Canton of Solothurn – not a university clinic. 'Crucial for me is the concern for my parents and my sister. In Münsterlingen I am so far apart from them that I feel obliged to make the attempt of an application.'[69] One factor that kept him in Münsterlingen was his friendship with Binswanger. He also enjoyed a freedom that he might have lacked elsewhere. Thus later in his autobiographical sketch, he declared that having always remained at the same isolated location had been an advantage. This allowed the psychiatrist to 'follow psychotic and psychogenic developments over a long time, to get to know family pathologies from his own observation over two or even three generations, and to comprehend the internal coherence of a clinical operation in all of its details'.[70]

After his postdoctoral qualification of 1957, Kuhn became an honorary professor at the University of Zurich. He fulfilled his teaching obligations on evenings, lecturing on daseinsanalysis. A handful of listeners, who frequently arrived from Münsterlingen, followed his challenging expositions. Kuhn highly valued his title as a professor.

## In the inner circle

Roland Kuhn worked in close association with Director Adolf Zolliker for thirty-two years. Interactions with the eight-year-older man were courteous and collegial, but the men always adhered to formal address, which was not unusual at that time. Zolliker features only in passing in Kuhn's autobiographical account; even in the extensive holdings of his private archive, Zolliker remains a background figure. He came from the Swiss Asylum for Epileptics in Zurich, where he had been the senior physician. The young secretary and trained nurse Agathe Christ came with him from the 'Epi' to Münsterlingen at the same time; she too would become a permanent fixture of the operation, remaining loyal to Münsterlingen until her retirement in 1975. She became a closely involved employee, well beyond her role as secretary; in particular, she organised the outpatient department.[71] The young senior physician Kuhn soon used her intensively for the dictation of his letters and reports; countless writings bear the abbreviation K/Ch at the top. Zolliker wound up on the margins of the emerging relationship of trust, targeted by the irony of the secretary, whose self-assurance bore witness to her roots in a good Basel family. 'And Herr Director is developing unimagined energies', she reported in autumn 1940 to Kuhn, who was away on official business. Zolliker was completing expert evaluations, making rounds, 'taking care of everything and showing much more interest than before'.[72] She could obviously count on Kuhn's tacit agreement with her characterisation of the 'boss' as a languid figure. Kuhn and Zolliker got along in that they respected one another and left each other alone. A hierarchical dependency can be discerned only in the early years, such as when Kuhn needed to wait for the 'boss's' approval for an article.[73]

Zolliker was more of an administrator; he handled the exchanges with the municipal and cantonal authorities, which also fell under his responsibility. That he neglected his rounds leaked out occasionally.[74] Sometimes he would simply disappear for a day; nobody knew where he was.[75] He stayed away from the asylum's challenging Monday reading and education group that Kuhn had organised for the doctors. Former assistant physicians remember him in remarkably contradictory terms, sometimes positively, sometimes negatively, like an image contrasting with the respective perception of Kuhn.[76] In one regard, Kuhn gave him the highest possible marks, namely, for setting up and maintaining a system of 'genealogical tables' that documented the familial circumstances of patients. 'A tool of that kind usually allows for more statements about the familial burdens with mental disorders than those that the sick persons themselves and their relatives could make, completely leaving aside the tendencies to hide corresponding occurrences in the family from the physician.'77 Biological inheritance definitely received more attention than any other type of determination.

The senior physician was a hard worker with ascetic traits. Extravagant culinary delights and alcoholic beverages were not his thing. Nor did the living arrangements encourage the cultivation of hospitality. This improved once he was married, whereupon the weekly education group was spoiled with a dessert. Tall, gaunt, and stiff-postured, Kuhn had been exempted from military service because he was physically unfit for duty. That said, he performed auxiliary services for the air force, where he used Rorschach tests to examine flight crews for their suitability and, as always, demonstrated full commitment. He also expected the same dedication from his subordinates; he was strict in this regard. But, in contrast to Zolliker, one could learn an enormous amount from him, as a former assistant of 1959/1960 recalled.[78] Residual papers from the early years include individual documents that testify to the affection of his subordinates, such as a message from 'King Roland's orphaned coffee roundtable' sent to Kuhn in Paris, telling him that everything is topsy-turvy at the clinic but that he need not worry.[79] The instigator was probably Agathe Christ, who was the first to sign the note, immediately followed by the young assistant physician Verena Gebhart. A photograph from the asylum's popular Carnival celebration shows 'King Roland' in 1954 in a white doctor's coat with a crooked paper crown on his head.[80] There is no evidence of such moments in later years.

Verena Gebhart came from neighbouring Kreuzlingen. She was nine years younger than Kuhn and stemmed from a respected family of rural doctors; her father and grandfather were doctors. Ernst Gebhart had once worked with Eugen Bleuler at the Burghölzli clinic, and thereafter in the private clinic in Zihlschlacht, before starting his own practice as a family physician in 1909. As a long-serving district physician, however, he later also repeatedly dealt with psychiatric issues.[81] His daughter found her professional path within a supportive family network. She studied in Zurich, living with the family of her uncle Wilhelm Löffler, who was not only a doctor but also the director of the polyclinic and a professor at the university.[82] She joined Münsterlingen as an assistant physician in November 1947 at the age of 26. Her new supervisor, Roland

Kuhn, played an important role in her choice of a dissertation topic. It dealt with the elaborate production and assessment of 500 Rorschach protocols of children – she was granted leave for this project in 1949 – which appeared in 1952 in the *Monatsschrift für Psychiatrie und Neurologie*, referee Manfred Bleuler, co-referee Roland Kuhn.[83] At the same time, she advanced to the position of senior physician. Children remained the focus of her work.

A small inventory of handwritten letters shines light on the evolving relationship between Verena Gebhart and Roland Kuhn. In Verena Gebhart's very first letters – his are missing – one can discern her interest in the senior physician, whom she patiently wooed.[84] He hesitated and stubbornly adhered to formal address. Complicating matters was that Kuhn had acted as an advisor to the Gebhart family in a case of illness in 1948/1949.[85] He remained on the fence until spring 1957, by which time Kuhn and Verena Gebhart had known each other for almost ten years (Figure 1.2).

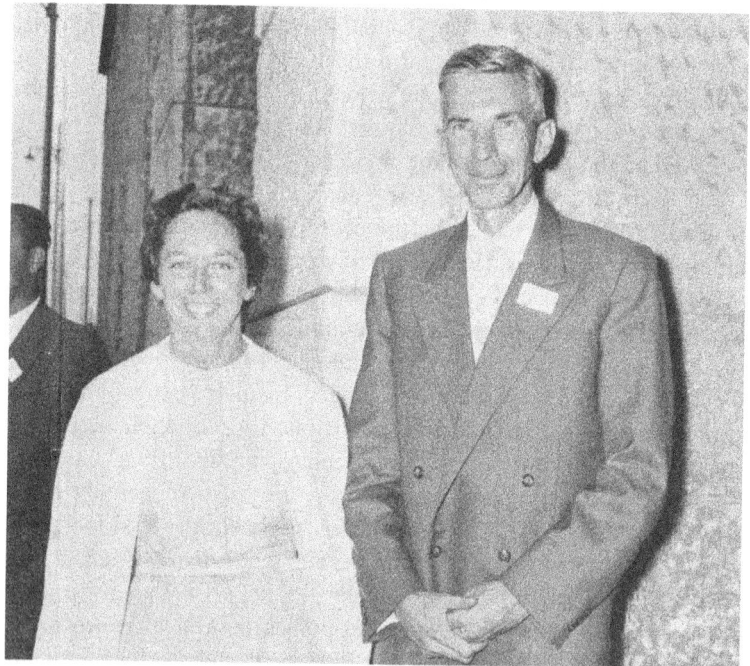

**Figure 1.2** Roland and Verena Kuhn at a congress in Rome, 1958

The turning point came at precisely the same time that his professional success with the antidepressant imipramine became apparent. The two of them married in February 1958. There was no lack of gossip; the staff occasionally made fun of the new couple.[86] Even after giving birth to three daughters, Verena Kuhn-Gebhart kept working at the clinic without change.

## Before psychopharmacology: The chemical industry of Basel

Until the 1940s, industrial pharmaceutics had little to offer psychiatric institutions; even at the companies, nobody would have come up with the idea that they might be a potentially massive market.[87] Isolated contacts between Münsterlingen and the Basel pharmaceutical producers are documented from the 1920s. In 1922, for example, Ciba offered Münsterlingen two ovarian extracts from the early period of the company's hormone research.[88] The top priority, however, was the psychiatric need for sleep medicines and sedatives, including opiates, which were indeed older than the pharmaceutical industry itself. Opiates were considered problematic because of their addiction potential. The most important manufacturers in Switzerland were the Basel companies Hoffmann La-Roche,[89] Ciba, and Sandoz. With regard to opium derivatives, Roche's range of products was particularly wide. After 1930, the company was working on much stronger morphine alternatives.

During the early twentieth century, Ciba and Roche had risen to become important manufacturers of various pharmaceutical products.[90] They were joined by Sandoz after 1920 and Geigy in the 1950s. Ciba, Geigy, and Sandoz were originally dye manufacturers; medicinally useful preparations could be developed from coal tar dyes (aniline) – an important discovery of the late nineteenth century.[91] Roche did not emerge from the dyestuff industry but rather from the industrial pharmacy sector. It achieved early successes with alkaloids, organic extracts such as opium or digitalis. People at Sandoz engaged in similar work on the basis of ergot. Important research had been developed at Ciba since the 1920s on recently discovered hormones, which at first were hard-won from organic substances (offal) and later synthesised.[92] Emerging from hormone research was cortisone, which was recognised for its dramatic effect in 1948; it was psychiatrically tested as early as 1950 in Great Britain, but with negative results.[93] The process involved the first so-called double-blind study in psychiatry, a testing method with two comparison groups that Roland Kuhn would always reject.[94] Developed by Albert Hofmann at Sandoz from the group of ergot substances, LSD came into play in 1943, an enormously powerful psychoactive substance that was already being tested in 1947 at the Burghölzli clinic in Zurich – on sick persons as well as in self-experiments on healthy people.[95]

Around 1935, pharmaceutical research and production at the Basel corporations and their German competitors underwent a powerful upsurge.[96] Promising new product families came into view: sulphonamides and then antibiotics during the war – now in England and the United States. Roche grew powerful with the synthesis of vitamin C, which at first was still considered a potential medicine. The new substances fascinated specialists and the public, even though exactly how useful they were remained somewhat unclear. During the war, when Roche and Ciba had already moved part of their research to the United States, the demand in the dye industry collapsed, which further increased the economic importance of the pharmaceuticals. Around 1950, pharmaceutical sales surpassed that of dyes at both Ciba and Sandoz, then in 1953/1954 also at the latecomer Geigy.[97] Science, medicine, industry, and the public interacted ever more closely, even though the situation was still very far removed from 'big pharma' – the giant globally active conglomerates of today.

The partnership between Geigy and Roland Kuhn would be immensely important not merely for Kuhn. The cooperation with the Münsterlingen psychiatrist also proved to be central for the rise of the company's young pharmaceutical division. The senior management of Geigy, the oldest of the Basel dye factories, had only decided in 1938, following the example of Ciba and Sandoz, to broaden its production program. The agrochemical division succeeded quickly thanks to the development of DDT. Pharmaceuticals, which at first produced only deficits, took much longer. Geigy entered the market in 1940, but dissipated its energies with marginally successful small-scale products. As late as 1947, the company reckoned it would not get out of the red before 1955. It was elated when, thanks to the successful rheumatism remedy

Butazolidin, this turning point was already reached in 1951. 'As a result, the period of losses of our pharma division should be over, a period that lasted ten years and that could only be sustained because the pharma losses could be covered by the dyestuff profits',[98] noted Robert Boehringer, who had joined the company after the war as an experienced consultant. He had previously worked for the German pharmaceutical company Boehringer Ingelheim, to which he had family ties, and then for Roche from 1919 to 1930. Another Roche alumnus was the German chemist Hans Stenzl, whom Boehringer had recruited in 1939. He had been responsible for the pain-reliever Saridon and was now developing the rheumatism remedy. With Boehringer and Stenzl, as well as the physician and pharmacologist Robert Domenjoz from Lausanne, and the young chemists Franz Häfliger and Walter Schindler, Geigy's pharmaceutical division had assembled a capable team.

## Parpanit: Geigy arrives at Münsterlingen

The key figure who brought Geigy to Münsterlingen and Münsterlingen to Basel was the previously introduced Ernst Grünthal, Roland Kuhn's teacher at the University of Bern and at Waldau. Driven out of Würzburg, the famous brain anatomist came to Bern in 1934, where the new director, Jakob Klaesi, wanted to expand scientific research.[99] Grünthal was one of the very few immigrants of Jewish origin who found entry into Swiss psychiatry. Although there was hardly any money to be had from the canton, the Rockefeller Foundation donated a research laboratory for brain anatomy at Waldau. In 1941, Geigy's new director of pharmacology, Robert Domenjoz, took note of a recently published article by Grünthal. In the *Schweizerische Medizinische Wochenschrift*, Grünthal had introduced his procedure for measuring the sensation of pressure and pain, which he had earlier developed in Würzburg. At Geigy they were deliberating on the profile of the freshly formed pharmaceutical division. Pain-relievers and sleep medications stood at the fore – everyone made those. Grünthal seemed to be a good contact because very little was understood about clinical trials. Thus this liaison included two outsiders. The practical work began in 1943, when Grünthal started testing morphine derivatives for Geigy.

This suited him just fine, for the funding from Rockefeller had since run out. At Geigy's expense, he hired a lab assistant and over the next few years tested several dozen substances on a handful of mostly healthy people. The substances had first been tested on animals and classified as toxicologically harmless by Domenjoz. Grünthal's reports were now regularly arriving in Basel.

Parpanit, the substance G 2747, was announced to Grünthal as an anticonvulsant – the letter G referred to the company name Geigy and the number to the sequence of the chemical tested, marking it as a research substance. Domenjoz was hoping for positive effects for movement disorders such as those associated with Parkinson's disease. But Grünthal described strange, narcotic-like effects: the healthy probands lost the sense of the position of their limbs; sometimes they felt like they were floating. In light of the strange effect on muscle tension, a subsequent phase focused on people who suffered from encephalitis lethargica (also called European sleeping sickness) and exhibited Parkinson's-like symptoms. This disease had frequently appeared during the interwar period, with many of those affected becoming so helpless that they spent the rest of their lives in asylums. Grünthal observed significant recovery, even though one 'cannot speak of a complete disappearance of Parkinson's signs under the effect of the remedy'.[100] Prior to any possible marketing of the substance, an in-depth clinical trial was now required.

The first contact with Münsterlingen is not documented. However, in late March 1946, Robert Domenjoz showed up at the clinic to call on Director Zolliker and his senior physician. This must have been preceded by Grünthal's intercession. Now everything moved quite fast. A few days later, Kuhn received the first delivery of test substance G 2747; he was given a summary of the pharmacological report, and Grünthal appeared in person. The project proved to be very successful, both with regard to the substance but also and especially as pertained to the emerging form of collaboration. Kuhn's first positive responses reached Basel as early as mid-May 1946. Although he also reported unpleasant side-effects, he added, 'The patients gladly put up with them if in return they at least subjectively do somewhat better, and sometimes they obviously also do substantially better objectively.'[101] In summer, Kuhn travelled to Basel, visited the Geigy laboratories for the first time, and gave notice of his final report, which is dated 10 September

1946. The trial had lasted five months, and had involved six women and eight men. Eight of the fourteen people suffered from encephalitis lethargica, associated in part with psychotic conditions; in addition, for the purpose of the comparison, there were various individual cases of other types of organic brain damage.[102]

The expert evaluation of Parpanit consisted of thirty-five pages; it was carefully elaborated and more clearly structured than some later reports.[103] The well-documented trial proves to be valuable in our context; influenced by Ernst Grünthal's preliminary work, Roland Kuhn for the first time developed a trial method for test substances, which he would later often replicate in a similar form. Kuhn had Zolliker approve the report, a move that for later years is no longer documented. The first section listed the persons being treated – they were anonymised with a method unusual for Kuhn[104] – and described the individual course of the experimental treatment. In his own copy, Kuhn added the real names by hand to keep track of things. The second section reported on accompanying examinations – pulse monitoring, respiratory rate, blood pressure measurement – and delivered a summarised assessment. Writing samples were pasted into the report, compelling evidence for a change in hand movement.

> With regard to method, it must still be said that we often visited the patients ourselves. We also questioned them and we kept a record of this. In addition, however, the nursing staff was instructed to observe them especially well and to write a written report about this. The processing occurred on the basis of these observations.[105]

The increased attention, according to Kuhn, had naturally influenced the patients and raised expectations of betterment. But with the long observation period, he noted, one had been able to reduce this suggestive effect. To create greater certainty, in one case a different approach was used; no explanation was given to the patient, who simply received the tablets from the nurse as a matter of course. 'We also did not concern ourselves with him afterwards, and, only after a longer period, we asked once in passing how things were going. Since this patient has no contact with others, we believe that in this case the effect is actually just caused by the preparation.'[106]

Parpanit was not a psychotropic drug, and patients were sometimes resistant to the intervention. In one case, it failed to sedate a particular patient who believed that the doctors were trying to poison her. She refused ever more fiercely to take the tablets – and ultimately succeeded.[107] Nevertheless, Kuhn confirmed the narcotic-like effect described by Grünthal and also pointed out unpleasant presentations such as headaches, dizziness, and in one case epileptic seizures. In many cases, although there was no healing, the treatment substantially alleviated the symptoms. This also applied to the one person who was administered the remedy as an outpatient. In this case, Kuhn obtained the consent of the patient's relatives and the family physician to set up an appointment for him again at the clinic. 'It is a completely new medication', Kuhn told the patient's father.

> It is the first remedy we know of that is supposed to work for conditions like those of your son. But first we want to gain some experience with the remedy and therefore have been using it in our asylum for around fourteen days. It is completely harmless and in certain cases actually has a surprisingly good effect.[108]

Numerous letters went back and forth. For later tests, we no longer found any evidence for this kind of practice of providing information.

Two patients died after the trial of 1946 – under the continued application of Parpanit, which was approved in late 1946. A 29-year-old man died in June 1949 from a pulmonary embolism in the presence of tuberculosis, according to the autopsy. Upon his transfer to Münsterlingen in 1948, he was given Parpanit right away, evidently without anyone recognising his severely frail health. A second patient who had participated in the trial of 1946 – also rather young, at only 35 – died in February 1947. Kuhn told the company about these cases, but could not see a connection to the administration of the preparation.[109] This assessment may be accurate, but other questions remain unresolved. In an expert evaluation for Geigy in 1949, Kuhn retrospectively referred to marasmus (malnutrition) as the cause of death.[110] Although the patient's name was noted, doubts as to his identity inevitably arise, for the medical history and nursing records register – quite differently – a sudden deterioration combined with a heart attack and pulmonary oedema. The man was given Parpanit until his death or just before. He had repeatedly protested against the tablets and complained about severe headaches.

Kuhn continued treating the same patients with Parpanit until 1949. Although the remedy was now approved, the company was still interested in additional information on optimal doses and long-term effects. In late 1946, Geigy went to the medical public with news about the new medication in three articles published in the *Schweizerische Medizinische Wochenschrift* – one by Robert Domenjoz, another by Grünthal, and the third from the University Polyclinic for Nervous Diseases in Zurich, where tests had been conducted in parallel with Münsterlingen. In Zurich, too, five of the sixty patients being treated had died during the eight-month duration of the trial without the report mentioning anything more than the mere fact of their deaths.[111]

Parpanit significantly enhanced the prestige of the Geigy company, which for the first time could present itself to the public as a capable newcomer. However, it could not provide for major profits because sales were too small.[112] The medication also quickly reached the United States. Starting in autumn 1947, it was being tested in Boston's Massachusetts General Hospital. Kuhn received a photocopy of a report in 1949. As mentioned in the article, one of the mandatory requirements for such tests was the comparative use of a placebo without informing the patients or their relatives.[113] But Kuhn was unwilling to do this, even in later years.[114]

The people at Geigy were grateful for Kuhn's work, regretting at most that he never published his precise reports (a second had followed in 1949). With his publication in 1946, Grünthal had made his connection with Geigy public; Kuhn evidently did not want to do so. The negotiations regarding his remuneration claims continued, which he conducted with diplomatic prowess. 'The observation of the effects of the medication actually amounted to a very major job, both for the patients themselves and for the nursing staff and me', he wrote in September 1946. 'But I do not want to issue an invoice for my report', he added. 'Instead, I would like to recommend that you pay something to the asylum according to your discretion. We would use part of it in a way such that it benefits the patients and the nursing staff. Another part we would use for the scientific work in our asylum.'[115] When questioned, Kuhn explained that the 'greatest desire' was 'to receive an electroencephalograph'.[116] In addition, he extended the prospects of further services for which the device might be helpful. 'Perhaps sooner or later there will be another occasion when we can also conduct investigations for you in other fields on the clinical effect of a new substance.'[117] In the end, Geigy paid 3,000 francs for the acquisition of the device, which became available in Münsterlingen in 1950.

In June 1950, Geigy once again knocked at Kuhn's door, asking whether he was willing to test the pain-reliever and rheumatism remedy Irgapyrin for an additional indication for the treatment of depressive states. Such a use may seem surprising, but evidently Geigy reckoned with the possibility of a shock effect, an approach that also was the basis for the use of convulsant substances. Kuhn said he was willing, but noted as a reminder that no medication had yet been found that could change the depressive mood, except perhaps the opium cure. He would need a lot of time for the investigation 'since we do not take in all that many depressive patients and probably multiple tests must be done to get something of a picture'.[118]

While the long-term trial of Parpanit was still underway in Münsterlingen, the Geigy research laboratory was already pursuing new objectives. In spring 1948, the director drew the attention of the chemist Franz Häfliger to iminodibenzyls as compounds of potential pharmaceutical interest.[119] They were related to phenothiazines, which were of great interest at the time. Originally known from older dyestuff chemistry, they were a recently rediscovered group of substances, which would give rise to chlorpromazine; marketed under the name of Largactil as of 1953, it became famous as the first neuroleptic drug. This is where our story begins to move towards a focus on the discovery of the psychopharmacological effectiveness of certain substances. In late 1948, the chemist Walter Schindler took over part of the work; soon there was an array of iminodibenzyl derivatives, with the first two going to Grünthal. Based on recent success with Parpanit, one was hoping for a preparation for Parkinson's. In summer 1949, Schindler synthesized G 22150 and, a little later, G 22355.[120] They had an antidepressant on their hands, but nobody knew it yet.

## Notes

1 StATG, 9'10, 1.1.0/60, ARM 1957, 3–4.
2 *Ibid.*, ARM 1958, 5.

3 On laboratory studies, see Latour and Woolgar, *Laboratory Life*; Rheinberger, *Experimentalsysteme*. On the consideration of further sites for the production of knowledge, see Galison and Jones, 'Factory'; Gooday, 'Placing or Replacing'; Schillings and van Wickeren, 'Towards a Material'.
4 For basic deliberations on the determination of effects depending on the setting, see Gomart, 'Methadone'. On the non-linear paths of scientific facts and things, see Dumit, *Drugs for Life*, 98; see also Jasanoff, 'The Idiom of Co-Production'.
5 A modern history of the canton is lacking; but see *HLS*, Thurgau Canton.
6 See the map in Bersot, *Fürsorge*, 20.
7 Ammann and Studer, *150 Jahre Münsterlingen*, 64, 115.
8 Overview of the development of patients and staff at Swiss clinics 1910–1935 in Bersot, *Das Pflegepersonal*, 14–27.
9 Figures according to StATG, 9'10, 1.1.0/60, ARM; detailed discussion of nursing staff using the example of Basel, Braunschweig, *Zwischen Aufsicht*.
10 Kuhn, 'Geschichte', 108.
11 *Ibid.*, 108.
12 *Thurgauer Arbeiterzeitung*, 11 January 1946; enclosed in copy in StATG, 9'40, 3.1.22/0, correspondence between Kuhn and Agathe Christ.
13 Kuhn, 'Geschichte', 108.
14 StATG, 9'40, 3.1.22/0, Agathe Christ to Kuhn, 17 September 1945.
15 StATG, 4'840'33, supervisory commission minutes, 8 February 1962, 8.
16 Precise information in Bersot, *Das Pflegepersonal*, 64–70.
17 StATG, 9'10, 1.1.0/60, ARM 1976, 4.
18 All information based on the annual reports.
19 Conversation with former trainee nurse, 18 April 2018.
20 StATG, 9'10, 1.1.0/60, ARM 1963, 8; 1979, 24. All persons who appear or are cited in this book have been anonymised. Exceptions are public figures, executive personnel (including important specialists) of the pharmaceutical industry, the Münsterlingen Psychiatric Clinic (senior nursing staff, physicians at a senior level and higher, head secretary, and administrators) and other institutions, as well as contemporary witnesses who wanted to be referred to by name.
21 StATG, 9'10, 5.4/9229.1, 29 March 1941.
22 Bersot, *Das Pflegepersonal*, 56.
23 Kuhn, 'Geschichte', 100.
24 *Ibid.*, 106.

25 *Ibid.*, 102.
26 *Ibid.*, 110; see Chapter 6, 207–212.
27 An overview in Braunschweig, *Zwischen Aufsicht*, 195–202.
28 More in Meier, *Spannungsherde*, 320 f.
29 Assessment based on StATG, 9'10, 1.1.0/60, ARM. The annual report of 1968, 5–13, included an overview written by Kuhn.
30 StATG, 4'840'33, supervisory commission minutes, 1939/1940.
31 StATG, 9'14, 5.2.6.0/2, governing council resolution, 22 November 1966.
32 StATG, 2'30'331-A, 54/9–1, government council proposal for a law on the healthcare system, 8 September 1981.
33 Vollziehungsverordnung des Regierungsrates zum Gesetz über die Organisation der öffentlichen Krankenanstalten (18 December 1950), *Amtsblatt des Kantons Thurgau* (1950), 921.
34 Wille, 'Hundert Jahre', 125; Kuhn, 'Geschichte', 109.
35 See *HLS*, Heinrich Herzog; also Kuhn, 'Geschichte', 109.
36 On the task book of 1896, see Wille, *Münsterlingen*, 126; for later developments, see StATG, 4'840'33, supervisory commission.
37 Wille, 'Hundert Jahre', 101.
38 StATG, 4'840'33, supervisory commission minutes, 9 September 1954, 4.
39 StATG, 4'840'33, supervisory commission minutes, Tuchschmid, A few thoughts on the regulations, 2 June 1957; on Tuchschmid himself, see *HLS*, Walter Tuchschmid.
40 StATG, 4'802'153, Höppli to the medical services department, 14 June 1973.
41 See Chapter 2, 52, and Chapter 5, 178–181.
42 StATG, 9'40, 3.2.1/0, Kuhn to Klaesi, 10 March 1939; in Kuhn, 'Roland Kuhn', 223, the incident is recalled with less intensity.
43 *Ibid.*, 223.
44 This and further information in *ibid.*, 221–223.
45 The 'overcrowding risk in the medical profession' was a constant topic during those years; see Stupnicki, *Die soziale Stellung*.
46 See StATG, 9'40, 10.0/10, report on the first trip to the United States, lecture evening, 18 June 1958.
47 Pidoux, 'Expérimentation', 450; also Schoefert, 'The View', 123–124.
48 Kuhn, 'Roland Kuhn', 232.
49 StATG, 9'40, 3.1.22/0, Agathe Christ to Kuhn, 11 December 1941.
50 StATG, 9'40, 2.3/0, correspondence and notice regarding a discussion in 1966; also 9'40, 3.1.41.
51 StATG, 9'40, 3.1.11/0, Kuhn to Wolfgang Blankenburg, 17 December 1997.
52 Kuhn, 'Roland Kuhn', 228.

53 Kuhn, *Maskendeutungen*.
54 StATG, 9'40, 3.1.2/0, Kuhn to Gustav Bally, 2 November 1964.
55 Plenty of material on this in StATG, 9'40, 9.
56 Kuhn, 'Beitrag', 56.
57 StATG, 9'10, 1.2.8/0, Government Council of the Canton of Thurgau, extract from the minutes, 28 March 1939; for the cost-of-living allowances, see the *Amtsblatt des Kantons Thurgau* (1943), 1119 f.
58 Comparative data in König et al., *Warten und Aufrücken*, 140, 624.
59 Calculated using the consumer price index according to Ritzmann, *Historische Statistik*, 503; inflation in 1939–1944 amounted to 51 per cent, and the inflation allowance was 13 per cent.
60 Stupnicki, *Die soziale Stellung*, 125.
61 See, for example, StATG, 9'10, 1.05/5, Kuhn to Zweidler, 17 July 1989. See Chapter 8, 264–268.
62 See Chapter 5, 186–187.
63 StATG, 9'40, 2.3/19.5, Verena Gebhart to Kuhn, 3 March 1955.
64 StATG, 9'40, 3.0.0/6, Kuhn to the office of personnel, no date (February 1964).
65 StATG, 9'10, 1.2.8/0, Government Council Member Müller to Director Hermann Wille, 19 January 1939.
66 Thus for example, StATG, 9'40, 3.1.11/0, Kuhn to Wolfgang Blankenburg, 17 April 1978.
67 Kuhn mentions several contacts in his self-representation: Kuhn, 'Roland Kuhn', 223.
68 StATG, 9'40, 3.1.12/0, Manfred Bleuler to Kuhn, 19 March 1942.
69 StATG, 9'40, 3.1.47/0, Kuhn to Klaesi, 14 September 1945.
70 Kuhn, 'Roland Kuhn', 223.
71 StATG, 9'10, 1.1.0/60, ARM 1975, 4.
72 StATG, 9'40, 3.1.22/0, Christ to Kuhn, 22 October 1940; similar tone and content: *ibid.*, 22 January 1945; 30 May 1950.
73 StATG, 9'40, 3.1.47/0, Kuhn to Jakob Klaesi, 23 May and 31 May 1944; similarly, also in 1946, the first report on the trial of a test substance, which Kuhn had Zolliker approve.
74 StATG, 4'840'33, supervisory commission minutes, 15 November 1954, where this accusation is made. The clinical director was responsible for the entire administration. When Kuhn took over the directorate in 1971, medical and administrative responsibilities were separated.
75 StATG, 9'40, 2.3/19.5, Verena Gebhart to Kuhn, 15 August 1954; also *ibid.*, 3 March 1955, on the late arrival to a joint meeting.
76 A former assistant physician of 1959/1960 remembers him as an authoritative bureaucrat, interview of 6 March 2018; René Bloch has fond memories, interview of 14 March 2018.
77 Kuhn, 'Roland Kuhn', 227.

78 Interview with former assistant physician of 1959/1960, 19 September 2018.
79 StATG, 9'40, 3.0.0/3, 19 June 1951; similar in tone, *ibid.*, 19 September 1952.
80 A reproduction in Tornay, 'La gentille dame Largactil', 57.
81 Obituary for Ernst Gebhart (1877–1954), *Thurgauer Zeitung*, 25 May 1954.
82 Archive of the University of Zurich, enrolment card 48237, Gebhart Verena.
83 Gebhart, 'Zum Problem'.
84 StATG, 9'40, 2.3/19.5, letters of Verena Gebhart to Kuhn, 1953–1957.
85 StATG, 9'40, 2.3/19.6, correspondence 1951.
86 Interview with a former trainee nurse, 18 April 2018.
87 See Schoefert, 'The View', 176.
88 See Ratmoko, *Damit die Chemie*, 47–97; StATG, 9'10, 1.2.1/1, Ciba to Director Wille, 18 July and 26 July 1922.
89 Henceforth usually called Roche. An initial contact with Roche regarding the free delivery of Sedobrol in 1916 is mentioned in StATG, 9'10, 1.2.1/1, Roche to Director Wille, 3 August 1921.
90 An overview in König, 'Besichtigung einer Weltindustrie'.
91 Ciba and Geigy merged in 1970 as Ciba-Geigy. See Chapter 4, 138–139, and Chapter 6, 197–199.
92 See Ratmoko, *Damit die Chemie*.
93 Haller, *Cortison*; Cantor, 'Cortisone'; on psychiatric testing, see Healy, *The Creation*, 184, 185, 283.
94 The pioneer of the method was the British psychiatrist W. Linford Rees (1914–2004), a contemporary of Kuhn; see Rees and Healy, 'Clinical Trials'.
95 Tornay, *Zugriffe*, 33–46.
96 See König, 'Besichtigung einer Weltindustrie', 129–134.
97 *Ibid.*, 209.
98 CA Novartis, Geigy, PP 130, annual report of the pharmaceutical division, 1951, 1.
99 On Ernst Grünthal (1894–1972), see the valuable information in Schoefert, 'The View' regarding Geigy, especially 173–185.
100 Grünthal, 'Über Parpanit', 1287.
101 StATG, 9'40, 5.0.3/3, Kuhn to Geigy, 28 May 1946.
102 This pertained to epilepsy, Huntington's chorea, Parkinson's disease, imbecility, and cerebral palsy.
103 StATG, 9'40, 5.0.3/3, report dated 10 September 1946.
104 Kuhn used the correct initials of the surname but a fictitious first name; later, he no longer did this.

105 StATG, 9'40, 5.0.3/3, report dated 10 September 1946, 24. The mentioned reports are missing.
106 *Ibid.*, 24 f.
107 *Ibid.*, 12.
108 StATG, 9'10, 5.4/11201, Kuhn to the father, 16 April 1946.
109 See also the medical files, StATG, 9'10, 5.4/10205; 9'10, 5.4./11783.
110 StATG, 9'40, 5.0.3/3, Kuhn's report to Geigy, 20 June 1949.
111 *Schweizerische Medizinische Wochenschrift*, no. 50, 14 December 1946, 1282–1291; additional articles followed over the next few years.
112 Some information in Schoefert, 'The View', 184, note 670.
113 StATG, 9'40, 5.0.3/3, enclosed photocopy, Schwab and Leigh, 'Parpanit', 629.
114 For Kuhn's opposition to placebos, see especially Chapter 4, 115 f.
115 StATG, 9'40, 5.0.3/3, cover letter to the report, 23 September 1946.
116 *Ibid.*, Kuhn to Geigy, 1 October 1946.
117 *Ibid.*, Kuhn to Geigy, 8 November 1946. In addition, Kuhn also received a cheque for 400 francs; see Chapter 5, 182.
118 StATG, 9'40, 5.0.3/3, Geigy to Kuhn, 28 June 1950; *ibid.*, Kuhn to Geigy, 5 July 1950. The trial remained quite small and was only brief.
119 CA Novartis, Geigy, G_JU/V, ZF Recht, expired contracts no. 2219, English translation by F. Rupprecht of a memorandum written and addressed on 23 January 1958 by Franz Haefliger to Adolf Krebser (six pages). Haefliger sometimes quotes from older documents, which increases the value of his account.
120 An overview appeared in 1954; see Schindler and Häfliger, 'Über Derivate'.

# 2

# The 1950s: Testing frenzy with Geigy

In summer 1982, two years after Roland Kuhn, Paul Schmidlin retired as well. The medical doctor had worked for Geigy since 1945, and later for Ciba-Geigy, where he rose to become the head of clinical trials and the deputy director of the medical department.[1] He had supervised the trials with Geigy substances at Münsterlingen longer than any other company employee, regularly corresponding or telephoning with Kuhn, visiting him at the clinic, or welcoming him in Basel since 1955. In early 1960, he spent a 'month of practice' in Münsterlingen to become more familiar with the clinical situation.[2] At the beginning of 1980, the company archivist of Ciba-Geigy invited Schmidlin, in light of his official capacity, to arrange for important relevant documents to be transferred to the archive.[3] Schmidlin complied with the request, and the transferred material now lies in the Novartis company archive.[4] These holdings have been particularly valuable for this study, but at the same time they are noticeably patchy. Roland Kuhn's name appears among many others in the context of numerous trials in various places. This is enlightening, since even though other investigators hardly feature in Kuhn's private archive, he was not, of course, Geigy's only investigator. However, the fact that Kuhn's name is not found more often in the company archive puts his significance for Geigy into perspective. Moreover, the documentation does not start until 1960 and thus excludes precisely those records related to the well-known antidepressant imipramine/Tofranil, even though Schmidlin played a major role in this area. It seems especially strange that Schmidlin discarded not only all of the many letters and reports received from Kuhn but also Schmidlin's own letters and internal file notes on discussions or decisions related to Roland Kuhn. Without Kuhn's private archive, one would hardly be able to imagine the density of the communications between Basel and Münsterlingen.

A 1982 article in the Ciba-Geigy newspaper honouring Schmidlin hints at a reason for this strange state of affairs. 'A central aspect of his life's work', we learn about Paul Schmidlin, 'was probably the antidepressant "thymoleptic" effect of Tofranil, which was indeed first tested as an antihistamine and then as a neuroleptic. Subsequently, Paul Schmidlin managed to profile further important antidepressants (Pertofran, Insidon, and Anafranil) and develop them into an actual product line of antidepressants.'[5] Kuhn is never mentioned. To delete Kuhn from the history of the development of antidepressants and fully appropriate this narrative, Schmidlin and, concomitantly, the company's internal written records had reduced him to a mere footnote; it was a move that unmistakably paralleled Kuhn's own practice of minimalising the role of Geigy (along with all other industry contacts) in the clinic's public reporting.[6]

Earlier, Schmidlin had been more cautious; in a 1958 internal paper, he still clearly commented on Kuhn's role.[7] But the company had changed a lot since then. By 1982, hardly any of the key figures in the 1950s development of psychopharmaceuticals still worked for Ciba-Geigy. Kuhn would not become aware of the trick Schmidlin had pulled on him until he was quite old (and after Schmidlin had died) – that is, not until Schmidlin's perspective informed the first scholarly account of the development of antidepressants.[8] Incensed, Kuhn created a counternarrative and, in order to prove his pre-eminent role in this development, inquired at Novartis for written records from the old Geigy archive to supplement his own documentation.[9] But nothing he was wanted was still available.

The development of the first antidepressant thus leads to a battle over authorship and ranking orders, part of which included the compiling or elimination of documentation. From a scholarly perspective, however, the question of who deserves credit for 'discovering' the antidepressant effect of Tofranil leads us astray. A cognitive process such as the development of a potential medication involves an entire network of actors and things, including the many unsuccessful paths of research.[10] Therefore, this chapter focuses on the long-term multilayered interactions between substances, patients, clinic staff, and the pharmaceutical industry, which ultimately brought the first antidepressant to the market in 1958.

## From ineffective sleeping pill to potential psychotropic drug

When Geigy's laboratory chemists started synthesising iminodibenzyl derivatives in 1948/1949, expectations about their possible uses were very vague. There were hopes for spasmolytic – that is, antispasmodic – effects, for example, against asthma. Following on the success with Parpanit, Parkinson's disease was also under discussion. In summer 1949, the first substances from the group of iminodibenzyl derivatives made their way to Ernst Grünthal at the Waldau Brain Anatomy Institute. Extracts from his reports are found in Kuhn's private archive.[11] The Geigy chemist Franz Häfliger summarised their content at the turn of the year 1949/1950.[12] Grünthal was unable to say whether any effect could be achieved for Parkinson's. However, the first trial on healthy probands revealed a clear soporific effect. According to Grünthal, this was especially prominent in substance G 22150. Substance G 22355 from the same substance group interested him too because of possible effects on the sensation of pain. Robert Domenjoz, Geigy's lead pharmacologist, responded immediately and arranged for an in-depth trial of the substance as a sleep remedy. In February 1951, Grünthal received five additional substances from the series with the task of comparing them with G 22150 from this perspective.[13]

In October 1950, after a preliminary oral discussion, Domenjoz arranged for a test quantity of G 22150 to be sent to Münsterlingen with the request that the substance be tested for suitability as sleep medicine, but also that it be compared to Parpanit, a new package of which was promptly delivered as well.[14] How many people received this drug from Kuhn remains unclear; three handwritten names are included in a subsequent letter. He seems not to have made a comparison with Parpanit.[15] The first delivery of 500 tablets was consumed within two months; another same-size delivery arrived before Christmas. A phone memo by Robert Domenjoz noted in March 1951 that Kuhn had not yet written the promised report, but that he believed 'that a usable sleep medicine can be developed from G 22150. The preparation enjoys a certain popularity among patients and nursing staff.' In addition, it had become evident 'that, for agitated patients, a good sedation can be achieved with G 22150' – this observation, noted in passing, would become quite important later.[16] Habituation did not occur, Kuhn reported, nor were there any disruptive side-effects. German testers who had also received the substance were less optimistic in this regard. The effect as a sleep medicine, they noted, was 'irregular'; a 'relatively large number of failures [were] observed, likewise side-effects are quite frequent, especially side-effects in the morning (tiredness, light-headedness, dizziness, drowsiness, headaches, etc.).'[17] The trial in Münsterlingen ended during the year without any record of the actual end date; this too would later be a recurring pattern. In the end, Grünthal distributed the medication on an ambulatory basis to acquaintances – by his own account, with good success. However, he considered other substances from the iminodibenzyl series so unsuitable that they never even reached the clinical trial stage. Kuhn's report remained unwritten; communications by phone and in person sufficed; he too was ultimately no longer convinced by the quality of the substance.[18] Thus for the time being, G 22150 and the other iminodibenzyl substances seemed to have reached the end of the road.[19]

But then came reports from Paris, which gave good reason to rethink matters. At an annual meeting in June 1952, French psychiatrists reported that a pharmacological substance had been unusually successful in sedating schizophrenic patients at the Sainte-Anne Psychiatric Hospital in Paris.[20] The substance was chlorpromazine, from the phenothiazine series, originally developed in hopes of an improved anaesthesia for surgery. Soon thereafter it appeared on the market as Largactil. At the Friedmatt clinic in Basel, the new method was taken up in early 1953.[21] As Roland Kuhn later recalled, it promptly became a success.

> In the history of Swiss psychiatry, 21 June 1953 will always remain memorable, when physicians of the Basel Psychiatric Clinic reported on their first experiences with the Largactil treatment that came from Paris. Within the next few weeks, the then-new treatment spread to the institutions of the whole of Switzerland.[22]

The precondition for the rapid breakthrough of a still entirely unknown method were earlier experiences with physical treatments. They paved the way for the belief that there might actually be medication for treating schizophrenic disorders, which had long been deemed incurable. Another colloquium in November 1953 dedicated specifically to Largactil heightened the interest even more. Kuhn travelled to the colloquium with Verena Gebhart.[23] She was closely involved in the wave of testing of psychopharmaceutical substances at Münsterlingen from the very beginning.

By late July, Kuhn had written to John E. Staehelin, director of the Friedmatt clinic in Basel, explaining that they too were now using Largactil.[24] Largactil is regularly recorded in medical histories of Münsterlingen patients as of 1953; many of the patients treated early on with the drug were later also included in Kuhn's trials. In February 1954, Largactil was officially approved in Switzerland; Kuhn never wrote up a report about the early experiences. Shortly before he had told the medical services department in Frauenfeld about Largactil and applied for a supplementary credit of 12,000 francs because the new medication was not cheap. 'Our previous experiences show that we cannot forgo the application of the medication without robbing our patients of an essential relief that modern medicine is able to give them. Our staff too feels that work is easier when many patients, particularly the most difficult, are sedated by the medication.'[25]

For Kuhn, Largactil seems to have functioned as a catalyst that drew his attention back to the trials with G 22150. Years later, Kuhn would claim that he had suggested to Geigy as early as 1951 that the systematic testing of G 22150 be continued for schizophrenics, no longer as a sleep medicine but as a psychotropic drug. But, he noted, the company had showed such little interest that he dropped the matter in frustration. This account happened to dovetail with the highly self-flattering notion that, along with discovering an antidepressant, he had also nearly discovered one of the first neuroleptic drugs, for G 22150 was closely related to one such drug.[26] Scepticism is warranted, however, for the story of a drug trial thwarted by a mindless company only emerges and gradually takes shape in his writings as of 1970.[27] Back in 1954, when Kuhn had actually reached out to Domenjoz with a detailed letter, he did not refer, for example, to any earlier such suggestion that might have lent weight to his concerns at that particular moment. Instead, he merely reminded Domenjoz of his report that the substance had a sedative effect on agitated patients.

> But when the Largactil treatment of the psychoses came up, it immediately occurred to me that the Largactil treatment comes remarkably close to that of your substance. I therefore used the occasion

of a fortuitous telephone conversation with one of your employees to make him aware of this problem. In my opinion, it would be interesting to pursue this matter further. Elsewhere they are also certainly looking to test substances that have a similar effect to Largactil on psychoses, and naturally one hopes in this way to perhaps find an even more effective substance.[28]

With no lack of business acumen, Kuhn appealed to Geigy's interest in being able to meet foreign competitors with a Swiss and possibly less expensive product. But in this case, major powers of persuasion were unnecessary, for Domenjoz was obviously already clued in; he responded quickly and proposed a meeting in Basel.

## Psychotropics: The start of ongoing testing

In mid-April 1954, a shipment of G 22150 arrived from Basel.[29] The moment marked the start of a decades-long practice of testing new substances for their psychopharmacological utility. From then until into the 1970s, unapproved substances were almost continuously being tested and used at the clinic, usually several at once. In April 1954, when Domenjoz inquired about the possibility of further testing, Kuhn pointed out his facility's limited capacity. 'You will probably understand that this is simply not possible in a state institution. We do not have the necessary staff, neither in the medical nor in the laboratory sector. I do not want to take on an assignment that I cannot carry out with the necessary thoroughness.'[30] With 731 inpatients, the clinic reached its highest occupancy level in late 1954; for each of the clinic's four assistant physicians and two senior physicians, there were 122 people who required looking after. Moreover, there was a rapidly growing outpatient clinic. The small laboratory set up in 1942 employed one lab technician. The sound performance of trials required constant measuring (blood pressure, pulse, temperature), observation, questioning, and controls, along with the compilation of the corresponding written documentation. Kuhn's reticence was well-founded, but it soon gave way to a veritable frenzy of testing; he never again spoke about his personal reservations from the early period.

Geigy's test substances were especially prevalent during the first years. By 1960, at least fourteen had made their way to

Münsterlingen. The first Ciba product came as early as May 1954, namely, the extraordinarily successful medication Serpasil, which had been approved as an antihypertensive in 1953 and was being tested with a new indication for the treatment of schizophrenia. But the scope of this trial at Münsterlingen was very limited. A combined preparation of Serpasil and Ritalin followed two months later.[31] The designation and delineation of the new substances were still unclear; they were referred to alternatively as 'mental drugs' or 'neuroplegics'. Around 1957, the prevalent term in professional discourse for this type of substance came to be neuroleptics (known as 'major tranquilizers' in the United States).[32] One year earlier, another Ciba substance from this class, potentially with an effect similar to Largactil, had arrived at Münsterlingen, but nothing came of it.[33] Starting in 1958, the Sandoz company also actively sought contact with Kuhn and delivered a first test substance. Kuhn found it to have little effect, but made suggestions for changing the formula.[34] At Sandoz they decided to continue the correspondence, even though Kuhn was speaking 'as a layperson in this field' and his ideas were infeasible. 'Since the latter shows quite a great interest and is an excellent investigator and we have now properly established contact with him, I consider it desirable to use this method as well "to keep warm" this trial site.'[35] By then, Roland Kuhn was a well-known and sought-after man in the world of clinical trials; in spring 1958, Tofranil, which he had tested, was approved as an antidepressant, whereupon it quickly proved to be a major therapeutic and commercial success (Figure 2.1). By now the only major Swiss pharmaceutical company not represented at Münsterlingen was Hoffmann-La Roche. Introduced in 1960, Roche's sedative Taractan, a now-forgotten precursor of benzodiazepines, was not tested in Münsterlingen, but Roche too courted the well-known investigator. 'It would be very opportune for us if you could form a personal assessment of the qualities of the effect of "Taractan" already prior to the official introduction.'[36] They never worked together on this case; even later, their collaboration remained sporadic because Kuhn was always quite sceptical about the line favoured by Roche (benzodiazepines) since it quickly led to addiction.

It is worth noting, as an interim result, that the strong perception of Largactil's success induced all of Basel's important producers to

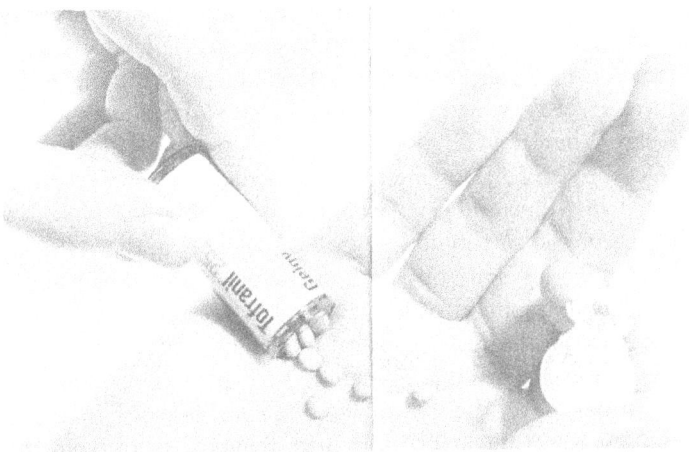

Figure 2.1 Advertising brochure for Tofranil, 1969

become active in this field. Geigy had gained a commercial lead that would not be challenged until the sensational ascendancy of Roche's Librium and Valium starting in 1961.

But let us get back to the beginnings at Münsterlingen, where the testing of G 22150 quickly got underway in spring 1954. The logistics were soon worked out with a system of storage, monitoring, ordering, and replenishment that would remain in operation for many years.[37] During the summer, the monthly consumption of pills increased to between 4,000 and 5,000. 'In our unruly wards alone, 130 tablets are administered daily', Kuhn wrote to Domenjoz in 1955.[38] The deliveries now each consisted of 10,000 pills, enough for roughly two months. In late July 1954, after a three-month testing operation, Kuhn delivered his first interim report. Shortly thereafter, Domenjoz told him they would henceforth be paying him a monthly 'trial fee' of 300 francs, retroactively from the start of testing in April. Kuhn agreed and provided his private account number; thus began decades of continuous financial earnings from Basel.[39] At the same time, he reported that he was now also able 'to test the new preparation about which we spoke last time'. It was G 22355, the future Tofranil. He asked for the new substance to be coloured 'so that these dragees[40] can be clearly distinguished from the others and no confusion can occur'. A second report on

G 22150 followed in March 1955, now in great detail. By this time the new substance G 22355 was also being used. The tablets were coloured red, and the drug was referred to internally as 'Geigy Red'. Substance G 22150, which would never receive a brand name, was now 'Geigy White'.

In October 1955, an internal 'Directive regarding Cures' was issued in Münsterlingen, probably written by Kuhn, which noted: 'The physician should himself keep a sheet in the ward, in which he enters his daily observations in key words, but legibly. The sheet should contain little, namely, the reason for the cure, short notes on the progression and on special incidents.'[41] The medical files, however, hardly ever include such physician notations, while information on the 'reason for the cure' is never found at all.[42] Roland Kuhn might possibly have removed them from the medical files to use them for his assessments and then disposed of them. But this seems to be an unlikely explanation for the scarcity of such notations, given that far less relevant documents were stored in great quantities. Especially since the directive was never renewed in later years, it is more likely that these notations were only made for around two years but were then forgotten.

The trial with G 22150 had new dimensions. In his first interim report of July 1954, Kuhn referred to forty-nine participating patients. He added their names in handwriting on the carbon copies, which he kept, this too a practice often followed in future. As per the second report of March 1955, the number of participants had grown to a total of 118 persons, whose names remain unknown (it probably included most of the original 49 participants).[43] Thus the trial involved approximately every sixth inpatient of the clinic. Among the 118 cases described by Kuhn in his comprehensive report of March 1955, 94 were schizophrenic patients, including, in his words, 'sixty-nine pronouncedly chronically sick persons. These have mostly been in the asylum for years and decades, so that for most of them the spontaneous course of their psychosis is familiar. Likewise, in these cases one knows the reaction to other treatment methods.'[44] Of these sixty-nine persons, a substantial share – namely, eleven – had been lobotomised, thus had undergone psychosurgery. But it should also be noted that Verena Gebhart, who also worked on the trial, used the substance quite differently in at least one case, in November 1954 giving it to a

16-year-old girl who was having problems in home economics and with her mother.[45]

The trial was a challenging undertaking, for it adopted a comparative approach; the key question to be answered was how well G 22150 performed compared with Largactil. The inclusion of G 22355 (Geigy Red) in the comparison in late 1954 further complicated matters. Kuhn addressed this in an aside in his report of March 1955, but wanted to 'express [himself] only very cautiously for now'. He could already say 'that the preparation G 22355 was ascribed with characteristics similar to Largactil, Serpasil, and G 22150. The substance seems to work in a similar way on psychoses.'[46] G 22150, too, was initially assessed as being very similar to Largactil. The patients became more sedate and slept better. 'They are less charged and above all largely lose their tendency to violence.'[47]

But this impression of a uniform effect soon dissolved, replaced by a more complex picture, which pertained above all to the so-called side-effects. More than eleven of the forty pages of Kuhn's first detailed report on G 22150 of March 1955 were devoted to them. The patients took the substance very reluctantly, finding it even more unpleasant than Largactil; the injections were particularly painful.[48] Decades later, Kuhn illustrated the difference between the two substances with his recollection of how, during Carnival back then, two patients had masqueraded as medications, as the 'good Lady Largactil' and the 'evil Lady Geigy'.[49] Kuhn found the occasional triggering of severe agitation to be especially problematic, and those affected found it very burdensome too.[50] Recent historiographical accounts cite the case of a patient in such a condition. Wearing a nightshirt and singing loudly, he supposedly rode a bicycle to the next village, which raised alarm among the inhabitants and at Geigy and almost called the continuation of the trial into question.[51] The very belated recollection of this event has high anecdotal value, but nowhere is such an incident mentioned in the dense records of the correspondence between Basel and Münsterlingen at the time. Nonetheless, there was no doubt about the excitatory effect. In March 1955, prior to the detailed report, Kuhn also wrote, 'Very unpleasant are the visual disorders, which, above all for people whose accommodation is no longer very good, in certain circumstances even forces the discontinuation of the medication.' In summer 1955, his concern grew to great uneasiness upon learning that testing with a Sandoz substance at the Friedmatt in Basel had led to the blindness of several patients – the two affected persons recovered with time. This prompted caution at Münsterlingen; numerous eye exams were subsequently carried out at the Cantonal Hospital Münsterlingen. They did not reveal anything serious, but the fright had a long-lasting impact and led to corresponding checks.[52]

As ambitious and inexperienced as he was, in autumn 1955, Kuhn recommended that Geigy quickly launch G 22150.[53] Back in a summarising report of March 1955, however, Kuhn had left no doubt that the substance was not quite as good as Largactil and Serpasil. Even so, G 22150 seemed to trigger fewer allergic reactions. 'This therefore raises the question, whether it would not be advisable to also conduct trials on a larger scale with a similar substance about which it can be assumed, due to its pharmacological characteristics, that the side-effects are fewer.'[54] Such trials had already started on a smaller scale – with G 22355, Geigy Red.

## The circuitous route to an antidepressant

Including G 22355 in the ongoing trials was an obvious step. Grünthal had singled out the substance early on, albeit for another indication, namely, because of a possible effect on pain sensitivity. In a second report, he had also mentioned an effect on schizophrenia. Roland Kuhn would later claim that he himself had played a part in the selection of G 22355 as the next substance to be tested because he had recognised the great similarity with Largactil from the structural formula, but he was mistaken.[55] He only received the formulas in November 1954, together with the first 1,000 tablets, and by then the decision had long been made.[56]

This test series, too, was conducted in the hope of finding a substitute for Largactil, thus a substance with an effect on schizophrenia. After just a few days, Kuhn confirmed that this was indeed the case.[57] But then the trials dragged on for months without producing clarity. 'I cannot yet tell you anything conclusive about G 22355', Kuhn reported after three-quarters of a year in September 1955. 'It seems to me that the substance is indeed tolerated significantly better than the other one. But it also seems to be rather less effective.'[58] But then in early 1956, when he nevertheless mentioned occasional incidents of 'real severe and unpleasant conditions of agitation', Domenjoz became increasingly sceptical. 'Your new experiences with G 22355', he responded by return mail, 'seem to indicate that this preparation, too, does not correspond to our ideal. Are you perhaps able to deliver an assessment today already, whether any further testing of G 22355 has any purpose at all, or whether it is only blocking your work opportunities that are so valuable to us?'[59] Discontinuation was imminent.

But Kuhn did not want to follow him. He firmly maintained that, even though he was still unable to properly grasp its specific character, the substance was better than G 22150, and he actually recommended an expanded trial. His prestige had grown so much in the meantime that Geigy agreed and ordered a larger quantity of G 22355. The commercial pressure on Geigy to finally bring a strong and successful new product to the market alongside its antirheumatic remedies was unmistakable. 'We are holding our position and enlarging it', said the consultant Robert Boehringer – an important player in the background – in September 1956, 'even though we are lacking new preparations. There's the rub! Until we can distribute a second preparation with a broad indication, our situation remains precarious.'[60] In the previous year, it was noted at the research and sales meeting that Kuhn would soon reach out to two suitable investigators in the United States.[61] Not yet having had much experience in the American market, the pharmaceutical manufacturer saw Kuhn as a useful helper, even though Kuhn hardly had any contacts there.

One of Roland Kuhn's long-term traits was that he was often very late in delivering his reports. This was the inevitable result of his increasing workload with multiple trials conducted in parallel and his tendency to repeatedly assess everything from one side and then the other. In light of Domenjoz's doubts, however, he now worked faster and in February 1956 delivered an extensive report on G 22355 to the company. The effect he ascribed to the preparation was quite similar to that of Largactil and Serpasil. 'It works on endogenous psychosis in the manner specific to these preparations, namely, not only sedatively but also transformatively on the thought process and on the secondary symptoms in schizophrenia.'[62] This aspect was paramount; in May, the minutes of Geigy's research and sales meeting summed up matters: 'There is a comprehensive report on G 22355 by Herr Dr Kuhn. This preparation seems to present advantages over Largactil for similar indications.'[63]

An almost incidental remark that would only become important in retrospect remained unmentioned. One had observed several decidedly positive results for depression, Kuhn noted.

> It is known that Largactil and Serpasil have a very uncertain and often hardly detectable effect on depressions. G 22150 already seemed to us to work quite well on depressions in individual cases. This became clearer for G 22355, such that we are asking ourselves whether it would be appropriate to recommend the preparation precisely for such cases and to try to carry out additional tests in this direction.[64]

Unfortunately, he noted, there were relatively few cases of depression in the clinic. For safety reasons, he had previously been unwilling to dispense the substance to outpatients; but he would abandon this reticence because the substance was hardly toxic. At Geigy they were very satisfied with this information and handed over the further testing, as per the usual procedure, to the medical department; Paul Schmidlin took over the management role. The committee for research and sales had already doubled Kuhn's monthly remuneration to 600 francs, effective 1 March 1956. The payments to Ernst Grünthal were increased from 700 to 1,000 francs.[65] For his part, Kuhn ordered 20,000 tablets of G 22355 and an additional 20,000 of G 22150, which was still being intensively tested; they were provided free of charge. Meanwhile, he had just recently started testing an additional substance, Geigy Green. Subsequently, the consumption of Geigy Red sharply increased, while that of G 22150 – Geigy White – gradually declined.

Thus the trials continued with heightened intensity. In April 1956, Kuhn now reported quite urgently to Domenjoz.

> Since, as is known, depression is not only the most common mental illness, but rather one of the most common illnesses that there actually is, and since the effect of Largactil on depressions, as is generally recognised, is modest and usually actually totally inadequate, substantial opportunities would now in fact open up here.[66]

Kuhn reported in July that they were presently using 400 vials and 12,000 tablets of Geigy Red a month, emphasising 'the often very good effect of G 22355 especially for depressive conditions. Today we are already compelled to provide test quantities to medical practitioners for the further treatment of released patients.'[67]

The tests seemed very close to delivering success, that is, the regulatory approval of G 22355 as a medication for the treatment of depression – but then they got bogged down. At Domenjoz's request, Kuhn issued a brief report in August 1956 that emphasised the dual effect on psychoses and depressions.[68] Domenjoz assured him that he was the most suitable person for orienting the envisaged additional investigators. The next day, Schmidlin submitted the study protocol, which he had received in July, to the research and sales committee for approval.[69] But in the subsequent implementation of the trials starting late summer 1956, Schmidlin never forwarded Kuhn's report and led the investigators – the records show seven names from Switzerland and two from Germany – to believe that the product was similar to Largactil and was to be tested for its effect on psychoses.[70] Half a year later, Kuhn received the results. The reports were clearly negative; the drug was hardly usable. When he realised that the investigators had not included depressions, he protested. On 15 February 1957, he travelled to Basel for a discussion. Schmidlin deferred and confirmed that the trial should now be 'expanded and intensified' to gather more experience and learn more about the effect on various forms of depression.[71] Kuhn himself was invited to propose new investigators, which he promptly did. In several cases, he personally established contact and introduced the medication, such as with directors of the university hospitals of Basel and Lausanne.[72]

In later years, Kuhn would bitterly complain that Schmidlin, with his approach, had almost wrecked the project.[73] David Healy, the British researcher who in the 1990s conducted numerous interviews with surviving psychopharmacology pioneers, also became aware of the strange delay and asked about the reasons several times. Nobody had a convincing answer. By then Schmidlin had died, but his widow, along with other persons closely affiliated with Schmidlin such as the Basel psychiatrist Raymond Battegay, turned the entire story around. Battegay claimed that it had actually been Schmidlin who had urged the reluctant Kuhn to also test G 22355 for its effect on depression after the failure to achieve success for the treatment of psychoses.[74] According to Battegay, Kuhn's failure to acknowledge this intervention had severely offended Schmidlin. But there is no evidence whatsoever for this version; it seems to be the product of resentment and self-aggrandisement.[75]

The recollections of Kuhn and Domenjoz, who were also questioned, were imprecise and mistaken about some aspects, which is unsurprising given how much time had passed and the age of the two men – when interviewed, Kuhn was 85 and Domenjoz 89. In one respect, however, Domenjoz left no question: 'But one thing is certain, Roland Kuhn was the person who discovered the antidepressant effect, without the shadow of a doubt.'[76] Kuhn declared Schmidlin the main culprit for the debacle. He might also have wondered about Domenjoz, who since February 1956 had repeatedly affirmed his special interest in the antidepressant effect but then authorised Schmidlin without arranging for the instruction of the investigators. This may have had something to do with the division of labour within the company and the lack of cooperation between mutually dependent departments.

Looking back in 2001, Kuhn conceded – in an unusual act of self-critical reflection – that his own view, too, had been inadequate in the 1950s: 'At that time we had no clear idea of the now obvious difference between the neuroleptic and the antidepressant effects! Above all, depressive symptoms in schizophrenics had confused matters.'[77] In fact, he himself had encouraged these misunderstandings because of the ambivalence of his first reports on G 22355, in which he repeatedly posited that the character of G 22355 was comparable to Largactil and then mentioned the worthwhile effect for depressions only as an addendum. Only later did he find that G 22355 was useless as a neuroleptic; originally, he saw this differently, but he no longer wanted to recall the earlier error of judgement. The unanimous negative assessment of the substance as a neuroleptic by unbiased investigators was sharper than his own, and it may actually have done some good when it came to the substance's ultimate assessment by helping Kuhn gradually free himself from the fixed notion that the substance had distinct neuroleptic characteristics.

Bringing another factor into play, Kuhn noted that it was only the intervention by Robert Boehringer that prevented Geigy from halting the trial.[78] The extent to which this was true must remain unresolved. But there is no doubt that Boehringer, who worked for Geigy as an important advisor, evaluated the emerging antidepressant effect of G 22355 in very positive terms. He obtained the substance himself and administered it to his wife, who felt better within just a few days. Boehringer's interventions are documented as of November 1957; they were striking. Boehringer evidently strove to neutralise the opposing forces in the company by starting very high in the hierarchy. This was also in keeping with his status at the company, where he was fully free to move about in the various departments. In late November 1957, he wrote to Carl Koechlin, for decades Geigy's powerful helmsman and the president of the supervisory board.[79] One month later, he turned to Carl's brother, Hartmann Koechlin, the technical director and supervisory board delegate, and told him he was expecting 'a sensational effect' from the new medication. 'I myself have observed how healing its effect can be for a depression, and how many families there are in which this malady arises.'[80] His 'Pharma-New Years'-Observation' of 30 December 1957 seemed clairvoyant. 'With this we are penetrating an area that previously was hardly accessible, whose scale is probably extraordinarily large.'[81]

## Breakthrough: Tofranil

In October 1957, Paul Schmidlin submitted the 'Circulation Dossier on the Approval Application' to the research and sales committee, compiled the now largely positive test results, and recommended a rapid market launch.[82] Despite the delays for which he himself was to blame, his reputation had not suffered; in June, the executive committee had promoted him to the position of an officer of the company.[83] In late August 1957, with the agreement of Domenjoz, Roland Kuhn had published an important article, 'On the Treatment of Depression with an Iminodibenzyl Derivative (G 22355)', in the *Schweizerische Medizinische Wochenschrift*.[84] In September, he had presented the new substance at the International Congress of Psychiatry in Zurich, at which point the preparation still had no name. However, the lecture drew only a very small audience – a dozen people, according to legend. All interest still focused on neuroleptics; nobody was expecting a medication of the type described by Kuhn. Schmidlin remained sceptical and advised caution.

With the introduction of G 22355, Geigy will enter a field of medicine that is new for the company; such an introduction therefore constitutes a special case. There are many – and, according to the view of the undersigned, important – reasons that speak in favour of the mode of introduction with a test designation.[85]

One still simply knew too little about the mode of action and its theoretical bases. 'If selling the preparation under a brand, however, the scientific prestige of the company will be much more strongly exposed than with the introduction under the mere designation with a number.'[86] Schmidlin therefore proposed the name 'Mental Drug G 22' and that promotional efforts be wholly restricted to clinics and mental institutions.

The restrictive line only partially prevailed.[87] The substance received its name just before it was approved: imipramine for the substance and Tofranil for the brand name. It was approved on 13 March 1958 in Switzerland, then at the end of the year in Germany, and in 1959 in the United States. In spring 1958, the newly married Kuhn, together with his wife and Paul Schmidlin, set off on his first trip to the United States, conducted for the purpose of promoting Tofranil. In 1960, a delegation travelled to the Soviet Union, which had bought Tofranil amounting to 380,000 francs.[88] 'The previous sales in Switzerland developed auspiciously above expectations', reported the pharma committee as early as July 1958. 'Unfortunately the delivery capacity available today of approximately one hundred kg per month is only enough for the additional introduction of the preparation in Germany and perhaps a few neighbouring countries.'[89] Boehringer Ingelheim, the German pharmaceutical company, provided assistance and temporarily took over production for the West German market.[90] In terms of the number of tablets sold, by the second quarter the new product achieved a share of 8.6 per cent of Geigy's total sales; in the fourth quarter, Tofranil widely outdistanced the company's previous bestsellers, the antirheumatic remedies.[91] Sales of Tofranil from the Basel location increased from 2.9 million francs in 1958 to 20.69 million in 1959.[92] No product from Basel had enjoyed such a huge success since Ciba had introduced Serpasil as a blood pressure medicine in 1953.[93] In 1959, Geigy was in third place compared to its main Basel competitors, Ciba and Sandoz; however, as was noted with satisfaction, the company was no longer all that far behind Sandoz and had higher growth rates. 'It seems that, with Tofranil, Research has given Sales its own long-expected second leg.'[94] Geigy's still-new pharmaceutical division had grown substantially. At the same time, the antidepressants moved to the fore and pushed the longstanding search for a Largactil substitute to the background.

In late summer 1958, the corporation's research director, Adolf Krebser, met with Roland Kuhn in Basel to discuss further collaboration. Kuhn agreed that he would not claim priority for *all* of Geigy's psychopharmaceutical test preparations, but he asked to be kept up-to-date on the experiences of other investigators. The pharma committee gave him immense credit. 'The committee therefore agrees to give him a special gratuity for a certain number of years, which will also be useful with regard to additional trials for which we will gladly involve Herr Dr Kuhn. These payments, which still need to be determined, would be made independently of the ongoing grants for trials.'[95] Emerging from the subsequent meetings was an agreement that promised Kuhn a bonus from the company for five years, starting with 30,000 francs for 1958, and 'in principle' the same amount in the following years, subject to the minor proviso that the amount of this payment would depend on the pace of business. This was accompanied by a provision that, from afar, brings to mind the typical prohibition of competition for highly skilled employees; thus in future, 'when working together with other companies, against which we raise no objections in principle', Kuhn would 'not carry out work on the specific area of endogenous depressions without a mutual written understanding'.[96] He had successfully fended off Geigy's initial effort to more tightly restrict his freedom by pointing out that other companies were already asking him to work with them.

> The processing of their preparations lies in part in the urgent interest of my patients and the asylum in which I work. At the same time, it also provides a comparative basis for the evaluation of your substances. It might be the case that I need to try such a preparation also for depressives, particularly also in cases where Tofranil does not work. Should a discovery be made in the process, I would inform you, as we have orally agreed.[97]

In late February, Kuhn received his first payment of 30,000 francs. It was much higher than his previous annual basic income, increasing it by two and a half times. The payment remained at this level for five years. In light of Tofranil's success, Geigy then increased the bonus to 50,000 francs annually as of summer 1964. Kuhn had received legal advice from a Bern lawyer for the contractual matters.[98] In this regard, he had one more important request for Director Krebser.

> May I ask you to draw up your letter of 15 January once more, and, in doing so, above all also in the address only write: 'Senior Physician of the Münsterlingen Sanatorium and Nursing Facility', since mixing up the directorate of the institution with this private matter should absolutely be avoided.[99]

Kuhn himself did not use the clinic's official stationery but rather wrote on his own letterhead this time; evidently, he typed the letter himself and did not – as was usually the case – dictate it to the secretary, Agathe Christ. However, this had nothing to do with Director Zolliker – Kuhn probably did not take this step out of a desire to circumvent him. But when it came to the cantonal authorities, Kuhn no doubt wanted to keep the financial remunerations for the trials, which he understood as a private matter, as inconspicuous as possible.[100]

## Pills of many colours: Kuhn as serial tester

In spring 1956, Domenjoz had reported on the status of the psychopharmaceuticals to the research and sales meeting. 'There are presently eleven substances available, of which eight were pretested for orientation purposes and three are in clinical testing.' *Pretested for orientation purposes* meant that the relevant substance had already been with Ernst Grünthal and found to be potentially worthwhile. The three substances in clinical testing were all at Münsterlingen: Geigy White, Red, and Green. The committee wanted an 'acceleration and expansion of the clinical trial' and asked Schmidlin

> to review with Herr Dr Kuhn the possibility of whether he could pretest a larger number of preparations in a short trial. The purpose

of this pretesting would be to obtain approximate information on effects and side-effects, which would enable us to do an initial evaluation of the preparation.[101]

In his new exploratory role as a rapid tester, starting summer 1956 Kuhn received one substance after another, while the main trials with Geigy White and Red were still underway. Schmidlin spoke about a 'pilot test trial'.[102] In autumn 1956, seven trials were being conducted for Geigy at Münsterlingen at the same time. There was also a Ciba preparation, which Kuhn had agreed to 'test for orientation purposes'.[103] Some of the Geigy substances were weeded out by the end of the year; in 1957, three new ones were added. For the purely experimental substances, the company now occasionally forwent the risk assessments by Grünthal and asked Kuhn to do them himself.[104] The company did not have enough of the substances on hand. Thus Kuhn agreed to test G 33679 Violet 'on a chronic case' for 'a possible toxicity'.[105] Meanwhile, the clinic's pharmacy needed to keep track of an almost unmanageable diversity of differently coloured tablets: green, white I and II, yellow, blue, orange/green II, black, violet, pink. Nurse Klara began sorting it all out in summer 1956 and gave Kuhn meticulous notes on the status of the inventory and where shortages loomed.[106] The situation only calmed down somewhat in summer 1959; the development of further iminodibenzyl variants seemed to have run its course.

However, the company's hope that the potential usability of new substances could be determined more quickly proved illusory. Kuhn's working method was by no means compatible with making quick determinations. As a tinkerer who loved experimentation, he was usually willing to prolong the testing. In his case, 'fast' meant from a few months to as long as half a year, but more often the trials dragged on for a year or more. Sometimes – and for reasons that cannot always be understood – Geigy revisited a substance that had already been rejected and sent it in for a second round of testing. Thus in 1959, Kuhn enthusiastically welcomed the return of Geigy Green (G 28568) in a slightly modified form (now G 31220). 'The substance is certainly psychopharmacologically effective. It is an excellent sedative, but the sedative-hypnotic qualities are clearly less strong than those of Largactil, not to mention those of Phenergan. The substance therefore causes less drowsiness.'[107] Kuhn's judgements tended to be more positive than those of his partners at the company; he always had patients on hand for whom, in his opinion, a substance showed a therapeutically positive effect. Ultimately, however, the complicated and difficult-to-produce compound substance was similarly discarded because of the lack of convincing effects.

The company let him keep going even after trials had been brought to a close. 'For now, we consider your preliminary trials with G 23746 and G 24415 sufficient for an initial orientation, such that at the moment we would like to desist from manufacturing additional test material. However, we strongly welcome having you continue the testing with the material that is still available', wrote Schmidlin in October 1956, for both tests were completely unproductive.[108] G 23746 Yellow caused vomiting and was unusable for this reason alone. But there was also little to report on G 24415 Blue. 'We have given up on these trials', wrote Kuhn in June 1957, 'because we have not been able to detect any influence whatsoever on the patients. However, here we never went beyond the initial tests with chronic patients.'[109] Only one recipient is documented. Despite the lack of effect, the severely ill man, who was isolated in a cell, received Geigy Blue for twelve months, the last two months being after the trial had ostensibly been abandoned. In his case, too, there is no documented effect of any kind or any justification for the continued administration.[110] Along with Largactil, he also received four test substances from the imino group. Only Largactil could sometimes sedate him.

A number of substances in the series were manufactured mainly for research purposes, the point being to compare them with each other to better understand a certain substance. In such cases, Kuhn proceeded independently and in some circumstances also continued testing after the company lost interest.[111] In this regard, hope for a healing effect was sometimes rather secondary; the purpose was more to understand interrelated effects and chemical structures and to refine substances. In accordance with the experimental nature of the substances, the number of probands in these cases was particularly small, often just a few individuals. On the other hand, in four of ten trials the documented numbers rose from fifty to one hundred. Occasionally other investigators were also involved, such as for G 28364 Black, which was also tested in seven other clinics. Kuhn received the reports on loan for perusal, but they have not survived. In his report of November 1957, he relied on the data of fifty-eight patients, forty-four of whom were diagnosed as schizophrenic; depressive illnesses were not included.[112] Nonetheless, he continued to make combinations with G 22355 Red, which was just about to be brought to market as an antidepressant. Whether the effect of a substance was presumed to be more antipsychotic or antidepressant – everything still seemed to be in flux. Kuhn constantly searched for the optimal supplement that still might have made Tofranil an effective remedy for the treatment of schizophrenia. 'The irregular successes of the medication for schizophrenia are based in part on its minor or lack of sedative-hypnotic effects', he conjectured in June 1957. The search took place along these lines. Sometimes here, sometimes there, he believed he had made a find.[113]

Apart from that, he deftly used the opportunity of such combination trials to secure for the clinic an ongoing free supply of Tofranil after the medication had been approved. This supply line functioned until 1961. Prior to the approval in 1958, more than 300,000 tablets had been delivered. The deliveries did not peak until later in 1958/1959, without there being any way to tell how many of the tablets went to the treatment of depression with Tofranil – now also often for outpatients – and how many went to new combination testing with substances that had not yet been approved. Basel only rarely admonished Kuhn because of his methodology. In late 1957, when he immediately started combining a newly arrived substance, G 31406 Pink, with Tofranil, Domenjoz pointed out to him the need to find out 'what G 31406 could do on its own, and then only at a later time address the question, whether this effect can be favourably modulated with suitable adjuncts or combinations'.[114]

Combining substances at his own discretion was one of the central features of Kuhn's testing method, and he would never give it up. He quickly assessed Geigy 31406 Pink as 'one of the most interesting preparations'. But he told Grünthal about incidences of states of agitation, as well as incidences of the 'most severe states of collapse ... that in fact seemed life-threatening' when G 31406 Pink was discontinued, while at the same time asking him not to forward this information to Geigy.[115]

Growing in conjunction with these serial trials was Kuhn's theoretical interest, his speculation about the connection between structure and effect, particularly with the variation of the dibenzyl sidechains. Were they the key to the puzzle of the effectiveness or non-effectiveness of substances with extremely minor differences? Did it have something to do with the addition or omission of chloride?[116] He was keenly interested in exchanging ideas with the pharmacologist Domenjoz and the Geigy chemists – much more so than in the views of his professional colleague Schmidlin. 'Since the core and sidechain for this substance', he wrote to Domenjoz in March 1957, 'are largely similar [to those of G 22355], there is the possibility that it also works for depressions or else particularly here it does not work like Largactil, which would then perhaps point to the significance of the chloride'.[117] Through his visits to Basel, he made contacts with the chemists, particularly with Walter Schindler, who had synthesised these substances.[118] Domenjoz wrote the following in February 1958.[119]

> For us and in particular for the chemist dealing with this work, however, it is of utmost importance to see certain speculations that are relevant to the synthesis of the preparation confirmed or refuted as soon as possible – since, after all, such clues are the precondition for our further conceptual constructions.

The deliberations of the pharmacologist and the chemist are not documented. For the moment, they went no further than a sporadic exchange of views, with Kuhn eagerly absorbing the new pharmacological knowledge. There was still a way to go before arriving at molecular models; not until the 1960s would Kuhn go one step further and put forward concrete suggestions on changing chemical substances.[120]

A Geigy employee retrospectively created an index of all the clinical trials carried out in the period from 1955 to 1962.[121] Even though he was still close in time to the events and had access to all the documents, the company's records were so disorganised that he had trouble determining the duration and end of many of the trials with certainty. A total of 117 substances – twenty-seven of which were psychotropic drugs, a share of 23 per cent – had been tested in various places. The number and names of the clinical investigators were not specified. Kuhn's predominant role emerges from his own documents; sixteen of the twenty-seven psychopharmacological substances passed through his hands. For him personally, the peak occurred in 1958, when he was involved in all eleven ongoing trials. Thereafter he was no longer as dominant, but he continued to be central. For the company, the peak took place somewhat later in 1960, when an unknown number of clinics were testing sixteen psychotropic drugs; Roland Kuhn was involved in nine cases. After that there was a big purge; by 1961, Geigy only had six substances left in the running, four of which were in Münsterlingen. In June 1957, Kuhn estimated that, in Münsterlingen since the start of testing in April 1954, 'approximately 500 patients ... [had been] treated with various substances of this chemical group'.[122] It is the only time he makes such a statement. Assuming his estimate was correct, calculations suggest that more than 25 per cent of all inpatients who stayed at the clinic between April 1954 and mid-1957 were involved in the early trials. However, the proportion of those involved must have been lower than this percentage at the start of this period and then grown substantially higher than this percentage over time. The maximum proportion would have been reached towards the end of the period in question.[123]

## Observing effects

Roland Kuhn worked very hard to make sure his determination of the specific nature of the tested substances was as precise as possible. His method concentrated on the individual case; the challenge lay in making careful observations and translating them into an appropriate linguistic form. Statistical systematisation was far from his mind; it only began in Switzerland in 1962, and he would not have been involved.[124] He faced many complications. On one side were the conditions of the illness, whose causes were anything but clear; on the other side were the substances synthesised in the chemical laboratory, which, in a way that was difficult to determine, intervened in the body's biochemical processes and triggered effects – sometimes blatantly obvious, sometimes barely perceptible. An effect was basically detectable through the external observation of behaviour, through measurable physical values, and then through the reporting of internal mental states. The latter required the patient's statements, which often only reached the investigator indirectly, mediated by the other physicians or by the nursing staff.

They were sometimes recorded in the individual medical files. Interim results and a final evaluation report provided for a written summary for the attention of the trial's sponsor.

The reports that made their way to Geigy varied in form and scope. Sometimes they were formulated as an extended letter, but often they arrived in Basel as independent documents with a cover letter. The Novartis archive holds a photocopy of one such report, which might have arrived there after the fact.[125] Some are individual reports and some are collective reports on several substances. The latter probably caused headaches for those processing the dossiers. Hence, from time to time a complaint would arrive from Basel, asking Kuhn to at least provide the information on G 22355 Red in a separate document. He could not be bothered; he decided on his own and did what he thought was right. The level of detail of his reports ranged from brief remarks on an individual test substance in a collective report to a forty-page treatise on his first trial with a presumptive psychotropic drug (G 22150) in spring 1955.[126]

The reports generally start by referring to the assignment, which is vaguely described ('whether it could come into question as a medication for the treatment of mental disorders').[127] This is followed by dry prose whose organisation and content have little in the way of a detectable system. Several brief statements about the group of test subjects (number, diagnoses, sex) are followed by sections on effects and side-effects, as well as a summary with a recommendation for further action. In keeping with his individualised approach, Kuhn additively arrayed individual treatments one after another or at most summarised them in small groups. Remarkably often, however, this penchant for making meticulous distinctions led to an air of indeterminacy: 'In a series of cases'; 'proves itself occasionally'; 'a certain effect'; 'seemed to have a sedative effect'.[128] Some statements were immediately partially retracted, for the opposite applied as well: 'it can further be said that it is a substance that belongs in the group that favourably influences schizophrenia to a substantial degree. ... But in many cases, the preparation leads to a deterioration for schizophrenics.'[129] However, such points of fracture also point to a certain quality of the reports, namely, that they did not hastily smooth out emerging contradictions to lead the sponsor to believe in certainties that did not exist.

The reporting style did not discernibly change in any substantial way over the years. Generally speaking, the depth of the reporting decreased with Kuhn's increasing load and his self-imposed commitment to carry out numerous trials in parallel. Kuhn's first detailed report of spring 1955 made very general observations on the 'suggestive influencing in a positive and negative sense', on the communications between patients and the nursing staff that could either bring a preparation into 'disrepute' or conversely make it look like a 'miracle medication'. But such statements later disappeared.[130]

One searches in vain for statistical overviews, even when large numbers of test patients are involved. A table – one with blood test results – appears but once, namely, in his article on Tofranil published in 1957. And the numerical precision of the following statement is rather exceptional: 'Thirteen of the 118 cases could take the medication only over fewer than ten days, mostly because of intolerance. They are included everywhere in the calculations and naturally worsen the success statistics, which without these cases would improve by around 10 per cent.'[131] In this first investigation of G 22150, Kuhn had by no means voiced any opposition to the large number of participants. 'Probably at least 100 cases should be processed, and nothing should be said about the effect of a substance sooner than after approximately one year.'[132] But in any event, numbers are usually interspersed in the text; they sometimes raise questions that are difficult to answer. 'The recounted experiences', Kuhn noted in the 1957 article that first introduced Tofranil to a broader medical audience, 'stem from forty cases with predominantly depressive clinical pictures that were treated with good results. But how many sick persons with similar disorders responded not at all or only very slightly? Our numbers are too small to offer reliable records for statistics.'[133] The method through which one arrived at a case 'treated with good results' remains unclear. Nor was the group of patients involved in a trial ever fixed and clearly defined at the outset; instead, it was gradually supplemented in terms of rolling planning. It was only when Kuhn evaluated his material and wrote his report that he performed the definitive selection until the number of cases was finally set, a process whose details remain inscrutable.

An inevitable and undiscussed point of departure for all reports was the distinction between effects and side-effects, or the therapeutic effect and the secondary responses.[134] It went hand in hand with the hope that the relevant substance would ideally develop, without major disruptive factors, a preferably specific effect on a certain clinical picture, that is, an effect that was both desired and also occurred in normal cases. To be sure, everyone concurred that the sought-for effect could not be entirely obtained without an undesired effect. 'The more effective the medication, however, the stronger are also the side-effects and vice versa', Kuhn noted in a lecture in 1961.[135] The arbitrary element inherent to the demarcation between effect and side-effect – a boundary that could be drawn in different ways – only came up for discussion in exceptional circumstances. 'We are getting to the discussion of side-effects', Kuhn wrote in a report of August 1958.

> If one ignores the states of excitement and the specific motoric pictures, as they appear with G 31406, and sees them as the actual effects of the preparation and not as side-effects, then one can say that, viewed as a whole, the preparation is extremely well tolerated and, in comparison to Tofranil, generally has even fewer side-effects.[136]

This statement, too, proceeds from the inseparability of the various dimensions of effect. Usually, however, the description was truncated at this point and gave the impression that the pertinent difference was inscribed in the substance by nature, so to speak, rather than being based on a researcher's decision.

When administered to human beings, the test substances triggered a variety of effects, some of which were welcome, others irrelevant or bothersome, and yet others unacceptable. If one considered the spectrum of effects as a whole, then the iminodibenzyl and iminostilbene derivatives appeared as hallucinogenic or narcotic-like substances, which occasionally also developed pleasant effects.[137] This emerged quite clearly in the description of so-called side-effects, without the concept of narcotic ever being mentioned. The reference to the 'very cocaine-like effect' of a new substance (G 33679 Violet) went in this direction, but remained isolated.[138] Kuhn always watched for signs of a possible dependency and was pessimistic about medications with a (presumed) potential for addiction.[139] Dependency, potentially also linked with pleasure, would have been diametrically opposed to his ascetic attitude. Even Tofranil, although deemed harmless, had its 'stimulating, euphorigenic, and intoxicating effects' when taken in sufficiently high doses, Kuhn noted in 1958.[140] He likewise attributed an 'occasionally even euphorigenic effect' to Geigy Black; it led to 'acoustic hallucinations', which he assessed as an 'increase of the psychotic manifestations'.[141] Much the same, he noted, was also observed for Serpasil (reserpine), which was already on the market. But, referring to its derivation from Indian snakeroot, he noted that Serpasil enjoyed 'a great advantage' because of 'the magical components of the age-old Indian healing plant'.[142]

Kuhn noted such actions to an even greater degree for G 31406 Pink, the most peculiar of which he felt was its motoric effect. 'In many cases, the patients begin to make distinctive affected movements. These can lead to actual dance-like motion sequences that are accompanied by song, which are obviously supposed to mean something.' Kuhn spoke about role behaviour, theatre, and stage to characterise the phenomena. 'Joining with this strange motoric behaviour is a pronouncedly elevated mood. The patients speak loudly, are jovial, feel good, seem to be content.' Then the eroticising effect, particularly for women: 'They became almost insistent toward men, but in part they also hugged, stroked, and pawed other women, and made indecent movements.'[143] Ernst Grünthal had earlier noted 'mild light-headedness of a pleasant kind', but without noticing any hallucinogenic effects.[144]

Preparations that could be linked in any way to sexuality had no chance with the sponsor Geigy.[145] The preparation was soon set aside in favour of the chemically closely related G 33040 Yellow II, which came on the market in 1961 as the antidepressant Insidon.[146] Emerging here, too, was a strange conceptual confusion around effect and side-effect. 'The substance seems to have a largely specific effect', reported Kuhn in his first report of June 1959. 'But for the time being we cannot yet say wherein the specificity exists in detail.' However, the side-effect turned out to be so dramatic 'for unsuitable patients' that Kuhn got carried away and elevated it to an 'effect': 'in an entire series of cases, it came to pronounced violence, which was not only very unpleasant for the patients but almost dangerous for the nursing staff. This was observed for half a dozen patients in various wards, whereby the staff of one [ward] knew nothing about the effect in the other ward.'[147]

Mixed effects were a nightmare for every commercial provider, for the approval authorities increasingly called for an unambiguous effect, even if this was wishful thinking.[148] Indeed, this was why Insidon (G 33040) never achieved approval in the United States. As result, its commercial success remained limited.

## The role of witnesses

The patients feared injections, which were often very painful. Hans Reimann, however, declared that the G 31406 Pink injections were simply 'wonderful'. 'He did not mean this ironically', notes his medical history.[149] Reimann was one of those 'model patients' who played an important role in the evaluation of new substances. 'He can vividly describe his state', Kuhn had noted when the 27-year-old diagnosed schizophrenic was admitted in 1954. The well-liked patient, who sometimes worked in the administration, lived permanently in the clinic until his tragic end due to an unexpected suicide. He was involved in an entire series of trials, which are not even completely recorded in his medical file.

To understand a substance's possible suitability as a medication, people were needed who could provide information. It was also by way of a 'model patient' that Kuhn claimed to have first recognised the antidepressant effect of G 22355 in late January 1956 – at least, this is how she made her way into the literature.[150] But Kuhn was not actually the attending doctor. On 21 January 1956, the responsible assistant physician, having been correspondingly informed by the nurse, noted as follows in the patient's medical history.

> For three days the patient has been transformed. All of her compulsion and unrest has faded away. The day before yesterday she herself noted, she had still been confused, she had never been so stupid. She does not know where it came from. She is only glad that she is now doing better again. It is not entirely clear to what extent the medication is supposed to have worked so suddenly within one week, or whether this depressive phase subsided spontaneously.[151]

Thus the 'discovery' was not the work of an individual; it was embedded in a social context with various participants within the framework of the clinical institution. Nor could what happened be seriously described as a healing, for the patient remained in the clinic almost continuously until being transferred to a nursing home more than twenty years later. But it was under the auspices of healing that the incident began its career; retrospectively in 2001, Kuhn described the incident as the decisive moment of discovery.[152] The temporary improvement evolved into a testimonial through which the new, unknown effect first entered the world. Back in 1955, Kuhn had declared that 'the subjective statements of the patient must be assimilated with much critique', noting 'there are numerous possibilities of error'.[153] On the issue of 'healing', however, he absolutely needed evidence in the form of patient statements or reactions from relatives.[154] 'Many times the relatives appeared in the physician's consultation hours with bright enthusiasm and declared, the sick person has not been this well for a long time', Kuhn wrote in his well-known article of summer 1957 that introduced G 22355 to the medical community.[155] Even in his internal reports to Geigy – in this case, August 1958 – the objective tone would suddenly become triumphal: 'In many places, the medication is described as a "miracle drug" and colleagues in the field of psychiatry repeatedly tell us that the successes are actually completely incomprehensible to them and that they would never have thought of the possibility of being able to treat depressions in this way.'[156]

## Death in Ward U

A set of files from the Münsterlingen clinic from 1958, which, under a list of names, documents the trials of the previous five years in the large Ward U ('Unruly Men'), has curiosity value. Written in meticulous calligraphy, the list was kept by someone – perhaps a patient – who neatly denoted the variously coloured medications with correspondingly coloured pencils. Twenty-two of the 244 listed names are followed by a cross, which was added afterwards and refers to the person's death during or shortly after the trial period. Two names appear twice (involved in two trials); thus this subset consists of twenty deceased persons, slightly more than 8 per cent, which raises serious questions.[157] Assuming that these deaths had something to do with the administered substances, G 28568 Green and G 22150 White appear to have been particularly dangerous.

Ten out of the fifty-two test patients from Ward U who received Geigy White and/or Geigy Green died after these substances were administered, which corresponds to approximately 19 per cent. By comparison, the three more experimental substances from the 'rainbow group' seem have been rather innocuous; even though they were tested on very few probands, none of the latter died. And the number of participants in the trial of G 22355 Red, which later became the successful product Tofranil, was high – the trial involved ninety-three people, two of whom died.[158]

Judging from the medical files, the deceased persons shared several features. First, most of them were elderly or very elderly (seven were 75 or older); second, they were generally in poor health – all were enfeebled and some undoubtedly near death. A large majority – all of those over 50 years of age – were diagnosed with senile dementia or arteriosclerosis. There were several cases of schizophrenia, but only among younger patients under 50 years old. Some had only been in the clinic for a short time but were given test substances nonetheless, in a few cases even just a few days before their death. And sometimes force was applied.[159] Reasons for the treatment with a test substance or why certain patients were selected are nowhere to be found. These patients no doubt belonged to that group of persons who could hardly express any information and who were included in trials for the general testing of physical and psychological effects.[160] Frequently one can also indirectly discern another factor, namely, the hope of sedating patients who were difficult to manage. That said, however, pure sedatives had long been available and were relatively inexpensive.

Not on the list is a young man, who at age 25 in 1956 had been in the clinic for three years. As a youth he had previously lived in the Asylum for Epileptics in Zurich, and he suffered from an unclarifiable organic brain disease with epilepsy and schizophrenic features.[161] Initially, he too was in Ward U, but he was then moved to an individual cell of a ward referred to as the *Hinterhaus* (rear building), where he was repeatedly restrained. 'He caused substantial difficulties there in that he was often loud and unruly, soiled and wetted the bed, spat.'[162] Apart from receiving Largactil, he was given an entire series of iminodibenzyl and iminostilbene derivatives, which at best sedated him temporarily. He has been mentioned earlier as the patient who was given G 24415 Blue for an entire year despite Kuhn having concluded that the substance had no useful effect. In early 1958, when it was decided to treat him with electroshock therapy, it became apparent that during his last shock treatment in summer 1957, after the discontinuation of Geigy Blue, he had suffered a two-sided fracture of the femoral neck, which had badly healed and left him completely stiff and unable to walk.[163] In light of this, the additional shock therapy was not applied. Instead, the patient was given Geigy Pink. After a severe collapse, he was put on Largactil again, the only substance he received that had a positive effect. One nurse took him on and helped him with walking exercises, and he did better for a time. 'The expression is calm and friendly, thankful for any attention.'[164] Further treatment efforts are not recorded; they had given up on the man. Even the protracted trial with Geigy Blue conveys the impression that the patient had been forgotten. The patient's medical history does not contain a single entry for the ten years after 1965; the final entry in 1975 records his death at age 44. The autopsy revealed severe brain damage, which was traced to the countless epileptic seizures. Roland Kuhn wrote to the father after the patient's death, giving him a nuanced and thoughtful account of how the illness may have occurred. Science too, Kuhn noted, had reached its limits here and ultimately could not provide any answers. The parents responded with a moving thank-you card. They had no idea what their son had gone through in Münsterlingen.

## Reflecting on depression

In late 1957, Jules Angst, the young senior physician from the internationally renowned Burghölzli clinic in Zurich, asked Roland Kuhn for information regarding his article on G 22355, which had been published the previous summer. Kuhn responded with a multipage essay. He refused to answer the question on the medical histories of the forty patients he had treated.

> I namely cannot quite understand how colleagues are able to represent the aetiology of depressive states so beautifully clearly that they can process them statistically. My experience must somehow be fundamentally different from those of these colleagues. Naturally, it is relatively easy, after perhaps one to three explorations, to say it

is an endogenous, a psychoreactive, or an exhaustion depression, in order to then, having been reassured, enter it into the statistics.

But in reality, he continued, when observing longer developments, one sees how often one state suddenly changes into another, which makes the supposedly precise terminological attribution useless. 'It may be that this looks very unscientific, but I must admit that I am of the opinion that it is more scientific to stand by these complications than to conceal them with a seemingly exactness of precise numbers.'[165]

In connection with the success of Tofranil, which went down in history as the first so-called tricyclic antidepressant, Roland Kuhn invoked the concept of vital depression, which he believed was optimally treated with this medication. He felt that a key element of this depression was the matutinal deterioration of the patient's condition, as he had already explained to Jules Angst. It took some time for what he meant by this type of depression to become clear in his publications. After the success with Tofranil's approval, he strangely stopped publishing; the testing of additional iminodibenzyls and iminostilbenes of the 'rainbow series' kept him extremely busy. Not until two years later did he start publishing new articles, which centred on Tofranil. Four years after the product was launched, he scheduled his first medical advanced training conference to formulate the concept of vital depression in detail.[166] 'I am of the opinion that this method results in an exactly definable and exactly determinable effect of a medication', he wrote to a colleague in 1966. He could not understand why hardly anyone followed him in this regard. Instead, one was content 'with quite vague terms that are poorly defined and, as per my experience, are also hardly suitable for the clinical determination of reality'. The psychiatrist countered that Kuhn's concept was not sufficiently workable to prevail. 'The only reason that we subsequently no longer use this term is because, outside the German-speaking area, this expression was either not understood at all or at least misunderstood.' Also, 'for didactic reasons', it was necessary to develop 'a schema of the spectrum of effects ... that can be used by students and doctors not specially trained in psychiatry'.[167]

Notwithstanding Kuhn's great enthusiasm about the new options for treating depression with Tofranil, he was not cut out for the role of a public prophet, as played, for example, by the psychiatrist Nathan S. Kline in the United States.[168] Kuhn lacked the necessary charisma; his texts, like his public appearances, were too unwieldy. He was ever the specialist who addressed specialists. Even so, he had clear expectations for the future. He assumed that the first psychopharmaceutically usable antidepressants would soon be followed by decidedly better and more specifically targeted ones.

> Our results, however, are not as good as the theory is beautiful, and we are therefore hoping for something different and better! We are hoping for medications with an effect of ever greater specificity that influence the psychotic process itself. One characteristic of this might be that the effect can be brought about or made to disappear depending on whether the medication is given or not. The (Tofranil) treatment of depression constitutes perhaps an initial breakthrough in this sphere of the chemotherapy of psychosis, even though it is only the start of a further development.[169]

Other reasons for Kuhn's public reticence are revealed by his exchange with Jakob Wyrsch, an old friend from his time as an assistant physician at the Waldau clinic. Kuhn reported almost apologetically in 1957 that he would be giving a lecture 'for the Geigy company'. The years of testing 'Largactil-like products' had led to useful discoveries that he now wanted to present at the International Congress for Psychiatry in Zurich. He meant this to explain why he was appearing there 'with such a topic, of all things'. Wyrsch was understanding, saying he was well aware that this was 'just a sideline' – there were greater things. When Kuhn asked Wyrsch in 1958 to write a brief exposition on the topic of depression for a Geigy publication, he apologised anew: 'I hope you do not misunderstand my request. I have not become a stockholder in Geigy and, apart from my honorarium for the clinical investigations, also do not have any involvement in the matter. I also do not want to help the chemical industry achieve exceptional successes.' Wyrsch subsequently made his debut as a Geigy author, but also occasionally jeered about the 'fat dividends' of the pharmaceutical companies. Thus the two men mutually affirmed their educated middle-class distance from the what they regarded as the despicable world of commerce.[170] He now hoped, Kuhn explained in 1959 to Jakob Klaesi, who had since retired from his position as director of the Waldau clinic, that he would soon find more time to 'occupy [himself] with something other than only with pharmacological substances'. He wrote much the same to Ernst Grünthal in 1961: 'The entire Tofranil matter does indeed oblige me to take part to some extent in the field of psychopharmacology. My actual interests, however, continue to be in the field of philosophy and psychotherapy.'[171] By this he chiefly meant his hobbyhorse, namely, daseinsanalysis.

The statistics of the diagnoses at Münsterlingen and other clinics recorded an increasing number of depressions since the 1950s. With the arrival of antidepressants, the diagnosis itself also generally underwent an upswing; in its modern understanding, the diagnosis first took shape during the postwar period.[172] Roland Kuhn wanted nothing to do with sociopolitical interpretations of this process, just as, in general, he rarely mentioned biographical, familial, or social factors in the development of diseases. His Basel colleagues Paul Kielholz and Raymond Battegay, on the other hand, went on at length with an expansive cultural-critical diagnosis of the times: 'The restlessness and uncertainty of our time, the loss of ties to religious, moral, and ethical values, and therewith the increasing encapsulation, isolation, loneliness and uprootedness of the individual, especially in the urban milieu, no doubt also play a causal role in the increasing frequency of depressions.'[173] Kuhn had nothing but derision for such arguments. That simply was not true, he wrote to Jakob Wyrsch, and brought up the horrific work hours and health burdens of the past. The phenomenon was receiving more attention today – he noted – and that was also why it was more conspicuous. Moreover, clinical statistics had previously used different terms. Jakob Wyrsch agreed – the contemporary concept of depression concealed many different things; 'the merit exists in that the name is better than back then and the statistics, however, are worse'.[174]

A manual on the 'Fundamentals and Methods of Clinical Psychiatry' appeared in the early 1960s. Swiss authors wrote many of the articles, and the introduction was by Jakob Wyrsch. The new 'psychopharmacotherapy', however, was not introduced by Roland Kuhn but rather by Frédéric Cornu from the Waldau clinic in Bern. Kuhn, on the other hand, introduced a different topic. 'Daseinsanalysis is difficult', he wrote, introducing his challenging and philosophically charged text.[175] The article was no doubt much more in keeping with his intellectual self-image than were the Münsterlingen trials, even though the latter had long dominated his everyday life.

## Notes

1. CA Novartis, Geigy, FB 1, material on Dr Paul Schmidlin (1917–1984).
2. CA Novartis, Geigy, PP 12/5, pharma production, medical department, minutes of a subject discussion, mental drugs, 5 February 1960, 3.
3. The invitation of the company archivist is in the referenced holding; CA Novartis, Geigy, FB 1, Paul Schmidlin.
4. As per said notice, the holding CA Novartis, Geigy, PP 12/5 is from Schmidlin.
5. CA Novartis, Geigy, FB 1, Paul Schmidlin; Ciba-Geigy newspaper, 6 July 1982, 10; quite similar, an earlier article on Schmidlin's twenty-fifth anniversary at the company, in: *Geigy Nachrichten*, 1 April 1970.
6. See Chapter 1, 18–19.
7. CA Novartis, Geigy, G_JU/V, ZF Recht, expired contracts, no. 2219, Fritz Rupprecht, The Invention of Tofranil, 4–5, with the summary of a 1958 paper by Paul Schmidlin (unavailable in the original), in this case dated 1953 because of a typo; see also StATG, 9'40, 5.1.0/0.2, Paul Schmidlin, Observations on the Clinical Testing of Mental Drugs. Experience with G 22355 (undated manuscript, presumably material for a lecture at the annual meeting of the American Psychiatric Association, San Francisco, May 1958).
8. Namely in the publications of Shorter and Healy; see also Chapter 8, 270–271.
9. Reference in StATG, 9'40, 12/71, Kuhn to Dr Raymond Battegay, 30 January 2001. The 'counternarrative' appeared in Ban et al., *From Psychopharmacology*, 282–352, the so-called imipramine dossier, which contains numerous relevant documents.
10. See Fleck, *Genesis*; Pignarre, *Psychotrope Kräfte*.
11. StATG, 9'40, 5.1.0/0.2, previous clinical trials with G 22150, undated (autumn 1950) and unsigned but clearly a carbon copy stemming from Robert Domenjoz; with extensive quotes from reports by Grünthal from 23 December 1949 to 25 September 1950.
12. CA Novartis, Geigy, G_JU/V, ZF Recht, expired contracts, no. 2219, memorandum Häfliger, attention Director A. Krebser, 23 January 1958.

13 Archive of the Psychiatric Museum Bern, private archive Grünthal, Kiste 1, 1_B: Geigy, Domenjoz to Grünthal, 9 February 1951.
14 StATG, 9'40, 5.1.0/0.1, testing of various Geigy preparations, Domenjoz to Kuhn, 25 October 1950.
15 Ibid., Kuhn to Domenjoz, 17 February 1954.
16 RA Novartis, clear plastic folder G 022150, letters, Kuhn-Geigy (Local 65, M26, G022150), previous experiences and findings with G 22150: file note Domenjoz of 27 March 1951: 'Regarding: clinical trial of G 22150. Telephone with Herr Dr Kuhn, Münsterlingen, of 22 March 1951.'
17 Archive of the Psychiatric Museum Bern, private archive Grünthal, Kiste 1, 1_B: Geigy, notable reactions after hypnoticum G 22150 (Dragée à 20 mg). Cases compiled from various German reports, 28 November 1951; cover letter by Domenjoz, 30 November 1951.
18 This is at least suggested by Kuhn's retrospective of 1954. See StATG, 9'40, 5.1.0/0.1, Kuhn to Domenjoz, 17 February 1954.
19 Ibid., Grünthal to Geigy, 1 December 1951.
20 Brief survey in Shorter, A History, 248–251.
21 Braunschweig, Zwischen Aufsicht, 210; Meier, Spannungsherde, 279–281.
22 Kuhn, 'Probleme', 319.
23 StATG, 9'10, 9.5/0, Kuhn to Paul Kielholz, Basel, 30 September 1953.
24 StATG, 9'40, 3.0.2/3, Kuhn to Staehelin, 25 July 1953.
25 StATG, 9'10, 9.5/0, Kuhn to the medical services department, 13 January 1954, 2.
26 StATG, 9'40, 5.1.0/0.1, file note of Kuhn, 18 September 2000: '... that I almost would have discovered not only the antidepressant but also one of the first neuroleptics'.
27 Kuhn, 'Beobachtungen', 210, suggests this course of events. In his autobiographical account, he omits this alleged episode; see Kuhn, 'Roland Kuhn', 238. In 1986, it appears in expanded form; see Kuhn, 'Clinique', 153. In his well-known 1957 article on Tofranil, he made no such claims; see Kuhn, 'Über die Behandlung', 1135.
28 StATG, 9'40, 5.1.0/0.1, Kuhn to Domenjoz, 17 February 1954.
29 The documented delivery of G 22150 of 26 April 1954 must have been preceded by an undocumented delivery; on 22 April 1954, Kuhn mentions that he had already treated five patients; see StATG, 9'40, 5.1.0/0.1, Kuhn to Domenjoz, 22 April 1954. The very first delivery occurred in 1950.
30 StATG, 9'40, 5.1.0/0.1, Kuhn to Domenjoz, 22 April 1954.
31 The preparation was never marketed.
32 Healy, The Creation, 117.

33 This was Ciba 17040.
34 StATG, 9'40, 5.0.8/1.
35 CA Novartis, Sandoz, H 205.006, 1959–1960, Cerletti to Renz and Jucker, 13 August 1959.
36 StATG, 9'40, 5.0.7/2, Roche to Kuhn, 22 March 1960, 2.
37 See Chapter 5, 169–172.
38 StATG, 9'40, 5.1.0/0.2, Kuhn to Domenjoz, 5 January 1955.
39 StATG, 9'40, 5.1.0/0.1, Domenjoz to Kuhn, 12 August 1954; *ibid.*, Kuhn to Domenjoz, 30 August 1954.
40 Medical definition of dragee: candied or sugar-coated pill to disguise the taste of bitter medication.
41 StATG, 9'10, 0.4/1, Directive regarding Cures. For doctors, 6 October 1955.
42 Physician records of this type are found in StATG, 9'10, 5.4/14298, 11 April 1957; StATG, 9'10, 5.4/12616.2, 23 February 1957.
43 However, 122 names could be determined from other sources, that is, four more than mentioned by Kuhn; not every identity could be clarified.
44 StATG, 9'40, 5.1.0/0.2, report for the attention of Domenjoz, 17 March 1955, 6.
45 StATG, 9'10, 6.2/6687.
46 StATG, 9'40, 5.1.0/0.2, report for the attention of Domenjoz, 17 March 1955, 39.
47 StATG, 9'40, 5.0.1/0.1, Kuhn to Domenjoz, 31 July 1954, 3.
48 StATG, 9'40, 5.1.0/0.2, report for the attention of Domenjoz, 17 March 1955, 8.
49 Tornay, 'Largactil', 58–59; this probably referred to the Carnival of 1955.
50 StATG, 9'40, 5.1.0/0.2, report for the attention of Domenjoz, 17 March 1955, 27–29.
51 Originally mentioned in an interview by Alan Broadhurst, a former Geigy employee of British origin; see Healy, *The Psychopharmacologists*, vol. 1, 116; repeated by Broadhurst in Ban et al., *The Rise*, 73; adopted by Healy, *The Antidepressant Era*, 51, and Tornay, *Zugriffe*, 133.
52 StATG, 9'40, 5.1.0/0.2, report for the attention of Domenjoz, 17 March 1955, 8.
53 CA Novartis, Geigy, PP 12/1, pharma committee, 13 September 1955, 2.
54 *Ibid.*, Kuhn's report, 17 March 1955, 38.
55 See the diverse statements of persons involved in Healy's interviews of the 1990s.

56 StATG, 9'40, 5.0.1/0.1, Domenjoz to Kuhn, 4 November 1954.
57 StATG, 9'40, 5.1.0/0.2, Kuhn to Domenjoz, 5 January 1955.
58 Ibid., Kuhn to Domenjoz, 8 September 1955.
59 Ibid., Domenjoz to Kuhn, 3 January 1956.
60 CA Novartis, Geigy, PP 12/4, Geigy-Pharmaka, 6 September 1956, 3.
61 Ibid., research and sales meeting, 1 July 1955, 3.
62 StATG, 9'40, 5.1.0/0.2, report for the attention of Domenjoz, 4 February 1956, 17.
63 CA Novartis, Geigy, PP 12/4, research and sales meeting, 25 May 1956, 2.
64 StATG, 9'40, 5.1.0/0.2, report for the attention of Domenjoz, 4 February 1956, 8.
65 CA Novartis, Geigy, PP 12/4, research and sales meeting, 2 March 1956, 4. The decision was conveyed to Kuhn that same day; see StATG, 9'40, 3.0.2/4, Domenjoz to Kuhn, 2 March 1956.
66 StATG, 9'40, 5.1.0/0.2, Kuhn to Domenjoz, 18 April 1956.
67 StATG, 9'40, 5.0.3/6, Kuhn to Domenjoz, 10 July 1956.
68 StATG, 9'40, 5.1.0/0.2, report by Kuhn, experiences with G 22355 on approximately 150 patients, 11 August 1956.
69 CA Novartis, Geigy, PP 12/4, research and sales meeting, 15 August 1956. The study protocol has not been preserved.
70 StATG, 9'40, 5.0.3/7, list of the G 22355 investigators, 4 April 1957. Ernst Grünthal was not included.
71 StATG, 9'40, 5.1.0/0.2, Schmidlin to Kuhn, 19 February 1957.
72 StATG, 9'40, 5.0.3./7, Kuhn to Staehelin, 26 March 1957; ibid., Kuhn to Steck, 9 April 1957.
73 Ban et al., *From Psychopharmacology*, 303–305 (the so-called imipramine dossier).
74 Healy, *The Psychopharmacologists*, vol. 2, interview Battegay, 376; on his proximity to Schmidlin and his wife, see 378–380.
75 Equally nonsensical is Alan Broadhurst's version, namely, that he himself, Schmidlin, and the Geigy employee Dr Kym had persuaded a reluctant Kuhn to also test G 22355 for depression. See Ban et al., *The Rise*, 73–74; Kuhn's statement on this matter in Ban et al., *From Psychopharmacology*, 302.
76 Healy, *The Psychopharmacologists*, vol. 3, interview with Domenjoz, September 1997, 366.
77 Ban et al., *From Psychopharmacology*, 303, Kuhn in the so-called imipramine dossier, English translation of his German text; by 'we', he means himself.
78 Healy, *The Psychopharmacologists*, vol. 2, interview with Kuhn, September 1996, 104–105; Ban et al., *From Psychopharmacology*, 304, imipramine dossier.

79 CA Novartis, Geigy, P 22/6, Boehringer to Carl E. Koechlin, at the time in Yonkers, United States, 28 November 1957.
80 Ehrenbold, *Samuel Koechlin*, 58; letter of 31 December 1957, supplementation of the quote as per information from Tobias Ehrenbold. See also Healy, *The Psychopharmacologists*, vol. 3, interview with Domenjoz, September 1997, 368.
81 CA Novartis, Geigy, 22/6.
82 CA Novartis, Geigy, PP 3, circulation dossier regarding approval application, dated 27 September 1957, 4 October 1957.
83 CA Novartis, Geigy, GL 11, executive committee, 20 June 1957, 2.
84 Kuhn, 'Über die Behandlung'.
85 CA Novartis, Geigy, PP 3, circulation dossier regarding approval application, dated 27 September 1957, 4 October 1957, 16.
86 *Ibid.*, 16–17.
87 The records of the minutes of 'Research and Sales' cease in November 1956. However, see CA Novartis, Geigy, GL 11, executive committee, 25 October 1957, 6: 'Antidepressant. The research and sales meeting has resolved to bring this preparation to market immediately.' The company followed Schmidlin's recommendation insofar as it focused advertising exclusively on psychiatrists and clinics.
88 CA Novartis, Geigy, PP 12/1, pharma committee, 22 June 1960, 2; 20 July 1960, 5.
89 *Ibid.*, pharma committee, 9 July 1958, 3.
90 CA Novartis, GL 11, executive committee, 26 August 1958, 9–10; 3 September 1958, 8.
91 CA Novartis, Geigy, PP 9/2, pharma production, quarterly reports 1958.
92 CA Novartis, Geigy, PP 130, Geigy pharmaceuticals, annual reports (written by R. Boehringer), 1959, 31.
93 CA Novartis, PP 12/1, pharma committee, minutes, pharma business Ciba-Sandoz-Geigy, attempt at a comparative analysis, 21 April 1960; quote from: pharma research, subject: business reports 1959 Ciba-Sandoz-Geigy, 25 April 1960, 2.
94 König, 'Besichtigung einer Weltindustrie', 210.
95 CA Novartis, pharma committee, 3 September 1958, 4.
96 CA Novartis, Geigy, G_JU/V, Verträge, Geigy to Kuhn, 26 February 1959. This letter records the results of an oral discussion of 9 January, as well as of an exchange of letters that is not available. The actual contract is not present.
97 *Ibid.*, Kuhn to Krebser, 16 February 1959, 2. This is one of the very few letters from Kuhn preserved in the Novartis archive.
98 StATG, 9'40, 5.0.3/2, Kuhn to Bern lawyer, 5 February 1959; the letter concerns the confirmation of the meeting on 7 February with

the enclosure of the contract; documents regarding the content of the advice are missing.
99 Ibid., Kuhn to Krebser, 16 February 1959, 3.
100 See Chapter 5, 185.
101 CA Novartis, Geigy, PP 12/4, research and sales meeting, all quotes 25 May 1956, 2.
102 StATG, 9'40, 5.0.3/6, Schmidlin to Kuhn, 29 October 1956.
103 See StATG, 9'10, 9.5/2, Kuhn to Kaufmann, Ciba, 14 November 1956. This concerns Ciba 17040, which was hoped to have an effect similar to Largactil.
104 See StATG, 9'40, 5.0.3/13, Geigy to Kuhn, 9 June 1958.
105 Ibid., Kuhn to Domenjoz, 11 June 1958.
106 See Chapter 5, 169, 171.
107 StATG, 9'40, 5.0.3/11, Kuhn to Willy G. Stoll, 23 June 1959.
108 StATG, 9'40, 5.0.3/6, Schmidlin to Kuhn, 29 October 1956.
109 Ibid., Kuhn to Domenjoz, 26 June 1957.
110 StATG, 9'10, 5.4/12772. The patient's medical history does not contain a single entry for the relevant period, January 1956 to February 1958; only the enclosed fever charts point to the duration of the testing with G 24415.
111 StATG, 9'40, 5.03/6, Kuhn to Domenjoz, 16 July 1957, regarding testing with G 31002, which Kuhn wanted to continue with the available supply after Domenjoz on 26 June had told him of the discontinuation.
112 StATG, 9'40, 5.0.3/6, test reports for the attention of Domenjoz, 29 November 1957, 2.
113 Kuhn, 'Über die Behandlung', 1137. See also Healy, *The Creation*, 228; he considers the attempts to cleanly separate antipsychotic and antidepressant effects as futile, for they are terminological constructs.
114 StATG, 9'40, 5.0.3/11, Domenjoz to Kuhn, 27 February 1958.
115 Ibid., Kuhn to Grünthal, 15 February 1958.
116 See the exchange with Domenjoz in: StATG, 9'40, 5.0.3/6, 16 and 18 July 1957.
117 StATG, 9'40, 5.1.0/0.2, Kuhn to Domenjoz, 2 March 1957.
118 See, for example, StATG, 9'40, 5.0.3/11, Domenjoz to Kuhn, 27 February 1958, regarding G 31406 Pink: 9'40, 5.0.3/6, Domenjoz to Kuhn, 16 July 1956.
119 StATG, 9'40, 5.0.3/11, Domenjoz to Kuhn, 27 February 1958.
120 See Chapter 4, 117.
121 CA Novartis, Geigy, PP 50, Klinik-Präparate: 1955–1962, undated (1962).
122 Kuhn, 'Über die Behandlung', 1135.

123 For this estimate, all accruals until 1957 (only 75 per cent for 1954; 50 per cent for 1957) were added to the total number of inpatients at the end of 1953, so that the 500 treated patients stand opposite a total of 1,705 persons; of these 500, an estimated 15 per cent were deducted as outpatients, which left 426 treated inpatients, that is, 25 per cent of 1,705. In this early period, for one, there were still fewer outpatients and, for another, fewer were included in the trials. Thus one arrives at a proportion of a little more than 25 per cent. Without any deduction for outpatients, the proportion of treated patients becomes 29 per cent.

124 Tornay, *Zugriffe*, 178–182; see also Chapter 4, 148–149.

125 CA Novartis, Ciba-Geigy, PH 7.04, pharma division (files Gelzer), report on G 22355, 4 February 1956. This is the report that first recorded the antidepressant effect.

126 StATG, 9'40, 5.1.0/0.2, Schmidlin to Kuhn, 3 April 1957.

127 StATG, 9'40, 5.0.3/6, collective report on G 23746 Yellow, G 24425 Blue, G 28342 Brown, G 28364 Black, 27 November 1957, 1.

128 StATG, 9'40, 5.1.0/0.2, report on G 31406 Pink, 10; 9'40, 5.0.3/6, report on G 28364 Black, 27 November 1957, 1–2, 4.

129 StATG, 9'40, 5.1.0/0.2, report on G 31406 Pink, 6 August 1958, 9.

130 *Ibid.*, report on G 22150, 17 March 1955, 2–4.

131 *Ibid.*, 9.

132 *Ibid.*, 5.

133 Kuhn, 'Über die Behandlung', 1136.

134 See, for example, StATG, 9'40, 5.1.0/0.2, report on G 31406 Pink, 6 August 1958, 13; *ibid.*, report on G 22150, 17 March 1955, 12 and 21. In general on the problem of side-effects, see Meier, *Spannungsherde*, 216–219; Spiegel, *Einführung*, 17.

135 Kuhn, 'Medikamentöse Behandlung', 520.

136 StATG, 9'40, 5.1.0/0.2, report on G 31406 Pink, 6 August 1958, 13.

137 Decades later, the British psychiatrist Joanna Moncrieff (see *The Myth*) developed similar ideas.

138 StATG, 9'40, 5.0.3/13, Kuhn to Rothweiler, Geigy, 6 December 1961; it concerned a metabolite of G 22355.

139 This was especially prominent in his criticisms of the benzodiazepines of Roche (Librium and Valium).

140 StATG, 9'40, 5.0.3/11, Kuhn to Schmidlin, 5 November 1958.

141 StATG, 9'40, 5.0.3/6, report on G 28364 Black, for the attention of Domenjoz, 27 November 1957, 6.

142 *Ibid.*, Kuhn to Domenjoz, 26 June 1957.

143 StATG, 9'40, 5.1.0/0.2, report on G 31406 Pink, 6 August 1958, 4–5.

144 *Ibid.*, Grünthal's preliminary report, 9 July 1957.

145 See CA Novartis, Geigy, PP 12/1, pharma committee, 13 May 1959, 3–4.
146 The substance G 33040 was structurally closely related to G 31406.
147 StATG, 9'40, 5.1.0/0.2, test report on G 33040, 10 June 1958, 2.
148 Healy, *The Creation*, 281.
149 StATG, 9'10, 5.4/13473, 20 February 1958.
150 Thus in Healy, *The Antidepressant Era*, 53, as test with 'Paula J. F.'; in Shorter, *How Everyone Became Depressed*, 165, as 'Paula G.'; in Tornay, *Zugriffe*, 154–155, as 'Paula I.'.
151 StATG, ZA KAs 21502, 21 January 1956.
152 See Ban et al., *From Psychopharmacology*, imipramine dossier, 302–303.
153 StATG, 9'40, 5.1.0/0.2, report on G 22150, 17 March 1955, 3.
154 On this, see particularly Balz, *Zwischen Wirkung*, 187–247.
155 Kuhn, 'Über die Behandlung', 1136.
156 StATG, 9'40, 5.1.0/0.2, test report on G 22355 and G 31406, 8 August 1958, 2; see also 9'40, 5.0.3/10, casuistic examples regarding Tofranil effects.
157 Regarding the deaths noted in this list, see Chapter 7, 231–233.
158 StATG, 9'10, 9.5/1, list of various trials Ward U, 1953–1958.
159 StATG, 9'10, 5.4./14182, 3 June 1956.
160 See Chapter 3, 99–100.
161 StATG, 9'10, 5.4/12772.
162 *Ibid.*, 31 January 1954.
163 *Ibid.*, 19 February 1958.
164 *Ibid.*, 14 August 1958.
165 StATG, 9'40, 5.0.3/6, Kuhn to Angst, 16 December 1957.
166 See Kuhn, 'Medikamentöse Behandlung', 520–521.
167 StATG, 9'40, 3.1.60/0, Kuhn to Walter Pöldinger, 26 July 1966; *ibid.*, Pöldinger to Kuhn, 30 September 1966.
168 On Nathan S. Kline, numerous references in Healy, *The Antidepressant Era* and in Shorter, *Before Prozac*. Kuhn sometimes made fun of Kline, saying that he produced his supposedly brilliant ideas while in a permanent state of Marsilid intoxication; see StATG, 9'40, 3.1.73/0, Kuhn to Steck, 30 November 1976.
169 Kuhn, 'Probleme', 325.
170 StATG, 9'40, 3.1.93/0.1, correspondence between Kuhn and Wyrsch, 11 January 1957, 15 January 1957, 15 April 1958, 21 July 1958.
171 StATG, 9'40, 3.1.47/0, Kuhn to Klaesi, 15 December 1959; 9'40, 3.1.39/0, Kuhn to Grünthal, 20 February 1961.
172 See Hirshbein, 'Science'. For various explanatory approaches, see the Introduction, 4.

173 Kielholz and Battegay, 'Behandlung', 763.
174 StATG, 9'40, 3.1.93/0.1, Kuhn to Wyrsch, 19 August 1958; *ibid.*, Wyrsch to Kuhn, 20 August 1958.
175 Kuhn, 'Daseinsanalyse', 854. On daseinsanalysis, see Chapter 4, 152–155.

# 3

# Test patients

In the early afternoon of 28 June 1965, Franz Traber faces two drawing tests in the Münsterlingen Psychiatric Clinic. The nursing staff of Ward K have given him two sheets of paper. Apart from a header for name, date, and time, both sheets are divided into eight rectangles. The first test calls for a specified object to be drawn in each field: a house, a flower, and six other things. For the term 'face', however, Traber draws the profile of a female nurse; the term 'person' elicits the drawing of a doctor or male nurse with a giant needle in his hand. After fifteen minutes, he switches to the second test. This one requires that he continues the drawing elements – dots or lines – that are already present, but the subject is up to him. Traber lets his gaze wander and draws what catches his eye: the tower of the nearby monastery church; a fruit juice bottle with a glass, the clinic's shaving utensils, two syringes, Nurse Rosa's battered eyeglasses, Herr Mäder's bald pate, and a hospital cot that he describes as 'my holiday bed' (Figure 3.1).[1] The dot in upper-left field is enlarged and becomes a 'sore spot'. At the end, Traber signs this test as 'farmer & illustrator', whereas under the first test he has written, also in block letters, 'I am a farmer, not an illustrator'.[2]

Franz Traber was a person whose medical history and biography clearly differ from those of other patients. His sketches are unique, suggesting a man with a sense of humour, a talent for observation, and creative prowess.[3] Yet at the same time, they can be grouped with a long series of other drawings made by patients on such forms. As in many other Swiss psychiatric clinics, the drawing tests in Münsterlingen were part of a routine that lasted decades; although they were not generally analysed, they were kept in the medical files.[4] When admitted to the clinic, every patient was given

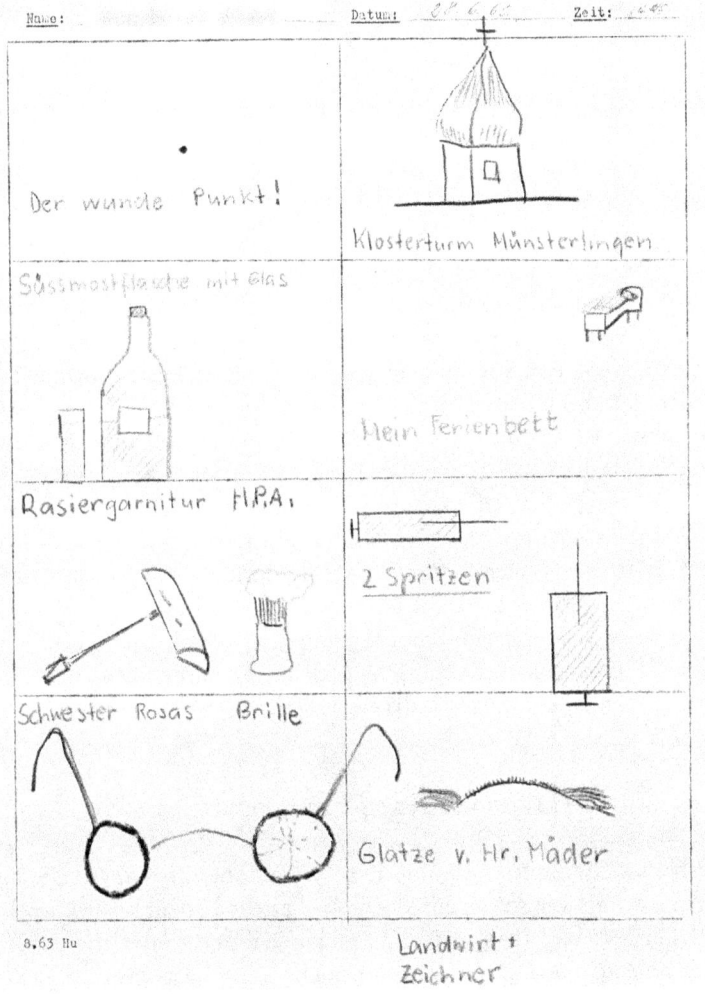

**Figure 3.1** Drawing test by Franz Traber, 1965

the task of writing a brief personal history and doing a drawing test. If readmitted down the line, they were given these forms again. Thus in this respect, Franz Traber was one patient among many. The anthropologist Emily Martin has spoken with regard to medicine about an 'empowered powerlessness'. Although patients are experiencing, active subjects,[5] the parameters of their agency are formed by diagnostic systems, scientific classifications, and the medical hierarchy.[6] The inseparability of knowledge from power is particularly conspicuous in the case of psychiatric patients like Franz Traber. In Münsterlingen, there was a clear asymmetry of power between patients and the clinic staff. But because very different types of patients were supervised, the spectrum of power relationships was wide, especially in the context of substance testing.[7]

Why did we process the dossier of Franz Taber, of all people? His name shows up in our corpus of sources in very different places, which gave us the opportunity to analyse his case from various angles. We first came across him in a test report that states he had severe adverse reactions to a substance – his name and that of another patient had been added by hand.[8] In addition, Franz Traber appears in Kuhn's private archive in three further places: a handwritten list of patients in Ward K who received G 35259 (ketoimipramine), a type-written list of discharged patients who had been given G 35259, and a list of patients who had received Ciba 32143 or 34276.[9] In the clinical archive, we found inpatient and outpatient medical files for Traber. His name was even found in the archival documents of a pharmaceutical company, which is quite exceptional.[10] As a rule, references to patients by name only appear in such documents if the trial involved incidents or fatalities.

## Münsterlingen's patient population

Traber's drawing tests of June 1965 were done three days after his second admission to the clinic – he had already spent several weeks in Münsterlingen the previous year. Three months later, the patient was able to leave the institution again, but he continued being treated as an outpatient. Thus Traber was counted twice in the clinic's statistics for 1965. He was one of 385 people hospitalised that year, and also one of 1,795 who visited the outpatient department. In the mid-1960s, the number of inpatients was just under 700. Since peaking at 731 in 1954, the number of inpatients had receded slightly and was now back at the average level for Kuhn's time at Münsterlingen.[11]

This decline coincided with another turning point. Whereas in the 1940s more patients tended to be admitted than released, the trend reversed in 1954. Occurring in many clinics, this shift can be traced to the introduction of modern psychotropic drugs. The new medications made it possible to release patients sooner and house the chronically ill elsewhere. 'The number of hospitalised sick persons declined', Kuhn wrote in a historical survey of the Münsterlingen clinic,

> since in many cases they did not become chronic. Chronic patients with regard to whom, based on previous experience, one had to reckon with the possibility that they would probably stay in the clinic for life, could be released to old-age and nursing homes, or even to their own families.[12]

As illustrated by the case of Traber, however, the psychopharmaceutical turn of the mid-1950s also entailed an increase in the number of outpatient treatments and readmissions. In the second half of the 1960s, Traber was hospitalised four more times; between clinic stays, he was continuously looked after at the outpatient department, which by then was treating almost 900 people a year. While the number of outpatients had already started rising in the 1950s, over the next decades it surged. In 1960, the outpatient department treated around 500 people; by the late 1970s, this number had tripled.

Franz Traber was a Thurgau farmer who owned a small farm, enjoyed his drink, and struggled with financial worries. Upon his first arrival at the clinic in 1964, he was diagnosed with depression; later, one referred to 'manic-depressive insanity'. In terms of his place of residence, social origin, and diagnosis,[13] Traber was a typical patient. The people treated at Münsterlingen were predominantly middle- and lower-class. They came from Thurgau and worked as civil servants or in industry or agriculture, or perhaps in skilled trades or in commercial enterprises. Affluent patients usually preferred one of the three nearby private clinics – Bellevue,

Zihlschlacht, or Littenheid. Although the largest group of inpatients (around one quarter to one third) between 1940 and 1979 suffered from schizophrenic, schizoid, and delusional disorders, the proportion with affective disorders, including depressions, grew most strongly during this period. While in the 1940s slightly more than 2 per cent – and in the 1950s just under 7 per cent – of the hospitalised patients had a diagnosis from this category, in the 1960s this group grew to 16 per cent and in the 1970s to almost 20 per cent.

What applied to inpatients was even more the case for outpatients. In the late 1970s, just under half of the women and more than one fifth of the men who visited the outpatient department were diagnosed with an affective disorder. A growing proportion of outpatients consisted of children and youth, which peaked in 1969 at 45 per cent. In the 1950s and 1960s, boys made up as much as 40 per cent of the patients, and girls accounted for as much as 25 per cent.[14]

The treatments varied broadly. Examinations and expert evaluations required only a few consultations. Independently practising psychiatrists or family doctors referred patients whose medications needed to be adjusted and reviewed. Some who received medical consultations at Münsterlingen came from other institutions and asylums. Former clinic patients and offenders on probation showed up regularly for monitoring; some patients visited the outpatient department every week for therapy. In the inpatient sector, the spectrum of people extended from those who were only briefly treated once through to those who were repeatedly hospitalised and to long-term patients who lived in the clinic for years. Some admitted themselves to the clinic on their own initiative; others were brought by their relatives or committed by authorities or physicians in private practice.

Apart from personal factors, what mattered most for individual patients was probably who looked after them and the ward to which they were assigned. As shown by Traber's drawing test, each ward was a world unto itself. The semi-open Ward K, where Traber stayed in 1965, had just under forty beds; other wards could be half or twice the size. Everyday life in a 'peaceful' open ward was substantially different from that in an 'unruly' locked-down ward. 'K patients', for example, were frequently allowed to hang out on the balcony or in the large courtyard because they did not need constant supervision, whereas the patients in the locked-down wards spent most of their days in the same room.[15] Thus in Ward P, a large dormitory simultaneously functioned as a work room; in some wards – for instance, Ward C for chronically ill and disabled women – the corridor also served as a day room.[16]

Traber's immediate contact persons were his fellow patients, the nursing staff, and the ward physician; he probably rarely encountered the director or a senior physician during his clinic stays. At the outpatient department he was treated for years by the same psychiatrist; only once, when the latter was away performing military service, did Traber sit across from Kuhn.[17] The likelihood of being treated by Roland or Verena Kuhn shifted over time. Both increasingly worked in the outpatient department, where Verena Kuhn specialised more in children and youth. Meanwhile, her husband, after taking over the clinical directorate in 1971, mainly continued to supervise patients who required an expert evaluation or contacted him personally.[18]

## Particularly affected patient groups?

Assuming that the entries in Franz Traber's medical files are complete and accurate, he was prescribed numerous approved medications – neuroleptic drugs, antidepressants, sedatives, and sleeping tablets. Along with these, he also received three test substances: G 35259 (ketoimipramine) for more than a year; Ciba 34276 (which later became Ludiomil) for just under two months; and Sandoz's IB 503 in 1965 for two days. Why was Traber given these test preparations? Let us look at IB 503. This substance was the prototype of a new substance class, whose effect was supposed to be both activating and sedating. Thus one wanted to test whether the remedy could be used for depressions and manic phases.[19] Kuhn started the trial with a depressive patient and Franz Traber, who was deemed manic depressive as of 1965. When the test began, the administration of IB 503 also seemed to follow a certain logic, wherein Kuhn selected two patients who – it was hoped – were suitable for the trial.

But why were these two particular patients chosen? Is it even possible to discern patterns in Kuhn's testing practices? Were the various substances administered to very specific patient groups?

Were the patients included at the beginning of a trial different from those included later? Were certain patient groups particularly conspicuous – for example, were some types of patients more frequently involved in tests than others? The analysis of the 167 medical files we examined produced a complex picture. The spectrum of patients who received test substances is broad. The affected persons varied enormously, whether with respect to categories such as age and social and geographic origin, or with respect to medical criteria such as diagnosis, symptoms, or length of treatment. Even so, there clearly were patients whom Kuhn deliberately used for certain types of testing. Thus to determine differences in the effects of closely related substances, for example, he preferred using patients who strongly reacted to substances and could also provide information. Testing with chronically ill patients, on the other hand, was more often intended to assess the tolerability of a substance or to work out two possible effect components – for example, sedation or stimulation. Such administration patterns, however, could also change again depending on the substance, trial phase, and temporal context.

The way the test substances were administered also varied. Whereas some patients only received one medication, others were given many. Certain preparations were dispensed only briefly, others for years, with or without interruptions. Rarely was a substance administered on its own at Münsterlingen without any additional psychoactive substances. As a rule, test substances were used together with other substances, usually in combination with approved medications, sometimes also with other test substances. There were many different possible combinations, which were used to pursue various goals. For some patients, the test preparations led to side-effects that were supposed to be combatted by other medications. Others, especially schizophrenic patients, could not, in Kuhn's eyes, have their standard medication discontinued, so they received the test substance along with their usual drug. Sometimes the attempt was made to increase the test preparation's effect through another substance or to achieve a desired mixture of different effects. Kuhn's marked tendency to combine substances, however, caused him assorted problems because it affected the reproducibility and the statistical analysis of the trials.

From today's perspective, Kuhn's test patients can be divided into three types, each with their own particular dependent relationship: long-term patients, children or adolescents, and nurses. The first group consisted of severely ill patients who lived in the clinic for many years and received several and sometimes large numbers of test substances. Frieda Vogt, the 'frontrunner' among the chronically ill, was given at least thirteen different test substances from 1954 to 1973. The patient suffered from severe catatonia, a form of schizophrenia with strong psychomotor symptoms. She was first admitted to Münsterlingen in 1936 at age 19, then readmitted in 1938 and constantly kept in the 'unruly' ward until she died in 1983. In the 1930s and 1940s, she was unsuccessfully treated with sleep and shock cures. In January 1954, she began being treated with Largactil, which soon thereafter was also approved in Switzerland; this treatment was discontinued after four months because of a strong drop in blood pressure. At the end of the year, she underwent psychosurgery, but her condition did not change. In the following years, Frieda Vogt was given numerous test substances: after Geigy White, Geigy Black, Geigy White II, Geigy Pink, and Geigy Yellow, in 1959 it was Geigy Blue's[20] turn. In 1961 the doctor in charge spoke, in summary, about 'varying success', but only linked this to the positively evaluated developments with the medication: 'At least the patient can be included now and then and stay in the day room, although she cannot be called on for any work. The catatonic phases have appeared less often, instead now and then there are short-lasting raptus-like agitations with grimacing, aggressive actions, and dance-like movements.' Apart from an X-ray report, her medical file contains no further entries for the next three years and the administered preparations are no longer mentioned. In 1964, Kuhn noted that there was 'actually nothing new from the last few years' to report on the patient.[21]

These trials focused on the substance; they were not therapy trials. Only this explains why Frieda Vogt was given numerous test preparations that were actually supposed to have an antidepressant effect. In the case of Geigy Blue, whose effect was still unclear, Kuhn wrote to Geigy in 1959 that the preparation had previously been given to schizophrenics to learn about its effect. 'After we had somewhat gotten to know the preparation on the very severely ill, we carried out a trial series with six chronically inhibited schizophrenics, whose reaction to the most varied types of psychopharmacological substances and to other treatment methods we already know well.' Kuhn admittedly pointed out that the effect certainly did not achieve the 'scope of the Tofranil effects for depressions'. Even so, he insisted that the substance needed to be better researched; thus far, it was very well tolerated and might actually be superior to G 33040 (which later became the antidepressant Insidon).[22] Indeed, Geigy Blue continued to be administered to the patient until 1961.

The number of chronically ill who received test substances without the awareness of anyone outside the clinic must have been quite a bit larger than the number of children in institutions and foster care who were involved in trials.[23] The latter group included Rudolf Ammann, who came to Münsterlingen in 1965. He had committed theft, skipped school, and repeatedly absconded from reform school, which is why the youth public prosecutor's office hospitalised him and called for a new expert evaluation. Verena Kuhn found the boy – who, among other things, complained of homesickness – to be 'very sensitive' and decided to dose him with G 35259 during his clinic stay. In the expert evaluation, she wrote:

> Today we would probably actually say that, along with the educational failure of the parents, one must also add certain abnormal character structures to explain the severe social failure of the child. Our medicinal treatment, too, has shown that, as a result, the boy has become more accessible and less passive. We therefore assume that, with regard to the difficulties that have emerged above all with the placement of the child, a slight depressive component played a role.

Thus in her eyes, the remedy's positive effect affirmed the diagnosis of slight depression, which is also why she felt the boy's problems could not be traced back solely to his upbringing. She recommended to continue giving the boy G 35259; other forms of therapy were not considered.[24]

However, there were also children from entirely 'normal' families who were given test substances with an antidepressant effect. The decisive factor was whether they exhibited forms of behaviour that, from the perspective of the treating doctor, might suggest depression. Thus Silvia Tobler, a 12-year-old, sensitive, somewhat anxious and underachieving girl, came to three appointments at the outpatient department between 1969 and 1972. Verena Kuhn presumed a mourning reaction because the patient's sister had died, but she nonetheless resorted to a test preparation (first G 35259, later Ciba 34276). Since the doctor and the mother felt the remedy had a positive effect, Verena Kuhn sent the family substances at regular intervals. Over time, other family members also received test preparations – an approach that can be documented for many cases. When the father reported at a check-up that the school grades of Silvia Tobler's brother had fallen, the latter too received Ciba 34276. The mother, who is described from the outset in her daughter's medical history as chronically depressive, was given a couple of Insidon tablets to see whether they would have a positive effect on her sleep disorders. 'She should probably also take Ciba remedies', Verena Kuhn noted.[25]

Hence, there are no indications thus far that institutionalised and foster children were treated any differently at Münsterlingen than children and youth who lived with their parents.[26] Neither did social origin play a key role in whether minors were given test substances. Instead, what is striking is how quickly psychotropic drugs were prescribed, how strongly any possible social factors or family problems were ignored, and how seamlessly clinical trials and the routine dispensing of test preparations merged. And this also applied to adults. Thus what most clearly distinguished the treatment of children and youth was the prioritisation of certain test substances, the decidedly lower dosage levels, and the pronounced dependency that intrinsically characterised the members of this group.[27]

The female nurses who worked at Münsterlingen and simultaneously received treatment there were also in a particularly dependent relationship. For some employees, the clinic's hierarchy itself already led to feelings of dependency and helplessness. A picture from the photo album of a former trainee nurse shows three female nurses scrubbing the floor on their knees (Figure 3.2). The woman explained that only auxiliary nurses had to do this job. Once, she reported, while she was cleaning the floor this way, Kuhn and the entire 'merry-go-round' (the people participating in the doctor's rounds) came by. For her, this was a key moment that clearly revealed the hierarchical order: 'One could not communicate eye to eye.'[28]

The dependency grew when employees were given treatment on-site. In psychiatric clinics, it was quite common for female nurses

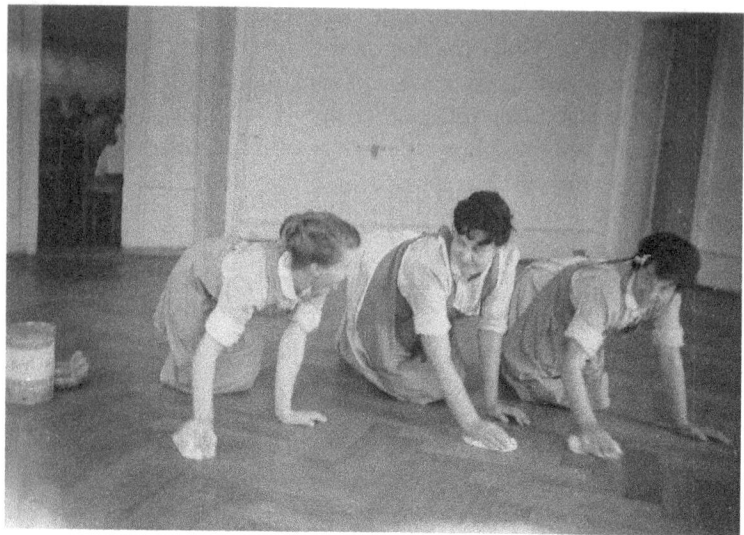

Figure 3.2 'Not eye to eye', trainee nurses scrubbing the floor, 1960

to be patients at the same time, not least because the clinics relied on patients when there was a staff shortage.[29] For Kuhn, it seemed only natural that clinic employees with psychiatric problems had a right to be treated free of charge.[30] Thus he conducted a series of psychotherapy sessions for female nurses for which they were to collect their dreams.[31] However, especially given that many employees also lived at the clinic, this offer meant that work and private spheres became incredibly intertwined.[32] Since everybody was acquainted, often spent leisure time together, and knew a lot about each other, the Kuhns as a couple received, through many different channels, much more information than that which merely pertained to the nurses being treated.

The medical history of Doris Huber, a nurse who received a wide range of test substances, provides a striking glimpse into the microcosm of the clinic. She was considered a valuable worker and for a long time was treated by Verena Kuhn, who seems to have looked after around the same number of female nurses as her husband. Even the very first entry of March 1958 shows how many threads came together at the Kuhns. 'The nurse wanted to quit, which is why the senior nurse spoke with her. She then found out that the patient is depressed and one needs to speak with her.' Information about Doris Huber was supplied not only by her superior but also by work colleagues and patients.[33] Informants even obtained and forwarded details about her sex life. Verena Kuhn saw no reason not to ask Doris Huber directly about certain particulars. Thus one entry states: 'A patient in the ward told me that the patient [Huber] is often severely upset and that this is clearly noticed. I ask her whether she is aware of this. She says, she thinks that the people can notice this. ... But I could rest assured that she will pull herself together as much as possible.'[34] Although Verena Kuhn stood by the patient with advice and support, she often interacted with her less as a psychiatrist than as a supervisor. Roland and Verena Kuhn evidently could not see that employees who both worked and received treatment at the clinic wound up in a two-fold dependency relationship and that they themselves also took on a dual role in such cases.[35]

## Information and consent practices

Whether female nurses knew more about their medication than other outpatients is difficult to tell. Some nurses evidently clearly understood that they were being given test substances.[36] Thus Roland Kuhn noted in a medical file, for example, that he was trying to 'teach' the nurse 'that an injection treatment with G 22355 is urgently indicated. ... I suggestively described several cases to her, above all to counter her objection that she is a guinea pig.'[37] On the other hand, other references suggest that 'new' remedies were mentioned without making it clear that they were test substances. Verena Kuhn, who always actively supported her husband in trials, noted in 1961 in Doris Huber's medical history that the patient was taking six tablets of Tofranil daily. 'I tell her, she should now, in addition, also have an injection of one ampoule of Geigy Yellow [later known as Insidon] for the night. She is in agreement.' If the doctor actually used the term 'Geigy Yellow' in this conversation, then Doris Huber, as a nurse, would surely have known that they were talking about a test substance because in Münsterlingen only test substances were designated with colours. In contrast, a few months later Verena Kuhn noted: 'We [Verena Kuhn] explain to her that there will soon be a new medication to try, which she will then get, which works faster, on the one hand, and more intensely, on the other. She would be grateful if that were to help.'[38]

When the substance arrived – it was G 35020, the later Pertofran – the nurse not only regularly reported on her condition and the effect of the preparation but also gave a urine sample each week, which was sent to Basel. Since the patient complained about swollen feet, Verena Kuhn looked into whether the problem could be related to ingesting the preparation. Even though the suspicion was not confirmed, six weeks later she suggested changing to a different substance.

> Even though patient finds she is doing very well, I think she should be doing even better. It should be better for her with eating, she should be able to do more and also to read something. She admits this. We agree that we then want try something after the holidays, to try the new American remedy on her.[39]

Such notes show that nurses were ideal test patients because they could continually and knowledgeably provide information on a preparation's effect. But whether they always knew they were participating in a trial often remains unclear.

Along with the female nurses, there also were other outpatients who were more precisely informed about the medication. This group included persons who searched Kuhn out from other parts of the country or even from abroad. Most were educated, affluent people who hoped that the 'discoverer' of Tofranil could help them; they even included psychiatrists, pharmaceutical industry employees,[40] and their relatives. The fact that test substances were given not only to female workers, small-scale farmers, housewives, and teachers but also to private outpatients and inpatients reinforces the impression that social status did not play a decisive role in the dispensing of test substances.[41] Kuhn rarely saw his outside patients, whose treatment was often limited to the administration of psychotropic drugs and occurred mostly by mail. Even so, he evidently found it easy to build up trusting relationships; his private patients were important to him, which no doubt also positively influenced the therapy.

Initial contact frequently took place through colleagues. Heinz Renz, for instance, approached Kuhn at a conference. At age 17, Renz's son began undergoing psychoanalysis and somewhat later failed his school-leaving exam. Since then he had been taking Tofranil at the advice of his analyst, but he was unsatisfied with the medication. At first the two doctors communicated by mail; a few months later, the son, Bruno, also contacted Kuhn. Therapy started in early 1962 and would last for several years, taking place primarily through correspondence. Originally the treatment was supposed to be limited to the medication, but it soon also addressed psychotherapeutic issues. Kuhn felt that the young man's analyst was incompetent, and after just the first consultation he wrote:

> Quasi in passing, I noted that obviously the psychotherapist is very far from being able to cope with this situation... . But I said nothing about the psychotherapist. At the end, I suggest to the patient to give it a try with the Tofranil metabolites. He is very much in agreement, he feels that, despite everything, there must be something that works, he does not have a negative attitude at all towards the medications.[42]

Bruno Renz tried the Metabolite III, the third conversion product of Tofranil, but, as Kuhn noted in summer 1962, Renz was hoping there would soon be 'new remedies': 'I explained to him that I have none for now, but that perhaps in future some will still be found that help him too, for there is much to indicate that he can be helped in many respects.'[43] Over the following months, they searched for the proper dosage and combination of medications. In early 1963, Kuhn reported to the father that he had not yet been able to clarify whether the patient's sporadic 'spectacular betterment' was due to biology or psychology. But either way, the treatment should be continued 'with a total dosage of the medication of around 225 milligrams daily'. Metabolite IV, which Kuhn considered very promising, might then provide the ideal solution. 'I am still hoping to soon receive the Metabolite IV from the Geigy firm, which possibly has a direct relation to depression and perhaps helps in cases where the usual medication does not fully lead to the objective.'[44]

Renz was surely one of Kuhn's favourite patients. He came from a similar milieu, was on the same page as Kuhn, and actively participated in the effort to find a medicinal solution. In Renz's case, Kuhn clearly acted with his knowledge and consent; even his father knew about the test preparations. From many other outpatient medical files, however, it is not evident whether the patients knew that they were receiving test substances. And hospitalised patients hardly had any idea at all about what they were being given. After his retirement, Kuhn wrote that the patients in Münsterlingen were 'never asked for their consent to taking a test preparation',[45] which dovetails with his recommendations to make certain substances look identical. Thus in 1960, for example, he suggested making a new test substance the same colour as Tofranil 'so that the patients do not notice when they receive a different preparation'.[46]

According to her own statement, one former inpatient we interviewed was told in 1970 that her proposed medication was a test preparation (Ciba 34276). Despite being very sceptical of antidepressants, she consented to the treatment and is fully convinced that she could have easily turned it down.[47] But thus far there is no written evidence that patients were systematically informed about test substances and that their consent was obtained and documented in writing prior to the 1980s.[48] The earliest surviving consent declarations we found were from 1987; they pertained to Kuhn's tests with levoprotiline, which took place in his private practice.[49] Thus everything suggests that the vast majority of Münsterlingen patients were not explicitly told about the test substances.

From the period's general psychiatric perspective, for a long time there was no reason to thoroughly educate patients about their illness and therapy. Therefore, inpatients rarely learned that they were being given test substances. Outpatients were more likely to be informed, but they usually gained this knowledge in passing – for example, when someone needed new drugs and requested a prescription by mail or phone, they might be told that the drug was unavailable at the pharmacy because it was a test substance. A former outpatient said that Kuhn had simply told him that the administered substances would have a positive effect on his condition. Only when asked what the substances were called did Kuhn explain that they were still being tested.[50] If outpatients or their relatives never received such information, which often depended on chance, then they only knew that certain drugs did not cost anything and were identified with numbers or colours.[51] As a rule, however, test preparations were administered like newly introduced medications. Clinical staff spoke about a new therapy, not about a test, and they referred to substances that were not yet on the market and therefore did not yet have a name.

## Agency and resistance

According to the nursing staff, regardless of whether patients knew what they were being given, they were accustomed to drugs and usually took their medication. Some did so without objection, and others required a little prodding. But there were also those who vigorously resisted,[52] as illustrated by the 1954 nursing records of a patient who was given G 22150.

> Fräulein Wild energetically refused the injection at 8 o'clock with the words: 'Now they are simply giving me injections so that I can't even go to church on Sunday. Here they are making you even sicker than you already are if you have the will to get well. I am not a test animal, I am a human being. I want to leave!' Only after the appearance of the ward nurse did she allow the administration of the injection.

Seven years later, a nurse wrote, 'Fräulein Wild does not seem to be enthusiastic about the injections, she says nothing, but shakes her head each time.' A few weeks after that, it was noted that the patient was still afraid of injections, and another time she cried after the injection.[53] Covert or open, loud or quiet, verbal or physical – the nature of the resistance varied strongly. And so did the response of the staff.

The tighter patients could be controlled, the less likely their resistance paid off. On one side of the spectrum were those who received injections or had substances mixed into their food. One nurse, who from 1957 to 1964 worked day shift and afterwards night shift for a long time, told about how they administered the preparations in a cup or on a spoon. Sometimes tablets were also crushed, dissolved in coffee or soup, or wrapped in pastries. If patients did not want to swallow the substance, one resorted to injections, which were often perceived as painful.[54] Another nurse explained that when patients fought back against taking substances, the staff used a special hand grip to give them the drug.[55] One long-term senior nurse, on the other hand, reckoned: 'The doctor gave the order, and the patient swallowed it or had to be made to swallow it. That is, we did not have any kind of coercions, but now and then one simply had to sit down next to the patients and try to convince them until they swallowed it.'[56]

Additional measures are found in the written sources. Thus one medical history notes in 1958 that the female patient did not want to take the medication (Largactil, in this case) and the senior nurse therefore temporarily moved her to the 'unruly' ward. After she returned, she 'willingly' swallowed the tablets.[57] Some inpatients did not openly resist the medication but liked to make them disappear. One nursing report, for instance, repeatedly mentions that a female patient hid her tablets in her pocket.[58] Clinic staff were aware of the problem and took countermeasures, but they could not control everything. One former patient explained, for example, that he spit the tablets into the toilet when no one was watching.[59] Resistance against taking medicine could have various reasons. Some patients refused not only to take their preparations but also to eat or to work, or they basically rebelled against the order of the asylum. Others rejected medications because they considered taking them to be an admission that they were ill and had problems. Still others probably refused because they believed the substances would harm them or they even incorporated them into their systems of delusion.[60]

On the other side of the spectrum were the outpatients, who took their medications at home, at least until depot injections arrived.[61] Here one needed to rely strongly on the cooperation of patients, relatives, or other individuals. Thus after being examined in the outpatient department, Franz Traber would bring his preparations home in paper bags. His wife took charge of them, regularly reported to the doctor on her husband's condition, and changed the dosage when she felt it was appropriate.

> The wife reported to us today by telephone that her husband is doing quite satisfactorily. She is a reliable reporter and also sees to it that the patient always takes the proper dose of medication; she is, so to speak, a private psychiatric nurse. As soon as the mood deteriorates somewhat, she gives a little more of the white Geigy, or the other way around.

The Münsterlingen staff therefore considered Traber's wife to be a 'reliable administrator of medications' whose judgement could be trusted.[62]

In other cases, the doctors were less confident that the medications were being properly taken. As shown by medical histories and interviews with contemporary witnesses, this scepticism was quite warranted. Outpatients seem to have often discontinued their medications on their own, taking them irregularly or stopping altogether. Occasionally, nobody at all had any proper knowledge about how the substances were being used. In 1974, Verena Kuhn noted with regard to a boy from the St Iddazell children's home:

> According to our medical history, the boy is supposed to take 3 x 10-mg Ludiomil. He claims, however, that he has half a white tablet in morning and evening. I do not know what is true here. The supervisor also did not inquire into the medications, so we do not know what he actually has and why he has something different to what we recommended.[63]

That said, if the doctors trusted someone to self-assess the situation, they had no apparent problem with handing over responsibility. One long-term ambulatory patient said that Kuhn never got angry if he changed the medication on his own initiative. 'At the beginning I got many, many, medications. Professor Kuhn taught me how to deal with these medications. Therefore after half a year I could then do quite a lot by myself.' The patient noted that Kuhn undoubtedly viewed him as a scientific case and was no less interested in the substance's effect on him than the patient was himself.[64]

This contemporary witness believes that Kuhn took great notice of his opinions – however, the opportunities for patients to exercise influence in this regard varied considerably. If people could clearly express themselves linguistically and describe how a substance worked, they attracted Kuhn's attention. A test report of 1964, for example, describes a patient as 'very critical, very intelligent' and as having 'experience in the observation of the effects of medicines'.[65] In other cases, however, clinic staff themselves determined whether a preparation achieved an effect. The decisive factor in these cases was whether something manifested in the behaviour or on the body of the patient that could be linked back to the substance. Statements such as those of a man who declared he had burned himself with a cigarette to burn away the poison of the ingested medication were at most seen as symptoms of illness.[66]

Franz Traber eventually spoke quite a bit about his condition; his reports are reproduced – in indirect speech and probably abridged – in his medical history. Yet how the farmer perceived and assessed the preparation's effect is barely discussed. Thus it is all the more striking that his complaints regarding IB 503 – the aforementioned

Sandoz substance that he received in 1965 – are recorded in multiple sources. On the first day of treatment, a nurse noted in a report that Traber had worked diligently in the morning, but then in the afternoon he told her

> that he has a strong muscle pain in his thigh, every few minutes or so. The effect was such that his legs were pulling strongly backwards, then around half an hour later he came again and said he now also noticed it in the upper-arm muscle, and this too was a twitch. He noticed this only after he has now had these new tablets.

Traber lay down, but the next day he immediately went to bed again after breakfast. The report then noted that the patient was complaining about trouble walking and that he could not see clearly. He was given a muscle relaxant again and was almost continuously asleep; IB 503 was not given to him in the evening.[67] Three days later, Kuhn wrote to Sandoz that he had so far tried IB 503 on two cases. In the case of one patient, 'after just the first tablet, such side-effects emerged that at first we did not dare to continue the treatment. The patient complained that he was blacking out, he felt groggy and dizzy, and he moved around very strangely, oddly stiff, Parkinson's-like, and he had dyskinetic seizures.' Since Traber had previously reacted similarly to other medications, it was unclear 'whether the disorders originate only from your new preparation. But it seemed to us that the new preparation strongly increased the disposition to such reactions.'[68]

## The patient's perspective

What does one do with Traber's statements? Can such sources be used to access his experiences and opinions? Or, in the final analysis, do they say more about the institution and the clinic staff? Ever since the British historian of medicine Roy Porter called for a history of medicine written 'from below' in 1986, one that no longer ignored the patient's perspective, historians have vigorously discussed this demand.[69] Apart from tackling questions regarding sources and source criticism, the debate has also focused on theoretical and methodological problems. For example, how does one deal with the fact that so few egodocuments of patients – such as autobiographical accounts and personal testimonies (letters, for instance) have survived? How does one cope with the problem that, in most sources, the patient's point of view is filtered and indirectly reproduced? Even if egodocuments are available, does not the context in which these sources were created decisively influence their content? The fact that many psychiatric patients remained mute or went unheard cannot be dismissed out of hand. Therefore, how does one mitigate the risk of distorted results when more statements survive from certain types of patients than from others? Can subjective experiences be reconstructed? What does one do with the voices of patients if one wants to do more than simply replay them?

We can only touch on these questions here. 'The' patient – as this chapter has shown – does not exist, nor does 'the' test patient, or 'the' patient perspective. Since the Münsterlingen test patients varied immensely, so too did the ways in which they assessed psychotropic drugs and dealt with them. This also applies to the former patients who told us their stories retrospectively from memory. Test substances played a central role in Münsterlingen for a long time and left their traces in countless sources. Even so, it is difficult to work out patient views on clinical trials or on a specific preparation – at least if one wants to go beyond isolated comments while also not wanting to settle for the many statements about their own condition that are at best only vaguely linked to the administered substances.

Although Franz Traber drew syringes in both of his drawing tests, 'the sore spot' that he drew on the one sheet was not necessarily a reference to his medication. Except for his complaints about IB 503 and a few requests for sleeping tablets, according to the files Traber hardly said anything about specific substances or psychotropic drugs.[70] Yet even so, these substances and drugs structured his encounters with the nursing staff and doctors.[71] He received drugs three times daily, at the clinic and at home. For a certain period, they were part of his daily rhythm and his life; they became part of himself without anyone knowing how he would have felt and behaved without them.

The concept of coercion and exploitation is too one-dimensional to accommodate the experiences of psychiatric patients.[72] Despite institutional hierarchies, a rigid opposition between doctors and patients and the associated idea of a history 'from below' is too narrowly defined, especially in the context of psychotropic drugs[73] and the increasing differentiation of psychiatry. That patients received a test substance tells us very little about how they were perceived, how they saw themselves, or how they perhaps see themselves after the fact – as a victim, as a passive reacting object, a subject, an aggrieved party, or a consumer, or as an actor in a multilayered dynamic process of negotiation in which psychoactive substances and other medications were assigned meaning.[74]

Franz Traber drew syringes and complained about ailments triggered in him by IB 503. Other patients integrated preparations into their stories, dreams, delusions, hopes, or fears. Thus patients too participated in the process of 'making sense of drugs'. When it came to the meaning and effect of substances, they played an important role. With regard to the administration of substances, however, they could usually only resist or cooperate. In this respect, they hardly had any room or power to act. The question of how patients confronted their treatment only became part of the therapeutic process once the new image of the patient, which emerged in the 1950s, slowly began to prevail in the 1970s.[75]

## Notes

1 The abbreviation 'H.P.A.' on Taber's drawing means Heil- und Pflegeanstalt (Münsterlingen). Herr Mäder is a nurse.
2 StATG, ZA KAs 18405.
3 The physician who later supervised Traber as an outpatient likewise attested to his 'dry humour'; see ZA KAa 18360, 20 January 1968.
4 On drawing tests as a research method, see Lemov, 'X-Rays'; *Dreams*.
5 In STS and actor-network theory, the issue of agency has been discussed predominantly in connection with objects and later with animals; see, for example, Callon, 'Some Elements'. In the human sciences, the focus has been more on the question of classifications and their effect on self-images; see, for instance, Hacking, 'The Looping'; 'Making Up'. For the diagnosis of depression, see Pignarre, *Comment la dépression*; Borch-Jacobsen, 'Psychotropicana'; Ehrenberg, *The Weariness*.
6 Martin, *Flexible Bodies*, 122. On the category of vulnerability, see Campbell and Stark, 'Making Up'. On diagnostic systems, see Horwitz, *DSM*.

7 On the patient's view, see Porter, 'The Patient's View'; Condrau, 'The Patient's View'; Bacopoulos-Viau and Fauvel, 'The Patient's Turn'; Hanley and Meyer, *Patient Voices*.
8 StATG, 9'40, 5.0.8/6, Kuhn's report to Dr Neff, Sandoz, 19 July 1965.
9 StATG, 9'40, 5.0.3/32, handwritten list Ward K, no year (presumably 1965); type-written list 'Released 1965–28 February 67'; 9'40, 5.0.8/6, 9'40, 5.0.2/4, list Ciba 34276 and 32143.
10 Clinical archive Novartis, Geigy, 7. BS 00024587–3; Kuhn to Frau Dr Meissner, 13 March 1969.
11 All calculations are based on the figures listed in the annual reports of the Münsterlingen Psychiatric Clinic. StATG, 9'10, 1.1.0/60, ARM 1939–1985. The information up to 1981 was used for the diagnoses.
12 Kuhn, 'Geschichte', 113.
13 For our calculations, we divided the diagnoses into the following categories: mental retardation; personality and behavioural disorders; neurotic disorders; schizophrenic, schizoid, and delusional disorders; affective disorders; organic disorders; disorders from psychotropic substances; developmental disorders. One problem was the many overlaps among the diagnoses. In our calculations, diagnoses such as 'depression schizophrenia' were counted as schizophrenic disorders, not as affective disorders.
14 The information on the outpatients pertains exclusively to the outpatient department in Münsterlingen. Information on the outpatient facility in Frauenfeld is found in the annual reports of the Hilfsverein für Gemütskranke; they are insufficiently differentiated for an assessment. In contrast to the proportion of children, that of youth increased only slightly over time. As per StATG, 9'10, 1.1.0/60, ARM 1968, 11, people under 15 years of age were considered children. For the youth, the upper threshold was 25 years of age.
15 See StATG, 9'40, 3.0.1/3, *Thurgauer Volksfreund*, 28 June 1973, insert 'Psychiatrische Klinik Münsterlingen'.
16 Interview of former senior nurse Ernst Wyrsch, 19 August 2016.
17 StATG, ZA KAa 18360, 19 October 1967. The outpatient treatment of the patient lasted around four years.
18 Interview with Kuhn's successor Karl Studer, 3 November 2016.
19 StATG, 9'40, 5.0.8/6, Sandoz to Kuhn, 11 February and 2 July 1965.
20 At the time, G 33006 was called Geigy Blue; thus it was not the preparation G 24415, which was also coloured blue and had been tested in 1956/1957.
21 StATG, 9'10, 5.4/9525, 12 January 1961, 9 April 1964 (quotes).
22 StATG, 9'40, 5.0.3/11, Kuhn to Geigy, 23 July 1959. See also Chapter 2, 68.

23 More recently, 'chronicity' has been discussed above all in social anthropology. See, for example, https://somatosphere.com/series_category/chronic-living/ (accessed 8 April 2024). On drug studies on institutionalised children in Germany, see Hähner-Rombach and Hartig, *Medikamentenversuche*; Wagner, *Arzneimittelversuche*; Sparing, *Medikamentenvergabe*; Kaminsky and Klöcker, *Medikamente*; Beyer et al., *Wissenschaftliche Untersuchung*; Lenhard-Schramm et al., *Göttliche Krankheit*. On the state of research, see Wagner, 'Ein unterdrücktes', 62–65. On the administration of test substances to infants in the St Iddazell children's home in Fischingen, see Akermann et al., *Kinder*, 150–157.
24 StATG, ZA KAs 17478, expert report for the attention of the youth public prosecutor's office of the Canton of Thurgau, 8 November 1965. When released, Rudolf Ammann was given the preparation G 35259 to take along. On 10 October 1966, the reform school was sent another 200 10-mg tablets of G 35259 for the boy.
25 StATG, ZA KAa 23412.
26 A study on Lower Saxony likewise found no evidence that institutionalised children were systematically selected for clinical studies; Hähner-Rombach and Hartig, *Medikamentenversuche*.
27 A dissertation on children and youth who were treated by the Münsterlingen Psychiatric Clinic's outpatient department is currently in progress; see Klauser, '"Schwierige Kinder"'.
28 Interview with a former trainee nurse, 18 April 2018. See also the interview with René Bloch, 14 March 2018.
29 StATG, 9'10, 4.0/3, Kuhn's notes on his discussion with Government Councillor Reiber of 12 October 1963, 22 October 1963, 1–2. Our sample included six female nurses who worked at the Münsterlingen Psychiatric Clinic and were also being treated there (9'10, 6.2/9856; 9'10,6.2/9857; 9'10, 6.2/11361; 9'40, 11.4/27; ZA KAa 13002; ZA KAs 24356), but only one male nurse (9'10, 6.2/16356).
30 StATG, 9'10, 1.2.8/6, Kuhn to Dr Bütler, cantonal physician, 19 July 1972, 3.
31 On Kuhn's interpretation of these dreams, see Tornay, *Träumende Schwestern*.
32 Along with the patients, for a long time many of the doctors and nursing staff also lived on the clinic grounds, and an especially watchful eye was cast on the female trainee nurses; see Chapter 1, 21–22.
33 StATG, 9'10, 6.2/9856.1, 4 March 1958.
34 StATG, 9'10, 6.2/9856.2, 1 September 1961.
35 The clinic staff also suspected that there were female nurses who were receiving treatment; see interview with the former nurse Marlies Verhofnik, 12 September 2016.

36 On the history of informed consent, see Weindling, 'The Origins'; *Nazi Medicine*; Reubi, 'The Human Capacity'; 'Re-Moralising'.
37 StATG, ZA KAs 24356, 1 June 1957.
38 StATG, 9'10, 6.2/9856.2, 5 May 1961; 8 September 1961.
39 *Ibid.*, 10 and 17 November 1961; 8 December 1961 (quote); 13 April 1962. The 'new American remedy' was probably Wy 3263 of the American company Wyeth.
40 References to employees in the pharmaceutical industry who were treated by Kuhn are found in his diary; see StATG, 9'40, 1.0.3/1, 17 July 1973; 25 August 1973; 19 April 1974.
41 The study on the Burghölzli in Zurich came to the same conclusion: Rietmann et al., 'Medikamentenversuche', 234. For private inpatients that were given test substances, see StATG, 9'10, 5.4/13473; ZA KAs 10859.
42 StATG, ZA KAa 13563, 20 January 1962.
43 *Ibid.*, 16 July 1962.
44 *Ibid.*, Kuhn to the patient's father, 15 January 1963.
45 StATG, 9'40, 5.1.2/2, Kuhn to an historian of medicine at the University of Hannover, 29 June 1989.
46 StATG, 9'40, 5.0.3/11, Kuhn to Rothweiler, 8 October 1960. See also 9'40, 3.2.0/3.1, Bein to Gelzer, Ciba-Geigy, 17 November 1976, which says that Kuhn wants the test substance to look the same as Ludiomil dragees. 'As a result it would be possible to replace Ludiomil with 49802 without it being noticed by the patient.'
47 Interview with former inpatient, 14 February 2017. The contemporary witness received treatment as an inpatient for two months in 1970. She suffered from a reactive depression and lived in Ward F, the admission ward for women. She says that she was told that the Ciba remedy was still in development and was therefore not yet on the market, but that the doctors had already had good experiences with it.
48 As of 1970, the (legally non-binding) guidelines of the Swiss Academy of Medical Sciences called for a consent declaration on the part of probands. On increasing regulations and the transformation of clinical testing, see Chapter 4, 121–124, 147–151, and Chapter 6, 202–207.
49 See Chapter 8, 257.
50 Interview with a former patient of Kuhn who was treated as an outpatient around 1970, 13 February 2017.
51 See, for example, the extensive correspondence between Verena Kuhn and a female patient from the 1960s in which several preparations are referred to by their trade names, but most of them are referred to by colour and size or by the test number. StATG, 9'10, 6.2/11474.
52 Interviews with former nurses Ernst Wyrsch, 19 August 2016, and Jürg Grundlehner, 23 August 2017.

53 StATG, 9'10, 5.4/13569, nursing report, 4 and 5 July 1954, 22 November 1961, 7 and 24 December 1961.
54 Interview with the former nurse Marlies Verhofnik, 12 September 2016. The fact that staff resorted to injections if someone refused to swallow tablets also emerges from the medical files. See, for example, StATG, ZA KAs 19817, nursing report, 23 February 1965.
55 Interview with a former nurse who worked in Ward K for six weeks in 1970, 11 November 2016. Comparable measures were applied at Burghölzli in Zurich; Meier et al., *Eingeschlossen*, 127–128.
56 Interview with the former senior nurse, Ernst Wyrsch, 19 August 2016.
57 StATG, ZA KAs 26098, 17 April 1958.
58 StATG, ZA KAs 19817, nursing reports, 18 July 1964, 23 July 1964.
59 Interview with a former patient who was hospitalised in the Münsterlingen Psychiatric Clinic for six weeks in 1967, 17 November 2016. StATG, ZA KAs 19817, nursing report, 18 July 1964.
60 See Majerus, 'Making Sense', 59.
61 Depot medications are drugs that form a deposit in the body – for example, in muscle tissue – and allow the substance to be released over a longer period. Depot medications became available in psychiatry around 1970.
62 StATG, ZA KAa 18360, 14 March 1967, 9 May 1967, 6 June 1967.
63 StATG, ZA KAa 30338, 2 September 1974.
64 Interview with a former outpatient of Kuhn, 21 July 2016.
65 StATG, 9'40, 5.0.2/2, Kuhn's test report on Ciba 34799 and 32143, 13 November 1964, 17–18.
66 StATG, 9'10, 5.4/14527, 4 May 1974.
67 StATG, ZA KAs 17160, report, 15 and 16 July 1965.
68 StATG, 9'40, 5.0.8/6, Kuhn's report to Dr Neff, Sandoz, 19 July 1965. Dyskinesia: dysfunction of movement process.
69 Porter, 'The Patient's View'; Condrau, 'The Patient's View'; Bacopoulos-Viau and Fauvel, 'The Patient's Turn'; Hanley and Meyer, *Patient Voices*.
70 See StATG, ZA KAs 18405; ZA KAa 18360, 17 April 1967.
71 Majerus, 'Making Sense', 56.
72 See Campbell and Stark, 'Making Up'.
73 See Meyers, 'Pharmacy'.
74 See Campbell and Stark, 'Making Up'. On the concept of the victim, see Goltermann, *Victims*.
75 See Meier, *Spannungsherde*, 262–274, 314–315.

# 4

# The 1960s: A flood of substances and new dimensions of testing

Along with letters, reports, and many other documents, Kuhn's private archive also includes a number of three-dimensional objects. A few in particular impart a powerful sense of the 1960s and can even stand as symbols for the decade: a construction set for the three-dimensional representation of chemical molecules, and three metal boxes filled with test substances.

During this time, Roland Kuhn meddled more and more in matters that were normally reserved for company chemists and pharmacologists. The construction set, given to him by Ciba in 1964, served him well in this endeavour. He built models and believed that they confirmed 'certain notions' about the 'connection between chemical structure and antidepressant effect'.[1] He contended that only by referring to the spatial model of the molecules was it even possible to say anything about effects: 'There are certain angles and spacings that are evidently decisive, and indeed more important than the number of atoms in a ring.'[2] He began to develop hypotheses about the interplay between structure and effect, and to suggest modifications of sidechains to find yet more variations of a base material. To help in the development of substances, he also sought out direct discussions with chemists. In the 1960s, Kuhn became an amateur pharmacologist – in part to the amusement of people in the industry, but also as a partner who was not to be underestimated and whose ideas occasionally met with success.[3] Always asking for a new substance's chemical formula, Kuhn also used to sketch the molecule structures by hand. Generally speaking, the psychiatric community was increasingly focusing attention on pharmacological mechanisms and how substances get converted in the body. The 1960s were entirely dominated by the mysterious relationship between chemical structures and specific effects. The overarching objective was to further develop and differentiate existing base substances to bring better, more specifically acting psychopharmaceuticals to the market.

The metal boxes, on the other hand, convey an impression of the sheer volume of test substances that flooded the Münsterlingen Psychiatric Clinic. It was a period of intensive testing, which followed on the heels of the discovery phase that began in the mid-1950s. Along with various small trials, the period also witnessed large-scale experiments involving huge numbers of patients. And with ever fewer suitable inpatient cases, they increasingly involved outpatients. The dimensions of the trials grew massively in terms of substance deliveries and case numbers. As an investigator now sought out by many companies, Kuhn became a small-scale pharmaceutical entrepreneur.

In this capacity, he also distributed more and more test substances. Packaged in small letters, the substances migrated from the metal boxes to the outpatient consulting sessions, the cantonal hospital, and family doctors, going out by mail to an ever-growing network of recipients. Kuhn and his wife became a distribution hub that forwarded test substances. The direct supply of outpatients by mail sometimes created some seemingly absurd scenarios. Thus a long-term outpatient wrote in 1969:

> Dear Frau Dr Kuhn! Of the tablets that I take at noon and in the morning, one in each case, there are only enough until and including Thursday. The white ones, after the new coloured ones, last week I received 2 x 100 of them…. Of those that I take two at night, there are still enough until I again need those that I [take] mornings and at noon.

Commenting in the medical file, Verena Kuhn wrote: 'There is a constant back-and-forth with the patient's medications. … One time she orders one remedy, then a different one again, then a prescription again.'[4] Along with the astonishing autonomy with which the patient managed her medications, it is striking how porous the boundary was between testing and therapy. The test substances she ordered were being treated as if they were licensed medications. This jumble of variously coloured test substances appears arbitrary with respect to method and therapeutic supervision; nothing suggests any orderly processes.

Yet, in the meantime, the world of clinical trials had changed. The 1960s were characterised by many parallel strands of development, which makes a linear history impossible to write. But with respect to Münsterlingen, a general picture of divergence nonetheless takes shape. While Kuhn and his employees continued their research as usual and relied on the proven method of case observation, elsewhere there were increasing efforts at standardisation, originating from the United States, and a stricter regulation of clinical trials. This oft-described transition attests to a new conception of objectivity in psychiatric and pharmacological epistemology.[5] The principle of tacit knowledge, to which Kuhn was attached, became less important. The direct medical gaze was supplanted by new methods. Placebo-controlled double-blind studies prevailed internationally, also because of an altered awareness of risks and side-effects.[6] In other words, the system of clinical experimentation was being reorganised.

## Thalidomide and the end of pharmacological optimism

The 1950s, especially the period directly after the introduction of Largactil, were characterised by pharmacological enthusiasm. This optimism was expressed with varying intensity in 1957 at the Second International Congress for Psychiatry in Zurich. People hoped that the problem of mental illness could soon be solved and believed they finally had a means to crack the mystery of the human mind and its disorders.[7]

This optimism towards all things psychotropic endured much longer in Münsterlingen than elsewhere. Around 1960, the giant waves triggered by Largactil, LSD, and related substances in the middle of the century subsided somewhat in many places. Optimism was joined by quiet doubts. Patients who had apparently been healed and then released showed up in the clinics again, and severe movement difficulties and other side-effects of neuroleptics were increasingly perceived as a problem.[8] Many psychiatrists came to see that the new psychotropic drugs did not heal a mental disorder like an 'antibiotic did a lung infection'[9] but rather alleviated symptoms. In addition, it was discovered that their effect often diminished after the drugs stopped being administered. Most substances had to be taken daily for a longer time.

Kuhn viewed this realistically, but nonetheless continued to believe in pharmacological progress. For him it was more a question of not-yet rather than a fundamental problem, and better medications seemed almost within reach. From his perspective, side-effects could often be cancelled out with sophisticated combinations of substances and dosage adjustments. He administered approved medications and test substances in finely tuned 'cocktails' based in part on his theoretical-pharmacological deliberations and on the patient's condition on the given day.

But then in 1961, the risks of psychotropic drugs suddenly came to light. Contergan, a sedative made by the German company Grünenthal with the substance thalidomide, had been available without a prescription in many countries. It had come onto the market in 1957 and was promoted as being as 'harmless as a sugar biscuit'. Four years later, it was discovered that the substance was responsible for severe embryonic deformations and miscarriages.[10] The problem was most serious in West Germany, with up to 5,000 affected children.[11] Suddenly the risks and dangers of medications consumed on an almost daily basis gained the attention of the public media: 'No healing without risks', read the front page of *Die Zeit*, while *Der Spiegel* spoke of a 'national tragedy', indeed about the 'pharmaceutical nightmare of the century'.[12] The thalidomide scandal would have major consequences for the pharmacological sector. Its scope highlighted the fact that medications had become mass consumer products, but that their approval occurred largely without the monitoring of risks and side-effects.[13] The population lost its confidence in medicinal safety, with the loudest calls for stricter regulation emanating from Germany and the United States.

This also abruptly brought up the question of the damaging effect of psychoactive substances on germ cells. After the English medical journal *The Lancet* reported on foetal deformities in rabbits, Geigy held a press conference in March 1963 to disarm suspicions of a 'teratogenic' effect on the part of Tofranil.[14] Geigy emphasised that Tofranil was not chemically related to thalidomide in any way.[15] However, effects on the unborn and on fertility henceforth remained a delicate subject. Animal testing was supposed to provide information about any possible damaging effect of Tofranil on germ cells, and the Intercantonal Office for the Control of Medicines (IKS) now also requested corresponding documentation of such tests.[16]

In summer 1963, Geigy postponed the launch of Tegretol because of findings from animal testing. In autumn that same year, the company for the first time felt itself compelled to post a warning against the substance's possible damaging effect on germ cells.[17]

In the United States, Senator Estes Kefauver started scrutinising the pharmaceutical industry in hearings as early as 1959, focusing initially on drug prices. Then in October 1962, the United States Congress passed the Kefauver-Harris Amendment to the existing Federal Food, Drug, and Cosmetic Act, which because of the thalidomide scandal shifted the main attention to safety and effectiveness.[18] It imposed substantially higher requirements for the approval of medications by the American Food and Drug Administration (FDA); effects, side-effects, and risks now had to be documented.

The pharmaceutical companies fell into turmoil. They had long been geared towards the global market and therefore strove for an 'internationally valid documentation' of clinical results so that America, an important sales market, as well as other countries whose authorities took their cue from the United States, did not fall away from the outset.[19] The Kefauver hearings radiated into other sales markets and also put pressure on drug prices. According to Geigy, the thalidomide affair had overshadowed the entire industry; it unsettled the population and led to tighter health and safety legislation. The company noted with concern that the information required for an approval was increasing enormously and now also had to include information 'on chemicals, production and monitoring processes, pharmacology and toxicology'.[20] Even for approved medications, their 'claimed therapeutic effect' had to be documented retroactively. Incidents now had to be systematically recorded and reported. In the following years, the FDA also demanded the reporting of all known side-effects of test and commercial preparations. In 1964, the Committee on Safety of Drugs (Dunlop Committee) in the United Kingdom also started its work, advising the authorities on the quality, efficacy, and safety of new drugs.[21]

As a reaction to the thalidomide disaster and the stricter FDA directives, in 1963 the requirements of the IKS approval authority were also increased in Switzerland. Effects and side-effects now had to be verified and the documentation requirements were increased.[22] In addition, an independent reporting office for injuries caused by medications was planned, although establishing it would be a long, drawn-out undertaking.[23] In the meantime, another procedure took shape. As stipulated by Geigy's medical department in 1965, 'cases worth reviewing' were to be reported to the Swiss Academy of Medical Sciences (SAMS). 'Trivial cases', on the other hand, went to the Association of Swiss Physicians (FMH). The SAMS undertook clarifications and issued recommendations to the affected company, the IKS, and the FMH. Geigy deemed this process to be 'worthwhile', for it gave drug makers the chance 'to intervene directly in the clarification of a reported observation. This can prevent unfounded measures from being taken and perhaps wrongs being done to the manufacturer.'[24]

Company documents vividly reveal the immense pressure that these changes put on the pharmaceutical industry. According to an internal Geigy annual report, 1963 had been the 'year of defence', and 1964 'the year of unease'. They were dealing above all with unproductive administrative work that had little to do with the clinical effect of a substance but rather pertained to incidents and side-effects. Staff shortages arose, and the pressure to have individual substances succeed heightened.[25] Over the decade, therefore, marketing became more and more important. In 1967, Geigy introduced network planning, a method for the schedule planning of interlinked processes. The marketing department was henceforth involved from the outset in establishing working objectives and priorities to ensure that there was a potential market for any products emerging from the laborious development process and that the investments paid off financially.[26]

Geigy had started reorganising internal processes right after the Kefauver-Harris Amendment was passed in 1962. Clinical trials were divided into stages A, B, C, and D, and an internal application for a trial approval now had to be made.[27] But confusion about this still reigned in early 1964. An employee therefore tried to clarify the 'repeatedly arising misunderstandings about the purpose of an application for clinical testing'. An application triggered the following procedures: inclusion of the necessary preliminary testing (toxicology, galenics); then the evaluation by competent personnel for chemistry, toxicology, and galenics, as well as by the responsible specialists and clinical workers; and finally an approval for initiating a stage-A clinical trial.[28] Trial stage A, also called 'clinical pharmacology' or 'human pharmacology', served in the first instance to search for effects and indications. Consequently, Kuhn was frequently used for these stage-A trials.[29]

However, this created a dilemma; comprehensive and elaborate clarifications were now supposed to occur prior to the start of any clinical trial. At the same time, from the company's perspective, such an immense outlay was only justified if a new effective substance could be expected to actually reach the market. Making such an assessment, however, required clinical trials.[30] Before one tackled the 'enormous requirements' of the registration authorities, one preferably would have an initial assessment of a substance's potential from clinical trials. This perhaps explains why in the 1960s some substances made their way to Kuhn for tests before the corresponding results of toxicity and tolerability testing were available.

At the same time, efforts were made to formalise these processes across companies; a pharmaceutical industry brochure published in 1964 on the 'clinical testing of new medications' referred to the new processes.[31] It explained that the path to new substances proceeded by way of pharmacological and biochemical preliminary testing, which, 'together with the findings from animal experiments' (toxicology), enabled conclusions about the 'spectrum of effects and tolerability'. If a substance held promise (which applied only to 1 in 3,000 substances), the active substance went to the galenic researcher, who would find a suitable form of delivery.[32] Next came the so-called tolerability trials, which usually included an 'initial experiment' with a self-experiment or with healthy volunteers.[33] Only then did the actual clinical trial start. The brochure further explained that one was increasingly adhering to the 'measurable', to the 'numerically' ascertainable, because this was stipulated by legislation. As a result, the state was compelling the doctor and investigator to perform 'scientific-experimental activity at the sickbed', which in many cases had an inhibitive effect. But particularly in Switzerland, the brochure noted, one was aware of the dangers of an all-too-rigid legislation. From Geigy's perspective, the IKS guidelines pursued the goal of meeting safety needs without overly hampering scientific progress.[34]

The 'demand of the registration authorities for "statistical evidence"' on effects and tolerability, however, led to complications in implementation: 'Neither the investigators nor we ourselves have assimilated this process yet, and above all we lack the specialised personnel with the appropriate biostatistical knowledge', noted a Geigy annual report of 1965.[35] In fact, many clinics did not begin to gradually adopt statistical methods until after the mid-1960s. Since the companies relied on investigators and needed to adapt to their preferences, the exact design of any test ultimately still remained up to the investigator.

Thus the pharmaceutical industry faced a completely new cost–benefit analysis. Since the journey of the substance out of the laboratory had slowed considerably, a bottleneck developed between chemistry and the clinic. The 'net time requirement' for preclinical toxicology and the clinical trial had grown to nineteen months, according to Geigy's pharma committee in 1965. After that came clinical trial phase/stage A, which took another one to two years – this referred to the testing on healthy volunteers. The costs for toxicological and pharmacological trials had skyrocketed. Bottlenecks also arose in animal testing, so it was outsourced to third-party animal testing centres and the company started building its own external facilities.[36] Recently constructed laboratory buildings were already quickly approaching their 'bearable limits' since the 'requirements of the experimental processing of new pharmaceuticals' had unexpectedly strongly increased. Because the time required for chemical development steadily grew, every commercial product needed between twelve and fifteen chemists, each of whom submitted around forty-five compounds annually for testing.[37]

Indeed, the number of new preparations generally declined in the following years; the big wave of innovation of the postwar period levelled out. The thalidomide scandal had generated pressure to change. In Switzerland, initially the pharmaceutical companies themselves introduced changes, which were needed for sales in the United States; they – and not the psychiatrists, politicians, or the public – brought them to the attention of doctors and clinics. As in other sectors, the industry relied on voluntary self-regulation and lean legislation. Thus at first, the methodical, documentary, and regulatory reorganisation contended with the issues of risk, safety, and cost efficiency.

Ethical problems, on the other hand, rarely explicitly came up in this context. Such questions were brought in by physicians.

With the Declaration of Helsinki in 1964, the World Medical Association created the first guidelines for ethical research in clinical trials, although they were not legally binding. This declaration also established 'informed consent' as a condition – that is, the informed, voluntary consent of probands to participate in trials.[38] In addition, a new distinction was introduced between scientific experiments (without therapeutic motivations) and therapeutic research (with therapeutic value for patients). In Switzerland, ethical issues related to clinical testing only began being addressed in the 1970s, above all in connection with the SAMS guidelines on 'research experiments on humans' published in 1970.[39]

### Geigy's man during the boom

Kuhn basically did not keep pace with the upheavals and the wave of standardisation that swept through the pharmaceutical industry. Even so – or perhaps for precisely this reason – he remained an important partner for the Basel companies, for psychopharmaceutical testing at Münsterlingen actually intensified during the 1960s. Trial series ran simultaneously or overlapped; while some patients were included in one trial and then the next, others received combinations of various test substances. Thirty-five trials verifiably took place during decade; although five additional test substances were delivered, we could not find any documentation to confirm that they were actually tested. Overall, under Kuhn's leadership the clinic entered into a veritable frenzy of testing. At times, almost the entire clinic must have been involved in the testing of medications. The situation became increasingly confusing even for the participants themselves; test substances from various manufacturers stood side by side, and colour coding – for example, 'Geigy Violet' – was central to keeping track of things in the everyday experimental routine.

Research continued to focus on antidepressants, where Kuhn had developed a certain reputation – but not exclusively; a few Basel companies were hoping to find a successor to Largactil with a less dulling effect. Geigy also wanted to launch its own tranquilliser, which never succeeded, however. These substances, too, came to Kuhn for testing. Fine distinctions between substances with similar effect profiles became increasingly important, especially for antidepressants, for which specific substance characteristics were worked out in clinic trials and through the marketing department.[40] Clinical trials could now also be conducted to serve marketing strategies, as expressed by a Geigy memo: 'Once ... the decision is made to seek the commercial introduction of a product, then the broad clinical work must occur under the sign of commercial realisation. It may no longer flinch and hesitate. It becomes purpose-oriented in the true sense of the word.' An expanded 'clinical trial' of a substance against contusions and venous diseases, for instance, had no purpose apart from 'making the product known to the largest number of practicing doctors. This not only generated a large amount of documentation ... but, at the same time, the product was introduced on a broad basis.'[41] Thus at least for the company, clinical trials could indeed be quite goal-oriented.

A number of psychopharmaceutical projects were underway at Hoffmann-La Roche as well. In 1961, the company launched amitriptyline; the substance was synthesised at almost the same time by Roche, Merck, and Lundbeck, which subsequently divided the market among themselves.[42] Amitriptyline was the second tricyclic antidepressant after Tofranil, that is, the latter's direct successor.[43] The new medication threw Kuhn into an agitated flurry. Having been able to try out the substance shortly after the trials were concluded, he considered amitriptyline superior to Tofranil. He immediately turned to Geigy's Director Krebser, who had asked Kuhn to contact him directly if something 'essential' happened. Kuhn felt the new Roche substance was indeed an important innovation. Like a spy, he immediately reported to his closest partner company. Fearing that the situation 'with regard to antidepressants could soon be completely transformed', he asked Geigy to swiftly patent a similar substance.[44] Thus the race had by now become quite palpable. Newer, potentially better products were challenging the first generation of psychopharmaceuticals.

Roche, in turn, associated Kuhn with the competition and called him 'Geigy's man'. Nonetheless, the parties began a hesitant collaboration in 1966, although without ever really warming to one another. All told, Kuhn tested five Roche substances in comparatively small-scale trials. None reached market readiness. Roche's distance to the 'discoverer of Tofranil' may also have been related to the fact that the company soon limited itself to preserving its market position and only engaged in 'defensive research'. It focused on tranquillisers, especially from the benzodiazepine group. The first appeared on the market as Librium, followed by Valium, so-called blockbusters for Roche that were later criticised for potential addictiveness. Kuhn had excoriated them early on, finding that they had a narcotic effect. At Münsterlingen, he repeatedly encountered dependent patients with corresponding withdrawal symptoms. There were regrets at Roche, too, that the company had been 'under the spell ... of benzodiazepines' and had failed to further develop its series of neuroleptics.[45]

## Searching for a successor to Tofranil

In the antidepressant sector, Geigy had kicked things off in the late 1950s and achieved a major market success with Tofranil. Now the company was developing successor and variant products based on this substance group. On the one hand, they were hoping for substances that worked faster with fewer side-effects, and on the other, they needed to prepare for the expiration of the Tofranil patent. Most Geigy substances of the 1950s were close chemical relatives of Tofranil; all originated either from the iminodibenzyl or iminostilbene series. With the onset of the 1960s, additional variations were developed, chiefly with modified sidechains. So there were chlorinated or demethylated Tofranil, five metabolites – that is, metabolic products – as well as many other numbered substances akin to Tofranil.

Three second-generation Geigy antidepressants came onto the market in the 1960s. Insidon was launched in 1961, followed by Pertofran in 1962 and Anafranil in 1966. These three substances were tested to varying degrees at Münsterlingen. Kuhn merely played a secondary role in the testing of Anafranil. Although he had received the substance in 1960, he only tested it on a few patients.

He played a bigger part in the testing of the later Insidon, which began in 1959 and more strongly captured his attention. At Kuhn's request, the substance was coloured yellow – this colour happened to be available and thus would avoid any confusion in the clinic. More than 100 Münsterlingen patients took part in the trial. As soon became apparent, Geigy Yellow had 'two faces'. Some patients became increasingly agitated and aggressive, such that their use of the substance was discontinued. In contrast, others became drowsy, which led Kuhn to use the substance for sleep disorders.[46] How could this difference be explained? When testing began in 1959, Kuhn used the substance not only for depressives but also for catatonic patients.[47] Geigy, too, initially had envisioned a 'middle position' for the preparation between Tofranil and Largactil. For Kuhn's catatonic patients, however, Geigy Yellow gave rise to many cases of 'pronounced violence', which was 'quite dangerous' for the nursing staff.[48] The trial was halted – albeit only due to inadequate supplies. Larger quantities arrived again in January 1961, whereupon Kuhn made a new attempt with seventy patients, here too with 'diagnostically very different groups' after the 'pre-trials' had already concentrated on 'very different chronically ill persons', of whom 'only several [were] depressive patients'. Somewhat later, people at Geigy would complain in a different context about his 'inhomogeneous patient material' because fewer than half of the cases could be included in the analysis.[49]

After four months, Kuhn suggested possible indications to the company. The substance seemed especially well-suited for the ambulatory treatment of depression, he reported. It worked really well, side-effects were minor, and the calming effect set in quickly. Also conceivable was an indication for children and youth. In fact, after Insidon was launched in October 1961, Roland and Verena Kuhn readily began using it on children, particularly those 'with light depression who also complained about sleep disorders'. From Geigy's perspective, Insidon was 'probably the most dazzling of our psychotropic substances'. For precisely that reason, it was popular with practitioners, but this was also why it fell into 'disfavour' with the FDA. The substance, namely, failed to clear the new hurdles for market approval in the United States because the indications were too broadly defined. At least as far the United States was concerned, Geigy had been unable give the product a sufficiently specific profile.[50]

Just a short time later, Geigy would raise the ante and in 1962 launch another antidepressant called Pertofran.[51] In contrast to Insidon, this time Kuhn was not one of the first investigators, who were in Geneva, Basel, and St Urban.[52] In September 1961, however, testing also began in Münsterlingen, where the substance was known internally as Metabolite III or G 35020. Kuhn tested the substance for probably more than half a year on around twenty patients. Just a few weeks after testing started in Münsterlingen, he reported to Geigy that the substance worked like Tofranil, except the effect occurred more quickly. Now Geigy wanted to pick up the pace. For 'known reasons', the company announced two months later, they had been forced to make a rapid decision on the substance. Geigy was alluding to the increased competitive pressure generated by amitriptyline. Moreover, the American company Lakeside had begun challenging the American patent for the substance. Within Geigy, they were already discussing possible brand names, and in order to more sharply distinguish their new product, they had decided against using the word fragment Tofranil. The trial was soon expanded to include seven investigators. In March 1962, while Kuhn was still knee-deep in extensive testing, the company made the internal decision to launch, once again explicitly mentioning the competitive situation due to amitriptyline and the patent dispute. The introduction occurred in record time in June 1962; Kuhn only learned about it indirectly.[53]

The increased tempo of this trial had given Kuhn problems. In January 1962, he reported that he was having difficulty finding appropriate cases, since most patients with depression were now being treated by general practitioners. He started developing a new group for clinical trials: the outpatients who came to his office hours. As he told Geigy, he was hoping 'in this way to nonetheless gather a few more cases'. In addition, he was evidently also looking for probands outside the clinic. Thus he wrote to a different Geigy employee about finding a suitable patient in the Cantonal Hospital Münsterlingen, but this patient had refused to come down to the psychiatric clinic.[54]

The new group of outpatients enlisted for testing Metabolite III also included five of the clinic's female nurses. They had already been receiving outpatient treatment under Kuhn. There was nothing new about nurses becoming patients and vice versa. A few had already been involved in the testing of Tofranil and Insidon or had received psychotherapeutic treatment from Kuhn for years.[55] Most had attracted attention for some reason or another in their ward, whereupon the senior nurse had sent them to Kuhn for therapy. Maria Bodmer's medical file, for instance, seems more akin to a personnel file than a medical file, for it primarily deals with performance issues and everyday problems in the ward. After half a year, Kuhn first prescribed her G 33040 against sleep disorders – that is, Insidon shortly before its registration in early 1962 – and then Metabolite III. The file contains no justification for this switch from a newly registered medication to a test substance, nor is there an explicit diagnosis. As an observation of effect, it states only that she is doing better now. 'She is less tired, can work better, and feels good.'[56]

The medication pattern for these nurses was basically the same. Four of the five initially received G 33040 (later Insidon), a few were also given Tofranil, and all five were subsequently included in the testing of Metabolite III, which in one case was combined with another test substance.[57] The trials of G33040 and Metabolite III were close to each other in time; in Kuhn's view, the substances had a similar effect and were primarily appropriate for depressive moods. The switching of the nurses to the metabolite might have been related to Insidon's market launch.

The spatial proximity to Kuhn, the regular consultations, and the observations of other people – for example, the head nurse – made the five nurses virtually ideal trial subjects. Were they better informed than other patients about what they were being given? In the medical file of one nurse, Kuhn in any case noted with regard to the later Insidon: 'The patient was angry for a time because one had told her Geigy Yellow is the same as Tofranil. I then explain to her the formula differences and it is striking how the situation is resolved and things improve.'[58] Noteworthy, too, is that the patients changed their doses or stopped taking the substances pretty much on their own accord, only to then be admonished by Kuhn during psychotherapy not to go off the medications. It is clear that the nurses had been given the same diagnosis as was needed for testing Metabolite III, namely, depression. Whether Kuhn only wanted to find probands or whether he also pursued healing purposes cannot be definitively answered.

Metabolite III, or Pertofran, not only provides insight into Kuhn's 'search for patients' but is also helpful in other respects. It was part of an entire group of metabolites that came to Münsterlingen. In contrast to Metabolite III, the others were tested only in Münsterlingen – and without success. Geigy never had any intention of bringing them to market. The testing was performed 'for scientific interests only with Dr Kuhn'.[59] At the same time, the company never bothered with thorough toxicological and tolerability pretesting, perhaps because it was clear from the beginning that such documentation would not need to be submitted.

The hypothesis behind the substance group was that, when breaking down Tofranil, the body produces metabolite substances that constitute the actually effective principle of Tofranil in its pure form.[60] Kuhn maintained close contact with Geigy's biochemical division and collected urine samples to help with the investigation of the breakdown of Tofranil in the organism. The first investigations pertained to Metabolite I,[61] but Geigy waived an 'extensive pharmacological trial' and the 'usual tolerability testing by Professor Grünthal'. However, the company said it would be happy for Kuhn to 'undertake corresponding tests on a few suitable patients'. He was supposed to tell them if he still wanted certain specifically targeted animal tests, but that only a small supply of substances was available.[62] Kuhn responded that he would test the toxicity on a chronic case. Only after that would he try to determine on a depressive patient whether the substance was effective. Kuhn's two-tiered process becomes visible here: an initial test on chronic cases, then the actual testing for the effect. Between 1958 and 1962, Kuhn then tested Metabolite I on 'approximately one dozen cases'.[63]

Between 1965 and 1966, Kuhn also tested the sixth metabolite.[64] In this case, toxicological tests had been carried out, but Geigy noted that a preliminary clinical tolerability test on healthy persons had not been done.[65] Kuhn soon reported 'downright unpleasant side-effects'; two female patients had become extremely agitated; the preparation was discontinued and he 'did not want to take any responsibility in this regard for the time being'.[66] As per the medical file, however, a chronically catatonic patient received the metabolite until August 1966.[67] If one considers that the metabolite was envisaged as an antidepressant, the inclusion of this diagnosis and the duration of the administration are surprising.

One Geigy executive was troubled by the fact that the substances were sent for clinical testing before the preliminary investigations were completed. Writing about a different preparation, he told Kuhn in 1964 that they were working on producing enough substance to be able to review the so-called subchronic toxicity, that is, the harmful effect through repeated ingestion. 'Without this toxicological test, it would hardly be responsible to give you the preparation for testing on humans.'[68] In practice, however, the approaches varied. In the case of the two metabolites, tolerability testing on healthy volunteers was omitted; in the case of other substances, Geigy did not perform an investigation of long-term tolerability. With regard to G 31531, for instance, the subject of a 'trial desired by Dr Kuhn', the subchronic toxicity was investigated, but the 'toxicological testing on the dog' was waived 'because a clinical trial is planned only with Dr Kuhn'. 'Practically no utility; of theoretical interest', the company noted before the clinical trial started.[69] And for other substances, toxicity in the event of repeated or long-term ingestion was evidently reviewed at the same time as the clinical trial itself.[70] During this period, Kuhn therefore also served Geigy by delivering early initial assessments of a substance's tolerability.[71]

## Keto: The trial that exceeded all boundaries

By far the longest and most comprehensive trial series conducted at the Münsterlingen Psychiatric Clinic began in 1963 with Ketotofranil. Officially, it lasted until the end of 1970, when, much to Kuhn's dismay, Geigy halted research on the substance. Despite the long-time efforts, the substance never came onto the market. The trial involved more than 1,000 Münsterlingen cases, including for the first time a larger number of children and youth, as well as many outpatients who came to psychiatric office hours with a wide range of concerns and complaints.

But what kind of substance was this, which so dominated the 1960s? Like most substances, it bore a number, G 35259, as well as the name ketimipramine or Ketotofranil. But it was known above all as 'Keto', an abbreviation that reflects the familiarity with the substance that must have developed over such a long trial. The longer names point to a second important point; Keto, too, was a successor to Tofranil, which explains why it was not treated as a completely new type of substance at the Münsterlingen clinic but rather as a variation of something they knew.[72]

Keto was probably first delivered to Münsterlingen as early as July 1959.[73] What happened next is unclear. The trial did not begin until around four years later, as a Geigy letter documented for the 'sake of form'.[74] The substance was supposed to be used for depression; the corresponding test quantities had already been handed over during a personal visit. In November 1963, Kuhn reported to Geigy on the start of the trial. The process occurred in stages; after a few 'preliminary tests', he administered the substance to a 'good test case'.[75] As Kuhn explicitly recorded, the preliminary tests were actually a tolerability and toxicity trial. The test case was to evaluate effectiveness. All of them had favourable results.[76]

But then Kuhn revealed what for him was an unusual caution; he still hesitated 'treating newly ill patients' with Keto, he reported to Geigy, specifically because of a bad experience with another Geigy substance that he had tested on at least eight patients in 1962.[77] The substance G 37329 had produced severe side-effects: desiccation and haemoconcentration, especially during the first weeks of treatment.[78] Geigy had then asked Kuhn whether he wanted to continue the trials or felt they were 'no longer defensible under the given circumstances'.[79] Kuhn voted to discontinue, whereupon Geigy then politely followed up, asking whether he might 'not still [do] a few tests' with the substances, since 'no new tests preparations are available' for the next few months.[80] Kuhn would later halt the testing with G 37329 on his own accord.[81]

Kuhn's comparatively cautious approach with Keto can thus be explained by the problems with G 37329. In mid-December, the Keto trial was expanded to eight additional patients. Kuhn now selected 'prognostically rather unfavourable' cases because, as per his justification, severe cases did not spontaneously recover, which meant that the effect of the substance could be distinguished without being obscured by the course of the illness. After around four months, he reported to Geigy that there still was 'something weird' about the trial. Some patients would sweat profusely, and when they were switched to Tofranil there had been 'strong neurovegetative side-effects' that were 'impactful' and 'created for us a quite disconcerting situation' for several days. They had reckoned with serious complications. Kuhn feared that the substance was not properly breaking down in the body and therefore wanted Geigy to perform metabolic investigations. During further testing, special precautions would need to be taken – by which he primarily meant that the testing would require 'a lot of personal experience and very good knowledge of the test subjects'. When patients were discharged from this first round of testing, they were switched to an approved medication – likewise an unusual precautionary measure compared to other trials. Thus far, he had not dared 'to let the test preparation leave one's hands'.[82] The experience with G 37329 must still have sat hard with him.

Despite these side-effects, he came to a positive evaluation; the results thus far were of 'very great significance', the substance was on par with Tofranil. For Kuhn, complications by no means indicated that the substance was unsuitable. Instead, this generally suggested to him that the proper dosage or the appropriate patient group had not yet been found. Thus in what would prove a decisive step, he decided 'after careful consideration' to include outpatients in the trial as well. The inclusion of outpatients was associated with 'increased risk', but the test would then advance much more quickly, for 'in all likelihood' Keto would have 'a very important future'.[83] Outpatients could not be monitored and observed anywhere as closely as inpatients. Nor could one respond as quickly to incidents. However, the advantages were obvious. Along with facilitating an acceleration of the trial (for the competition was palpable), the number of cases could quickly be increased. Besides, depressive patients – the target group – were increasingly being treated on an outpatient basis or in doctor's practices, a development Kuhn attributed not least to medications such as Tofranil.[84] The inclusion of a growing number of outpatients offered the chance to carry out a trial that would push all previously known boundaries. True, prior tests had included outpatients as well, but they were now joined by more and more cases that Kuhn did not already know from earlier inpatient stays.

By summer 1964, the Keto trial series had grown to forty patients. Kuhn's evaluation was even more positive; the substance was not only equal to Tofranil, he reported, but rather constituted a 'considerable advance' compared to the latter, and side-effects practically never occurred anymore. He began pressing for a market launch as soon as possible, for he had recently been supporting the hypothesis that, contrary to the opinion of many psychopharmacologists, the antidepressant effect was, in fact, not tied to side-effects. Hence the urgency, for it was only a matter of time before 'one eventually arrives at such ideas elsewhere too'.[85] Geigy basically agreed, but asked Kuhn for blind tests with Keto and Tofranil. Kuhn refused, arguing that blind testing was not practicable and they should let the matter rest; with time, Basel might realise Keto was effective even without it. Geigy then had a different clinic carry out the desired double-blind trial in 1965. According to an internal Geigy memo, such a double-blind test was a first for Switzerland and 'for reasons of time' was conducted 'prior to the completion of our toxicological documentation'.[86]

Kuhn kept testing. By late 1964, the trial at Münsterlingen already included 100 cases. Other investigators, however, failed to confirm his persistent positive evaluation of Keto, which surprised him. He found it very difficult to understand that 'Herr Colleague ... can hold it to be without effect', insisting to Geigy that the other investigator must have chosen the wrong patient group. Kuhn applied multiple strategies to buttress his high opinion of Keto. First, he emphasised his extraordinary experience as an investigator. Since fewer and fewer depressive patients were being hospitalised, clinics were accumulating cases that were 'atypical, difficult to handle, and even more difficult to evaluate'. To include these in trials, one needed 'very specific experiences'.[87]

Second, Kuhn cited the entire clinic staff as witnesses. Not just he, but also his medical colleagues and the nursing staff were 'absolutely convinced' by Keto. They included the 'older sisters and nurses who had participated in the introduction of Largactil to the asylum, who intensively collaborated in the working out of Tofranil, and who since then had repeatedly gathered experiences with the most varied psychopharmaceuticals.' No one would express even the slightest doubt about the substance. Quite the contrary; the staff was repeatedly recommending that patients be treated with Keto. And this actually 'told best of all whether a medication works or not'.[88]

Third, he began to comply with a request by Geigy to collect statistical evidence, at least to some degree. He compiled 100 cases on index cards and used them to create a tabular overview – albeit one that he repeatedly relativised: 'This would still need a lot of commentary'. The statistics, for instance, were influenced by the many substance combinations, although he felt the combinations led to better outcomes. And the ambulatory cases were especially problematic patients and hence a 'negative selection', for they had been referred to him by other doctors precisely because they were patients nobody could previously help.[89]

Keto worked superbly – that much was clear to Kuhn. But his approach and testing method depended so strongly on his person that the results could scarcely be replicated anywhere else or generalised. Combination treatments in particular diametrically opposed the goal of a systematic evaluation. However, Kuhn had confidence in his clinical gaze and was certain that he could sharply distinguish between known and unknown effects. 'I have always conducted the treatments such that I can make myself a pretty precise picture about what the new preparation does and where its limits are.'[90] Statistics basically did not sit well with him. 'One is much more likely to get a proper view of the mode of action of a preparation on the basis of the precise knowledge of individual cases than by means of large statistics in which much is inevitably distorted by the mutilation of the material.'[91]

Kuhn therefore reverted to his typical reports with detailed case descriptions. The next expert evaluation of Keto would in fact grow to seventy-five typewritten pages; the 100 cases from his report of August 1965 had all been treated with Keto for more than half a year. This long duration, according to Kuhn, had made placebos unnecessary since, with time, effective remedies were clearly distinguished from ineffective ones.[92] Of the 100 cases, 66 were receiving outpatient treatment. Kuhn now saw far more advantages than disadvantages to outpatient testing; moreover, nowadays antidepressants could only be properly assessed by including 'clinic and polyclinic patients'.[93] Kuhn reported that the condition of four-fifths of the patients had more or less strongly improved and that Keto marked a 'new, very important advance in psychopharmacology'. By means of combinations with Insidon, Pertofran, and other substances, he had also tried to treat other components that went beyond 'purely phasic depressions' – that is, to individually adapt the therapy.[94] Geigy continued to tolerate this approach for several years, even though it blurred the boundaries between the clinical trial and therapeutic application.

His expert evaluation of Keto also discusses the treatment of children. Kuhn therefore must have started such treatment no later than 1965. He found that children tolerated Keto better than Tofranil because it was less likely to induce vomiting. With respect to children, there were entirely new indications to be discovered for the substance across the board.[95] The small-dose, 10-mg tablets, which Kuhn then repeatedly ordered, were meant for this patient group.[96] Children were basically not treated any differently than adults, except for the lower dosage. The proportion between success and failure for children was pretty much the same as for adults, according to Kuhn.[97] Nor was Keto the only test substance given to children. They tended to receive the particular test substance that happened to be most popular at the time: first Tofranil, later Insidon and Keto, and finally Ludiomil, before and after their respective approval.

Kuhn's wife Verena, who at this time specialised in children and youth psychology, was primarily responsible for the treatment of young people. In outpatient office hours, she treated them for a variety of complaints, from difficulties at school to stuttering, bedwetting, and sleeping problems, behind which she often discerned subtle depressive components. Most of the children came to the outpatient department at their parents' request; others were referred for treatment or evaluation by other institutions or children's homes.[98] In 1966, Verena Kuhn – possibly together with her husband – wrote a manuscript on the 'Casuistic Study of One Hundred Children Treated with Antidepressant Medications'.[99] They also included Keto cases, while others were treated with approved medications, particularly Tofranil. At any rate, by April 1966 eighteen children were among the now 150 new Keto patients featured in the reports to Geigy.[100] The inclusion of children and youth occurred mainly with the expansion of the trial to outpatients, for they were primarily handled on an ambulatory basis.

Verena Kuhn seems to have shared her husband's penchant for pharmacological substances, for Kuhn wrote about the treatment of children with antidepressants in both of their names: 'It is increasingly incomprehensible to us that there still are child psychiatrists who believe that drug treatment, if it is proper and advisable, has drawbacks.'[101] But one rarely finds verbose justifications for the administration of a test substance or detailed descriptions of effects on her part. In her case, what typically crops up in medical files instead is the phrase, one wants to 'try it once with this substance'.

Hence, the reasons why a child received a test substance are often hard to follow. For example, parents sometimes also brought their children in for an appointment because of 'underachievement'; not more than a few consultations would be needed before a test substance was dispensed or sent to the home. Other children received Keto because they wet the bed.[102] While bed-wetting was at least a secondary indication for Tofranil, using the Keto test substance to treat children's underachievement, stuttering, or difficulties at school was quite far removed from any scientifically oriented clinical trial protocol.[103]

The Keto trial series was further expanded for adults as well. The test substance had come to be given out more like a standard therapy. In any event, the long treatment periods and the now carefree distribution to family doctors and patient relatives do not suggest a clinical trial. Neither was any actual question being pursued anymore; at most, the idea was now to verify the medication's positive impression with the greatest possible number of cases. In point of fact, at Münsterlingen Keto had supplanted the approved drug Tofranil by 1966. As Kuhn noted to Geigy, 'ever since we have access to G 35259, we hardly use Tofranil anymore'. Since Keto was no longer merely being used to treat clear-cut endogenous depressions, he also needed 'to be able to prescribe medications without restrictions'. By this he meant Keto. And thus the annual demand, which he repeatedly reported to Geigy while keeping anxious watch over his shrinking supplies, climbed accordingly in the following years.[104]

In mid-1970, Kuhn ordered his last resupply. Preferably, he wanted a six-month supply of 250,000 25-mg Keto tablets all at once. To his surprise, however, his request was denied.[105] Ostensibly, the reasons had to do with delivery formats. Geigy had already manufactured 40-mg capsules in 1968, but Kuhn felt the tablets were more effective than capsules, and he also preferred the 25-mg dosage.[106] But Geigy now reported that the 25-mg dosage was not part of the development program. 'The development of new formats without corresponding biochemical investigations is no longer justifiable today.' In a sudden reversal, Kuhn was also asked to stop using substance combinations and to limit the number of patients in future Keto testing.[107]

Internally at Geigy, a major operation was underway: the merger with Ciba.[108] Kuhn was told that he had not been forgotten, but that all projects needed to be put on hold because of the imminent merger. Confused, Kuhn turned directly to Hugo Bein at Ciba: 'Since at the moment I do not know whom to turn to at the Geigy company about ketimipramine, I would be grateful to you if you could tell me whether I can count on further resupply by early October.' Kuhn's approach led to 'alienation' at Geigy.[109] The supply line was cut off. Because of Keto's uncertain future, they could no longer promise him any test quantities, stated Geigy in October 1970. Then in December 1970 the axe came down. Ciba-Geigy decided 'to drop further plans with this preparation'; Bein told Kuhn about the decision at Christmas, explaining that many testing facilities had reported that Keto was no more effective than currently available drugs; another factor was the animal toxicology results. Presumably, as part of the merger with Ciba, the company also wanted to make several directional decisions and strategic choices between similarly active substances.[110]

Kuhn considered this a wrong decision with serious consequences. He wrote the following in response to Bein's Christmas letter.

> You write that you hope that I understand your reasons to halt the trials. For now I must say in this regard that our patients, at any rate, cannot understand how one could give up on such an effective and good preparation. It is virtually the stereotypical conversation in our consulting rooms. Our patients want to know why they should no longer receive a medication that has provided them the best of service, for years in some cases; the mothers are moaning, what are they supposed to do with their children if the old misery starts again at home and at school. For us it is quite difficult to justify the situation to the patients, since we ourselves are by no means convinced about the correctness of the decision.

The decision would adversely affect not only the patients, Kuhn went on, for it also confronted Kuhn and his employees with several practical problems whose scope he could not yet assess.[111]

The main problem was obvious. Many of the Münsterlingen patients now had to be switched to a new substance. Starting in 1971, most of the previous Keto patients were switched to Ciba 34276, which later became Ludiomil. But not quite all of them; the substance must still have been given occasionally, in one case as late as 1979.[112] By February 1970, some 1,214,000 dragees of Keto had been used, Kuhn reported. They had been tested 'on a patient material of slightly more than one thousand cases, about which something can be said regarding the results'. Children between 2 and 16 years old made up slightly less than one third of this group. Among the more than 1,000 total cases, over one third were treated as outpatients. There was also at least one fatality – a hospitalised patient died from a lung embolism after Keto injection therapy. Twelve had committed suicide, and one 17-year-old had attempted suicide. In addition, Kuhn reported, there had been two inadvertent Keto poisonings of small children who had access to the tablets, but without lasting consequences.[113]

Of the more than 1,000 cases referred to in Kuhn's report, only 346 patients are listed by name in Kuhn's private archive. The fatality does not show up in any other documents and cannot be associated with any patient known by name. However, the number of cases does not match the number of patients, for, as Kuhn himself wrote, sometimes he included patients who had already been part of a previous group, either because they reentered the clinic or because they started taking the substance again after a certain break.[114]

Notwithstanding the many gaps that still remain, Keto, like no other substance, marked the transition from inpatient psychiatry to outpatient therapy – it was intended for the latter market and it was also soon being tested there. The large numbers, the long treatment period, and the broad spectrum of patients shows that the transitions from clinical testing to therapeutic treatment were fluid for Keto. Whether the experimental or therapeutic interest stands out more strongly can depend on the particular source, even in one and the same case. In the course of the trial series, Keto was used ever more frequently as routine therapy, often without specific methodological measures, documentation, or analyses. Many aspects lay outside any kind of designed trial protocol – for instance, the continued use of the test substance even though the trial had already ended, the combination of Keto with various other substances, and the medication's heedless distribution. Keto was Kuhn's favourite substance, and he had invested so much time and hope in the medication that the trial's discontinuation affected him personally as well. The substance had become ensconced at Münsterlingen as a wonder drug well before the trials ended – despite the negative evaluations by investigators at other clinics and the fact that Kuhn's results were not confirmed anywhere else. In this respect, too, Kuhn and Münsterlingen appeared more and more as an island amid currents that ran in other directions.[115]

### FR 33: An exception with incidents

Parallel to the frenzied search for the optimum antidepressant and to the glut of potential Tofranil successors, an entirely different trial began at Münsterlingen in autumn 1962. The test substance of the Sandoz company was called FR 33. It was intended as a new neuroleptic, thus for the treatment of psychotic disorders. A new kind of chemical compound, it had never been used for psychoses before, but had shown a mood-moderating effect in a pharmacological test, announced Sandoz.[116] The first shipments arrived on 8 August 1962, and around three months later Kuhn reported that they had made 'several tests in the last few weeks' with it.[117] An earlier success had already been achieved in the butyrophenone substance group that included FR 33; a related substance – Haloperidol (Haldol) from the Belgian company Janssen Pharmaceutica – had come on the Swiss market in 1960. Later in 1963, Cilag would then introduce Luvatren, another neuroleptic from this substance group.[118] Sandoz, in contrast, would remain unsuccessful here – FR 33 never reached market readiness.

Ultimately Kuhn, too, issued a negative evaluation of the substance group. The preparations of this group worked 'in quite convoluted ways', he told Sandoz's competitor, Ciba-Geigy.[119] He wrote to Sandoz that FR 33 had a negative effect; indeed, the entire substance group was too 'uncertain and unspecific' in its action. Therefore, the tested substance held no therapeutic interest, but the 'experiences gained from it could still provide certain suggestions'[120] – meaning suggestions with respect to the interaction between chemical sidechains with a tranquillising or stuporrelieving[121] effect. Despite Kuhn's scepticism, the FR 33 test series at Münsterlingen continued until at least April 1964, with isolated references suggesting that the substance was still occasionally being used in 1965.[122] Scientifically interesting, therapeutically unspecific, and difficult to deal with in clinical testing – what exactly happened during the trial series?

We are aware of forty-two Münsterlingen inpatients who received FR 33 – a number that contradicts Kuhn's statements to Sandoz. Some were only given the substance a single time, others received it for months. Men were somewhat overrepresented compared to women (25:16, one case unknown); in addition, at least five of the patients involved had undergone psychosurgery in the early 1950s. While patients diagnosed with reduced intelligence or 'idiocy' were still included at first (five), the trial soon switched to schizophrenics (thirty-five). Because of its chemical relatedness with haloperidol, Kuhn initially assumed that FR 33 worked the same way: as a tranquilliser for 'agitated idiotic patients' and providing relief to stuporous schizophrenics. But as it turned out, the opposite was true. The test substance could lead to 'wild agitation' that only eased when treatment was stopped.[123]

The target group was 'chronic schizophrenic conditions': patients who were not helped by any of the conventional therapies; 'sick persons, who either through their unpredictability and through occasional sudden outbreaks of anger or acts of violence cause great difficulties for the nursing staff'; or the 'withdrawn, stiff, unapproachable and uninfluenceable catatonic stupor conditions', that is, patients who strictly refused to work, did not accept a greeting, and 'often for years simply [sat around] not doing anything'. Kuhn outlined this illness profile for FR 33 in a report to Sandoz, which he wrote around eighteen months after the trial began.[124]

The fact that he chose aggressive patients prone to outbursts, or stiff, mutistic ones, also had to do with the hypotheses regarding the substance's action. Proven medications were already available for the treatment of psychoses – for example, Largactil or Melleril. The goal now was to find preparations that 'clearly influence the psychotic occurrence, if possible without a dampening effect', meaning drugs that were less sedative.[125] Kuhn and Sandoz hypothesised that FR 33 was more tension-relieving and activating than dampening; the key indication for FR 33 'would therefore be the severe, chronic catatonic stupor'.[126]

Our patient group includes sixteen persons who, as per the documentation, only ever received FR 33 as a test substance – and by contrast, eight patients who verifiably received between six and twelve test substances. Thus some were used to try out many substances, whereas others consistently received one standard medication, such as Largactil. Most of the patients had already been staying at Münsterlingen for a long time when the trial began. In every 'sanatorium' there was 'a larger number of such sick persons', Kuhn noted, for whom no change could be attained; they were chronic schizophrenics whose condition had gradually deteriorated over the years.[127] For this patient group, it was especially difficult to discontinue the previous medication. Therefore, as in many other trials, the test substance was administered in frequently changing combinations with approved drugs, including with Melleril, Tofranil, Insidon, and Largactil.

That the substance also happened to be 'capricious' became clear within just a few months after the trial commenced.[128] In early February 1963, the company informed Kuhn about incidents at other clinics, namely, about three fatalities[129] that, according to Kuhn, could 'practically with certainty' be traced to FR 33.[130] 'In agreement with Herr Director Dr Zolliker', he decided to continue the testing anyway, for he assumed that further incidents could be prevented with more careful dosages.[131] That winter, many trials were interrupted at Münsterlingen, including that with FR 33, because a two-month flu epidemic broke out in the clinic. In mid-April, however, the trial series was resumed with more than a dozen new cases. Only eight days later, Kuhn told Sandoz about an initial success, but also about serious complications. One patient had severely collapsed twice during the first trial phase, but then had also recovered after the substance was discontinued.[132]

Kuhn was reporting here on an incident that had already occurred between September 1962 and mid-February 1963.[133] New incidents followed. Because of 'a combination of unfortunate circumstances and negligent actions of the staff', in one ward 50-mg tablets were administered instead of 10-mg ones. An older patient subsequently collapsed and became unconscious and lost his pulse.[134] Another patient collapsed after being switched from chlorpromazine to FR 33.[135] Both gradually recovered.

By contrast, in the case of a third patient, a 38-year-old woman[136] diagnosed with schizophrenia, Kuhn reported an 'astonishing' improvement. The woman was planning for the future again and had regained her spontaneity – possibly a new kind of substance effect, Kuhn speculated.[137] The nursing staff had noted that, after just a short time, it became apparent that the patient was doing much better after receiving FR 33. One could talk to her, she helped with work, she started knitting again as well as eating in the 'day room', and she was in a cheerful and positive mood.[138] Even so, on 6 February 1963, the treating doctor ordered an ECG – probably just after Sandoz had reported orally on fatalities.[139] Kuhn noted in the patient's medical file that the drug was rapidly reduced and gradually discontinued once they learned that 'FR 33 creates dangerous incidents'. In mid-April the substance was discontinued; in mid-May the patient was initially placed on leave and then released even though Kuhn felt she was not 'really healed in the actual sense of the word'.[140]

Thus for the 'success patient', FR 33 was discontinued as a precaution, while at the same time he started a new series of trials with the same test substance. In the near future, he would 'need a lot of the test substance' as long as 'no serious incidents arise that hinder our trials' – at least 5,000 tablets a month, Kuhn wrote to Sandoz in late April 1963.[141] However, his expectations did not hold up very long. In mid-May he reported the substance's arbitrary nature to a Vienna doctor, who was also testing FR 33: 'The effect apparently does not take place in parallel with the dosage.' Therefore, one needed to be able to dose with restraint and wait, because for a long time nothing happened, but then a lot occurred at once.[142] Although the dosage and effect did not clearly correlate, Kuhn's only lever for controlling risk still seemed to be the dosage. In autumn 1963, new 5-mg tablets were manufactured at his suggestion.[143] While at the start of the trial up to 150 mg were still being administered per day, over the course of 1963 he switched to smaller doses of between 10 and 50 mg.

Thus despite incidents, the FR 33 trial continued. Only after several months would it become clear that this also raised 'new problems'.[144] A 38-year-old patient diagnosed with 'idiocy (with frequent states of agitation)' received four tablets of a sleeping and tranquillising drug and two 10-mg tablets of FR 33 each day. His physical condition then deteriorated such that he effectively suffered from severe motoric symptoms and quickly became marantic, that is, undernourished. They started him again on anti-Parkinson's drugs and then discontinued all drugs in mid-August, but without success. The patient died on 31 August 1963.[145]

A 52-year-old female patient diagnosed with 'chronic hebephrenia' (schizophrenia) collapsed in April 1963 'on a single tablet of ten mg',[146] whereupon the treatment was discontinued. In mid-August it was noted that the patient continued to lose weight. Largactil was used to try to get her to eat more. In November, the patient suddenly broke out in a high fever and 'unexpectedly' died just a few hours later.[147] As well as a lung infection and meningitis, the autopsy identified marantic endocarditis.[148] Whether the patient's death can be traced back to FR 33 cannot be conclusively determined. It is revealing, however, that Kuhn mentioned the fatality in his test report to Sandoz but in a retroactive comment in the medical file denied any connection to the substance.

> What can no longer be decided is whether she ate too little because her physical condition deteriorated in the last months, or conversely, whether she was unable to eat because of her increasing catatonic stupor and therefore physically lost her power of resistance. What is certain is that the medications have nothing causally to do with the fatal outcome.[149]

Also interesting when considering whether Kuhn and Sandoz linked the substance to the death is their cooperation in writing a joint publication on FR 33. A draft still contains the following sentence: 'Fatalities did not arise with the very careful dosing that we used; however the incidents were at times threatening and very unpleasant.' But the publication itself does not contain the phrase on fatalities.[150] It must have been deleted during the editing process, which suggests a decision to avoid any explicit mention of the topic of deaths. Perhaps there were indeed suspicions that the fatality was linked to FR 33 and therefore the statement no longer seemed defensible.

However, the incidents did not mean the trial series was stopped, at least not in Münsterlingen. Sources show that, in the case of one patient, FR 33 was not discontinued until January 1964 and only after several collapses. For other patients, the continuation of testing is documented until mid-January 1964. In one case, FR 33 is still noted at the end of March, and in another in mid-April 1964.[151] In late September, Kuhn wrote to Sandoz that, when he read the draft of his text, the substance actually seemed 'very encouraging'. But the trials themselves had been 'very burdensome ... because one never knew what was happening, and it is very likely that a certain affective component was involved that motivated me to practically give up on the trials'.[152] To almost give them up, but not completely? In any case, the medical files we consulted suggest that the FR 33 trial was not suddenly aborted but rather slowly petered out.

Sources on the preparation of the aforementioned publication provide further insights into Kuhn's approach. An anonymous reviewer felt that Kuhn's passage on the clinical aspect had to be rewritten 'so as to be less impressionistic'. He noted that the reader is not told who made the observations, how these observations were made, and, above all, how bias was avoided.[153] Kuhn justified his approach by saying that the trial happened to have been very difficult and problematic. FR 33 had triggered such unpleasant side-effects 'that I therefore did not believe I could justify using it on patients on whom more complete clinical observations were possible. It is really just about gaining an orientation, in which direction, for example, the effect of this preparation goes.' He evidently tried to gain orientation with a specific group of patients: 'one can actually only justify carrying out such tests on very severely ill patients'. But this raised the problem that one had to rely fully and entirely on external observations without statements from the patients themselves.[154]

Kuhn thus started with two patient groups in mind. The first group – the so-called serious cases – only allowed for rough observations of the substance's effect. Patients in the second group, on the other hand, could provide detailed information. The severity of the illness was balanced against the risk of side-effects and incidents. Kuhn explicitly mentioned this balancing act; the substance was 'not non-dangerous' but 'also [had] positive traits'. One needed to clearly find out whether 'it was justified to take further risks or not'. In the case of FR 33, he ultimately felt the risk seemed too high and the prospects of success too small, which is why he gave up on the trial after thirty-three cases.[155] Around two weeks later, Sandoz paid 3,000 francs for the trial;[156] the joint article was ultimately published despite initial difficulties;[157] and, in May 1967, Sandoz decided to delete FR 33 from the list of test preparations.[158]

All in all, from the episode one gradually gains the impression of a situational, unstructured approach and a highly problematic substance that repeatedly resulted in incidents and, even in Kuhn's eyes, was risky and difficult to control. Although in individual cases he discontinued FR 33 or reduced the dose, for other patients he kept administering the substance despite collapses and reacted late or not at all. Thus in retrospect, one would probably concur with the anonymous reviewer; in the case of FR 33, he took an 'impressionistic', uncoordinated approach that accepted significant risks – and which might have been chiefly motivated by scientific interests.

### New testing methods, new paper tools

Roland Kuhn's status as an investigator changed over the 1960s. An internal memo of the Wander company from 1968 provides a pointed and illuminating outside view.

> Prof. Kuhn is still enthusiastic about imipramine and remains a proponent of this preparation. He is full of prejudices. It is pretty difficult to deal with Prof. Kuhn. Only our personal relationships with him can perhaps move him to properly test our substances. But one must actually presume that his trials will be limited. He will only test the preparations on a few patients (ten at most) and will try to formulate his verdict.[159]

The memo goes on to say that one could not 'expect detailed reports' from Kuhn, nor did he reliably adhere to deadlines. In the end, Wander in fact decided not to include his test results on an antidepressant in its analysis because he failed to follow the instructions.[160]

The reason that test protocols existed at all was because of new rules on pharmaceutical research. Wander, for instance, formalised its clinical trials towards the late 1960s. This therefore ruled out the kind of 'impressionistic' approach we saw with FR 33, at least theoretically. According to an internal document of 1969, every clinical trial required a clear and unmistakeable question. The duration, number of patients, required amount of substance, delivery format (for example, tablet, injection), fee, as well as the date of the next review had to be set with the investigator before the trial started. The relationship between the company and the clinical investigator was a sort of contract: 'Two equal partners agree on a trial mode and strictly adhere to the details stipulated therein.' The total quantity of substance was to be delivered at the beginning; discussions were supposed take place every two months; individual logs were to be kept and 'dropouts' and their reasons were to be listed in the statistics – that is, cases that were withdrawn from the trial because of 'release, death, intolerability, transfer'. The methodological goal was now objectivity and quantifiability. However, the document closes with a qualification: 'In general we will need to adapt to the capabilities and inclinations of the clinical investigator – but he must just as much accept our ideas, our desires within the limits of the possible.'[161] By the end of 1967, Sandoz too had similarly formalised its trial protocols. They now had to include information on the goal of the study, the selection of patients, the dosage format, the evaluation criteria, and side-effects. Sandoz also decided to demand the return of unconsumed test quantities after a preparation was abandoned.[162]

These new requirements brought with them new paper tools: case protocols, forms, and questionnaires. But such documents or references to them are rarely found in the holdings of the Münsterlingen clinic and Kuhn's private archive. Notably, the earliest form comes from an American firm, dated 1961, and lies in the dossier without having been filled out.[163] In 1962, Geigy tried to get Kuhn to record his cases with the later Pertofran 'according to our schema on a questionnaire'. Developed 'because of desires from the USA',[164] it was meant to facilitate direct comparisons with other clinics.

Kuhn was uncomfortable with such a schematic approach.

> I admittedly have already had inhibitions since the beginning, because I find that the diagnostic schema does little to meet my needs. But then it became apparent that the cases often proceeded differently than it appeared at first, so that I needed to start making corrections, and then I told myself again, if I issue this now then perhaps already in fourteen days it will no longer be accurate.[165]

Geigy countered that even though questionnaires were always coupled with controversial schematisations, 'in the end, however, in the form of the questionnaire, valuable material is available to us for statistical requirements'.[166] This time Kuhn allowed himself to be convinced for once, and for each of ten cases he delivered two filled-out, rather rudimentary questionnaires.[167] However, he did not change his basic attitude, and in its further collaboration with Kuhn, Geigy also did not bother with any more questionnaires.

Kuhn generally rejected the statistical approach. This method, he noted, only dealt with 'numbers, tables, and curves' and turned the sick person into a 'case', into just an 'object'.[168] Having recognised Tofranil's antidepressant effect through clinical observation, without forms and statistics, he adhered to this exploratory method for the rest of his life: open trials, which served more to find an appropriate indication for the substance effect than to purposefully test for a certain effect stipulated from the outset; trials that evolved over time, focused on changing patient groups and whose methodology was based on clinical observation. Kuhn's trial reports, which he sent to the pharmaceutical companies in the form of a letter, also then consisted mainly of descriptive case analyses, without systematic evaluations, but with summarising remarks.

Thus while Münsterlingen continued to rely on this method that had proven itself with Tofranil, the world had changed. The quantity of paper that had to be submitted for an approval had literally exploded. Internally, Geigy noted that it was known from the American company Eli Lilly that six pages had still sufficed in 1940 for an approval application in the United States; 'in 1950, sixty pages were submitted, in 1960, around six hundred pages, and in 1963, eight thousand pages'. For the drug companies, the famous Professor Kuhn, known as Geigy's man, now became a rapid or pilot tester who could help them relatively quickly gain an initial impression of a new substance's spectrum of effects but whose results could no longer even be mentioned in approval applications. In 1966, Geigy noted, for instance, that two substances were 'intended for a quick trial with Dr Kuhn', and afterwards 'possibly with Prof. Heimann'[169] – Kuhn therefore functioned increasingly as an initial clinical investigator before the substances were released for broader clinical trials. In this way, the companies themselves ultimately circumvented their own formal requirements.[170]

Such accelerated procedures were already envisaged in 1956, when Geigy searched for a way to achieve quicker results, as noted in the minutes of an internal meeting. One wanted to clarify whether Kuhn could perform preliminary testing on a larger number of preparations to 'obtain approximate information on effects and side-effects'; if successful, the substance would then be released for 'broader testing'.[171] Kuhn saw 'the possibility of being able to issue a somewhat reliable judgement, whether the further testing of a compound is worthwhile or not, after a test period of around six weeks. It is hoped that, thanks to this accelerated method, the testing of additional compounds will be accelerated.'[172] The background for these accelerated tests was the enormous competition for a successor to Largactil that followed immediately after the psychopharmacological turn in the mid-1950s. Towards the end of the 1960s, however, Kuhn became an outmoded investigator because he ignored the new methods. Nonetheless, now moving more firmly into a niche, he still had a role as a preliminary investigator in the roundelay of clinical investigators.

The statistical turn, which gripped American psychiatry above all,[173] did not occur at Münsterlingen. In contrast to clinics that standardised their diagnostic systems, trial documentation, and trial method during the 1960s, Kuhn stayed with clinical case studies (laboratory analyses such as blood or urine tests were added, depending on the substance; blood pressure and temperature measurements were standard). Switzerland's university clinics, on the other hand, began carrying out comparative trials and collaborative research: 'The number of new psychopharmaceuticals is so large', wrote Paul Kielholz of Basel, 'that it is no longer possible for the individual psychiatrist to test their effectiveness comparatively'. In comparative trials, new preparations were tested in comparison with already established medications. Thus there was a control group that received a standard drug; and the new effect would need to be better than that of the standard drug. By joining with other clinics, larger numbers of patients could be attained in less time and side-effects recognised more quickly.[174] A working group for methodology and documentation, which formed in the German-speaking world as of 1966, was meant to ensure that findings were gathered and progressions of effect evaluated according to roughly the same system – with standardised, statistically analysable forms.[175] The psychiatric clinics of Switzerland's universities deployed statistical methods from around the mid-1960s, but even there the trials often remained exploratory.[176]

Placebos added an additional level to controlled trials. To distinguish between a treatment effect – for example, an improvement that only occurred because the patients received a medication or more attention from the doctors – and the substance effect, one group was treated with a so-called 'empty preparation' without the substance. This could occur blind (only the patients do not know what they are getting) or double-blind (neither the psychiatrists, nursing staff, nor patients know whether a placebo or substance is being administered). In the German-speaking world, placebo controls were initially rejected and, in contrast to the United States, only slowly managed to prevail.[177] Many psychiatrists considered it unethical to administer a placebo to patients for a longer time since this kept them from receiving an effective medication.[178] Therefore, in practice, despite new regulations, the so-called randomised, double-blind studies – that is, studies in which placebos and substance are randomly allocated – only really began taking over towards the end of the 1960s.[179]

Kuhn always refused to administer placebos.[180] He found that, on the one hand, placebo effects could be ruled out with longer test periods; on the other hand, 'with very good observation and a lot of experience', so-called genuine effects could be distinguished from suggestive effects within just a few days.[181] In a retrospective interview in the late 1990s, Kuhn then also said that he never controlled double-blind studies with placebos, never used standardised 'rating scales', and also never statistically analysed the data from a large number of patients.[182] Indeed, the Münsterlingen archives contain no references to placebos or larger-scale statistical analyses. However, Kuhn applied his own form of blind study by having test substances coloured in the same way as approved medications that were already known, particularly to keep inpatients from knowing that their medication had been switched.[183]

Kuhn's attitude became more extreme as he grew older. In 1993, he wrote to a Swedish pharmaceutical company that double-blind studies with placebos could no longer be justified today

> above all also because one cannot be content with trials of three to four weeks but rather must necessarily conduct longer trials. This means, in practice, that, with regard to antidepressants, one will be unable to achieve any progress. But since the bureaucracy of the health authorities is not going down this track, it will probably take decades before one realises that this does not work. In any case, I will not live to see it.[184]

## Between daseinsanalysis and psychopharmacology

Kuhn relied on his experienced gaze, which he sought to bring to bear on every individual patient in precise observation. This self-image runs through all of his writings and was ultimately also in keeping with the daseinsanalysis approach.[185] At first, it seems contradictory that Kuhn in the 1960s – this peak period of clinical trials – undauntedly published on the subjects of daseinsanalysis and Rorschach tests. Although the many trials must have claimed a large share of his time and research capacity, they formed only a small part of his publication output.[186] He would not strive to publish more on psychopharmacology until his advanced age, when, with a nascent self-historicisation, he began to concern himself with fame and honour.[187] In contrast, during the 1960s he probably did not consider this field to be a branch of research that could decisively enhance his reputation among academic psychiatrists. In all likelihood, Kuhn felt that psychopharmaceutical research was too close to practice, and apart from the chance to hypothesise about chemical structures and modes of action, it offered very few opportunities for grand explanations and the formation of psychiatric theories.[188] Thus he continued to focus on phenomenological approaches and on daseinsanalysis, which led to close interactions with the psychiatrists Ludwig Binswanger and Henri Maldiney, as well as to sporadic contact with Martin Heidegger and Gaston Bachelard.[189] According to Kuhn, daseinsanalysis viewed the human being holistically: 'Therefore ... defective functions can be recognised in their significance for the whole. In this way, physical and psychic functions and their disorders, such as depressions, for instance, appear with regard to their inclusion in a unified whole.'[190]

Notwithstanding the apparent contradiction between publication activity and research practice, and despite the various hats that Kuhn wore depending on the milieu, there are substantive parallels between daseinsanalysis and his testing method. Both are in the tradition of hermeneutics, that is, empathetic projection and understanding.[191] This stands opposite empirical approaches based on questioning, experimentation, numbers, and statistics. Kuhn's hermeneutical approach also affected, first, the question of whether individual cases can be generalised, and second, his own role as observer and doctor. For in the hermeneutical approach, the observer remains just as central as the person being treated. In this approach, it is the experienced clinical gaze that first brings the decisive findings to light.[192] Conversely, empirical approaches seek to exorcise the observer where possible by means of placebos, random orders, and statistics, since they view the observer as biased and subjective.

In phenomenological-hermeneutical psychiatry, the individual case has a middle position. It does not stand entirely for itself and itself alone – thus it is not about understanding the patient solely in his specific uniqueness – nor is the patient, in a casuistic sense, merely an illustration of greater laws. Rather, it is much more about recognising the general in its individual manifestation, which after all is only visible in the latter. Or, in Heidegger's words to Kuhn: 'There are admittedly differences between the individual human beings, for example, in a farmer or an intellectual, but through daseinsanalysis the general structures of the dasein can very well be revealed; in contrast, for example, to the coarse psychology of a Bleuler, who only collects facts.'[193]

In Kuhn's writings and practices, however, the individual case remains strangely abstract. Thus in describing Kuhn's era at the clinic, one of his successors at Münsterlingen struck a 'contrast between the highest peaks of the intellectual dealing with psychoses and the comparatively rather barren and distanced dealing with concrete sick persons' who were 'often only "shepherded"'.[194] A similar divide appears in Kuhn's private archive. In his texts, he repeatedly declared his commitment to precise observation and to the close supervision of patients, but in medical files he seems oddly disinterested in the possible causes of their suffering, whether these were of a social or biographical nature.[195] His test reports illustrate this middle position of the individual case. Often he simply strung case descriptions together without any of them being informative in themselves or used for a higher-level analysis. In actual practice, thinking phenomenologically simply meant not looking for an underlying explanation but rather describing the dasein.[196]

In the gradually changing world of clinical trials, Kuhn vehemently defended his methodology. According to Kuhn, instead of using statistics and double-blind trials, he had always examined each patient individually, sometimes several times a day, and repeatedly questioned them. His colleagues and the nursing staff had also provided observations, which he took seriously and picked up on.[197] While in principle this approach was still feasible for small circumscribed trials, by the 1960s it must have reached its limits because many comprehensive trials were conducted in parallel. Precise observation was now plainly out of the question, even if Kuhn still claimed otherwise. The sparse entries in many of the medical files testify at the very least to neglectful recording practices in everyday clinic life.[198] The surviving trial documents, too, contain very little detail about individual cases; the lion's share consists of slips of paper and lists of names with plus and minus signs or key words such as 'better' or 'worse, too little'. The special reports written by the nursing staff, in which a brief entry on the patient's condition was usually made each day, seem more systematic.[199] Kuhn often drew from these reports to write his assessments for the pharmaceutical industry.

Individual cases were only given a lot of space in Kuhn's own notes if they aroused his particular interest. This extended from questions about the clinic's practical routines to dreams. Among the questions on practical routines, he was interested chiefly in internal clinic procedures, problems in the wards, and interpersonal conflicts. In addition, the 'functioning' of his patients in everyday life seems to have been important, which for him was revealed during work therapy, meals, or rounds – whether the patient 'accepted the greeting' on these occasions was always central. Kuhn assigned more significance to this 'functioning' than to sounding out the causes of the malady. Individual patients also received plenty of space if they had interesting dreams. As did his wife and other doctors, Kuhn conducted psychotherapy, which consisted above all in the recording of dreams. This generated large amounts of paper; dreams were recollected by patients, dictated by Kuhn, and typed out by his secretary – particularly if they concerned especially 'interesting' patients (usually depressive, ambulatory, and female) with vivid dreams. However, little was done with them; dreams were neither closely analysed nor picked up again during therapy.[200]

The trial documents also suggest an indirect and rather unsystematic view of substance effects and patients. Kuhn's observations joined with those of his spouse, the senior and assistant physicians, the nursing staff (Figure 4.1), and relatives. From these polyphonic

The 1960s                                       155

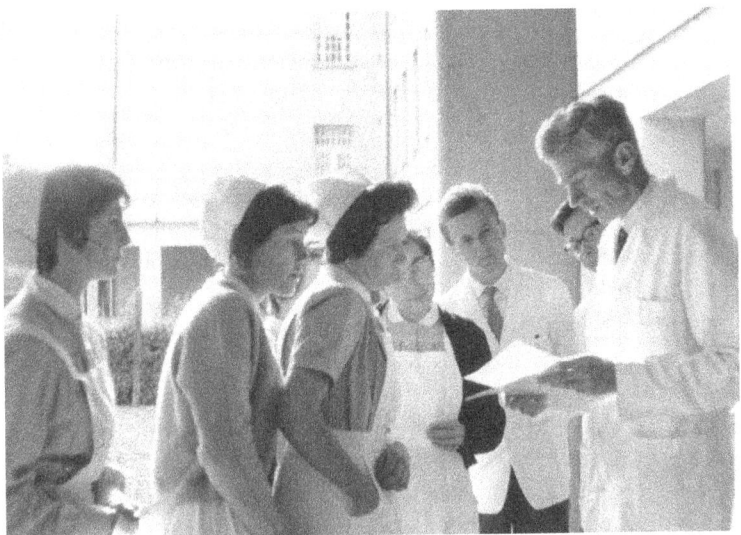

Figure 4.1 Roland Kuhn ('Daddy-Long-Legs') with staff, 1961

yet fragmentary and largely blurred impressions, Kuhn cobbled together his test reports. Intuitive and impressionistic? Or rooted in an old-fashioned, even paternalistic conception of the doctor's role? When it comes to how he was categorised by his contemporaries, a marginal note on a Ciba document from 1971 stating that Kuhn was 'an artist after all' is perhaps revealing.[201] Representatives of the pharmaceutical industry seemed to associate Kuhn more with the arbitrary but occasionally genius characteristics of an artist rather than with modern, serious scientificity. The sources suggest that even his self-image as wrought by his own hand never fully matched his clinical practices.

During the course of the 1960s, the psychiatrist's observing gaze generally suffered a loss of confidence. With the international alignment and standardisation of disease categories, an effort was made to reconcile regional differences (for example, so-called psychiatric schools).[202] Clinical trials were formalised and newly regulated, and psychiatric classifications, too, were standardised with the goal of making it possible to compare diagnoses and therapies. The new blind procedures and the formalised and statistical analyses served to eliminate individual bias and generate comparable, reproducible results.[203] Consequently, psychiatry moved closer to the methods of general medicine and experimental science.[204] Impulses for this transformation originated, on the one hand, from American science. As early as 1961, a Geigy employee reported internally on the new 'single-blind' and 'double-blind' approaches from the United States, which one now also wanted to adopt in Europe.[205] On the other hand, the innovations were due to the increasing economic pressure on pharmaceutical companies, which were developing far more medications than before. More and more drugs needed to be tested, while there were fewer and fewer suitable patients in the clinics – especially for testing antidepressants, which were now often being dispensed by general practitioners. 'Properly designed trial plans' were needed 'to be able to obtain more from the available patient material', noted the Sandoz company in 1962.[206]

The most powerful motor for these radical changes were stricter regulations and a new risk awareness in the wake of the thalidomide scandal, discussed at the beginning of the chapter. It was because of these international developments and the new regulatory mechanisms that Kuhn, given his hostility towards these processes, migrated over the 1960s from a central place in clinical testing to the margins. The hermeneutical approaches he espoused gradually lost importance. Kuhn, however, remained true to daseinsanalysis throughout his life and did not feel that it held any contradiction to psychopharmacological research. To be sure, he had become famous through discoveries in biological psychiatry, as he wrote to Heidegger, but 'I would not have succeeded with the pharmacological discoveries without the philosophical education and without daseinsanalysis'.[207]

## Notes

1 StATG, 9'40, 5.0.2/2, Kuhn to Kaufmann, Ciba, 27 February 1964.
2 StATG, 9'40, 3.0.2/6, Kuhn to Jucker, Sandoz, 20 June 1964.
3 The phrases 'Test desired by Dr Kuhn' (G 21302; G 31531; G 38038) and 'Substances worked out at his request' (G 31220; G 35570) are found in internal Geigy documents with reference to various substances. CA Novartis, Geigy, PP 12/5, pharma production, medicinal division, various subject-area minutes, 1960–1967.
4 StATG, 9'10, 6.2/11474, patient to Verena Kuhn, 17 June 1969; *ibid.*, 3, 30 March 1971.

5 On the history of objectivity, see Daston and Galison, *Objectivity*; on the statistical turn, see Bonah et al., *Harmonizing Drugs*; Gaudillière and Hess, 'General Introduction'.
6 On tacit knowledge, see Polanyi, *The Tacit Dimension*; on the changing awareness of risk, see Daemmrich, 'A Tale'; *Pharmacopolitics*. On the experimentalisation of medicine, see Marks, *The Progress*. On placebos, see Lakoff, 'The Right Patients'; Shorter, 'Brief History'.
7 Rinkel, 'Foreword', viii; Osmond, 'Chemical Concepts', 10.
8 On therapeutic optimism and its dissipation, see Snelders et al., 'On Cannabis'.
9 RA Novartis, AW 143076 & HF 1854, letters Kuhn and Wander remarks, file note, 9 September 1968.
10 Schwerin, 'Die Contergan-Bombe', 255. See also Stephens and Brynner, *Dark Medicine*.
11 Daemmrich, 'A Tale'.
12 Randow, 'Keine Heilung'; 'Gefahr im Verzuge', *Der Spiegel*, no. 49 (5 December 1962), quoted in Schwerin, 'Die Contergan-Bombe', 255.
13 Gaudillère and Hess, 'General Introduction', 4; Schwerin, 'Die Contergan-Bombe'.
14 Robson and Sullivan, 'The Production'.
15 CA Novartis, Geigy, PP 22/6, pharma production, psychopharmaceuticals: Tofranil, press conference of 26 March 1963.
16 CA Novartis, Geigy, PP 12/2, pharma committee, minutes 2/63, 6 January 1963, 1–2; minutes 5/63, 3 April 1963.
17 CA Novartis, Geigy, PP 12/2, pharma committee, minutes 8/63, 3 July 1963, 4; *ibid*., minutes 11/63, 2 October 1963, 7.
18 Tobbell, '"Who's Winning"', 430; Greene and Podolsky, 'Reform'.
19 CA Novartis, Wander, subsidiary companies file 1968, Spain, 2; Geigy, PP 42, pharma production, annual report of the medicinal division 1964, 6–7 on India, which in practice adopted FDA decisions.
20 CA Novartis, Geigy, PP 1a, pharma production, Geigy pharmaceuticals, annual report 1963, 1–2.
21 CA Novartis, Geigy, PP 12/3, pharma production, pharma committee, minutes 1/65, 14 January 1965, 6; Geigy, PP 1a, pharma production, Geigy pharmaceuticals, annual report 1963, 2; Geigy, PP 42, pharma production, medical department, annual report 1964, 9; *ibid*., annual report 1965, 10.
22 On the Intercantonal Office for the Control of Medicines, see Chapter 6, 202–203.
23 The private-sector Swiss Centre for Medicinal Side Effects (SANZ) was not established until 1979. Lüönd, *Rohstoff Wissen*, 139–141.

24 CA Novartis, Geigy, PP 12/3, pharma production, pharma committee, minutes 2/65, 2 February 1965, 5.
25 CA Novartis, Geigy, PP 42, pharma production, medical department, annual report 1964, 1.
26 CA Novartis, Geigy, PP 36, pharma research, quarterly report II/65, 25 June 1965, 1; *ibid.*, quarterly report III/66, 13 October 1966, 1–2; *ibid.*, quarterly report II/67, 15 July 1967, 6.; *ibid.*, quarterly report I/68, undated, 9–10; *ibid.*, summary of the annual report 1969, 24 February 1970.
27 Today's familiar phase models that distinguish between pharmacological and toxicological trials and tolerability testing on healthy volunteers (phases I–II), clinical testing (phase III), and market monitoring (phase IV) did not yet exist in this form.
28 CA Novartis, Geigy, PP 50, pharma production, pharmacological division, clinical preparations (1955–1966) and annual report 1963, 29 January 1964.
29 CA Novartis, Geigy, PP 42, pharma production, medical department, annual report 1964, 1.
30 *Ibid.*
31 Oberholzer, *Die klinische Prüfung.*
32 Very few substances could be without additives. Creating an ingestible, absorbable medication requires additives, preparation, and form. This is the task of a galenicist.
33 Geigy usually conducted these tolerability test with Ernst Grünthal in Bern. See Chapter 2, 37–38.
34 Oberholzer, *Die klinische Prüfung*, 7–11, 20–21.
35 CA Novartis, Geigy, PP 42, pharma production, medical department, annual report 1965.
36 For Geigy, 'Stamford Lodge' in England for chronic toxicology trials; in addition, an animal breeding program was established. CA Novartis, Geigy, PP 36, pharma research, quarterly report I/65, 2 April 1965, 1–2.
37 *Ibid.*, quarterly report III/1965, 3 November 1965, 1; Geigy, PP 12/3, pharma committee, departmental meeting of the executive committee with pharma committee, 4 November 1965, 4.
38 World Medical Organization, 'Declaration', 1448–1449.
39 See Chapter 6, 205–206.
40 For example, in the case of the Tofranil successors Insidon, Anafranil, and Pertofran.
41 CA Novartis, Geigy, PP 3, pharma production, pharmaceutical department, founding, history/chronology, 1939–1950, note on two memoranda, 26 July 1965, 2. This also applied to psychopharmaceuticals;

see, for example, Geigy, PP 42, pharma production, annual report of the medical department Geigy Basel 1965, 134.
42 CA Roche, RDR, internal report Dr Bruderer, VI/Chem., H. W. Roth, VI/ZS, Present State and Prospects in the Field of Antidepressants, 23 May 1975, 23. See also Healy, *The Antidepressant Era*, 75; Lopez-Muñoz and Alamo, 'Monoaminergic', 1571–1572.
43 With iproniazid (Marsilid), a Roche antidepressant belonging to the MAO inhibitor group of substances came to market at almost the same time as Tofranil. In Switzerland, concerns about possible toxicity were voiced early on; see Rietmann et al., ' "Wenn Ihr Medikament" ', 216; CA Novartis, Geigy, PP 12/1, minutes pharma committee, 11/58, 14 May 1958; *ibid.*, 4/59, 2 April 1959.
44 StATG, 9'40, 5.0.3/23, Kuhn to Krebser, 5 December 1961.
45 CA Roche, RDR, report no. 71'49 9, Dr Blum, Vergleichende Beurteilung von Benzodiazepinen in verschiedenen pharmakologischen Tests, 4 January 1968, 2; *ibid.*, internal report Dr Bruderer, VI/Chem., H. W. Roth, VI/ZS, Present State and Prospects in the Field of Antidepressants, 23 May 1975, 7; *ibid.*, report no. B-53'543, Interner Forschungsbericht. Ein Bericht über Neuroleptika, Dr Kyburz, 29 September 1975, 6; StATG, 9'10, 1.2.11/3.2, Kuhn to Foglar, Hoffmann-La Roche, 13 June 1969.
46 StATG, 9'40, 5.0.3711, Kuhn to Geigy, 22 October 1958; 9'40, 5.0.3/11, Kuhn to Geigy, 9 January 1961; CA Novartis, Geigy, PP 12/5, pharma production, medical department, subject-area minutes, brief remarks on the status of the trials, 21 April 1960.
47 Meant here is catatonic schizophrenia, which is characterised by psychomotor disorders – for example, a strong tension in the body.
48 StATG, 9'40, 5.0.3/11, Geigy to Kuhn, 16 February 1960; 9'40, 5.1.0/0.2, Kuhn's test report to Geigy, 10 June 1959.
49 StATG, 9'40, 5.0.3/11, Kuhn's test report to Geigy, 20 April 1961; CA Novartis, Geigy, PP 12/5, pharma production, medical department, subject-area minutes 1/64, 18 and 20 March 1964, 1–2.
50 StATG, 9'40, 5.0.3/11, Kuhn's test report to Geigy, 20 April 1961; 9'40, 5.0.3/26, Kuhn to Geigy, 6 November 1962; CA Novartis, Geigy, pharma production, annual report of the medical division 1964, 4; Gaudillière and Thoms, eds, *Marketing*, 173.
51 Desipramine, desmethylimipramine, Metabolite III, or G 35020.
52 Brodie et al., 'Preliminary'.
53 StATG, 9'40, 5.0.3/13, Kuhn to Geigy, 3 October 1961; *ibid.*, Geigy to Kuhn, 22 November 1961; CA Novartis, Geigy, PP 12/2, pharma production, pharma committee, minutes 11/61, 19 July 1961; *ibid.*, minutes 19/61, 20 December 1961; *ibid.*, minutes 4/62, 7 March

1962; StATG, 9'40, 5.0.3/13, Geigy to Kuhn, 26 January 1962; *ibid.*, Kuhn to Rothweiler, Geigy, 22 May 1962.
54 StATG, 9'40, 5.0.3/13, Kuhn to Rothweiler, Geigy, 12 January 1962; 9'40, 5.0.3/16, Kuhn to Pulver, Geigy, 20 January 1962.
55 On nurses as patients, see also Chapter 3, 101–103; Tornay, *Träumende Schwestern.*
56 StATG, ZA KAa 13002, 15 March 1962.
57 'Wy 3263' of the American Wyeth company, known in Münsterlingen as the 'American remedy'.
58 StATG, 9'40, 11.4/27, 25 January 1961. For further examples, see Chapter 3, 101–103.
59 CA Novartis, Geigy, PP 12/5, pharma production, medical department, minutes, psychopharmaceuticals subject-area conference, 1/1964, 18 and 20 March 1964, 1, 4; *ibid.*, minutes, psychopharmaceuticals subject-area conference, 3 July 1964, 1; minutes, psychopharmaceuticals subject-area conference, 29 September 1964, 1. On the metabolites, see Theobald et al., 'Zur Pharmakologie', 187–197.
60 Brodie et al., 'Preliminary'. Six such substances were developed; two, however, were biologically inactive (Metabolites II and V) and, although very promising, Metabolite IV could not be adequately stabilised chemically. The remaining three were trialled by Kuhn.
61 G 33679, Geigy Violet. See Chapter 2, 67.
62 StATG, 9'40, 5.0.3/13, Geigy to Kuhn, 9 June 1958.
63 StATG, 9'40, 5.0.3/13, Kuhn to Geigy, 11 June 1958. See also Chapter 2, 67.
64 G 36526.
65 CA Novartis, Geigy, PP 12/5, pharma production, medical department, minutes 1/1964, 18 and 20 March 1964, 4.
66 StATG, 9'40, 5.0.3/31, Kuhn to Geigy, 9 December 1965; *ibid.*, supplementary report on female patient, undated.
67 StATG, 9'10, 5.4/9525. This long-term patient was given a total of twelve substances, including Metabolite IV for just under a year.
68 StATG, 9'40, 5.0.3/32, Stoll to Kuhn, 4 August 1964.
69 CA Novartis, Geigy, PP 12/5, pharma production, medical department, minutes, psychopharmaceuticals subject-area conference, 1/1964, 18 and 20 March 1964, 3.
70 *Ibid.*, 2–3.
71 The sources on toxicity and tolerability testing for other companies are significantly poorer. For Ciba, there is evidence that the company gave a test substance to Kuhn before having precisely tested its tolerability ('also on a dog') in the case of repeated application. The

## The 1960s

reason given for not doing the test was a shortage of the substance. See StATG, 9'40, 5.0.2/2, Bein to Kuhn, 11 November 1966.

72 On the subject of successor substances, see StATG, 9'40, 5.0.3/32, test report G 36259, Kuhn to Geigy, 29 October 1966.
73 *Ibid.*, three confirmations regarding the receipt of the substance, 26 July 1959, 5,000 units.
74 *Ibid.*, Geigy to Kuhn, 15 August 1963.
75 *Ibid.*, Kuhn to Geigy, 4 November 1963.
76 *Ibid.*, report of 28 February 1964, 2.
77 *Ibid.*, 4.
78 StATG, 9'40, 5.0.3/13, Kuhn to Geigy, 3 February 1962.
79 *Ibid.*, Geigy to Kuhn, 27 June 1962. Geigy then also started to investigate the side-effects in animal experiments.
80 *Ibid.*, Kuhn to Geigy, 17 July 1962; Geigy to Kuhn, 23 July 1962.
81 The company did not issue its official discontinuation notice until December 1964; CA Novartis, Geigy, PP 50, preparation clinic stage A, annual report 1964, 12.
82 StATG, 9'40, 5.0.3/32, report of 28 February 1964, 5–15.
83 *Ibid.*, 15–17.
84 *Ibid.*, Kuhn to Geigy, 2 December 1964.
85 *Ibid.*, Kuhn to Stoll, Geigy, 30 July 1964.
86 *Ibid.*, Kuhn to Geigy, 2 November 1964; CA Novartis, Geigy, PP 50, pharma production, preparations clinic, stage A, annual report 1964, 11.
87 StATG, 9'40, 5.0.3/32, Kuhn to Geigy, 2 December 1964.
88 *Ibid.*
89 *Ibid.*, Kuhn to Geigy, 2 December 1964; Kuhn to Geigy, 2 February 1965.
90 *Ibid.*, Kuhn to Geigy, 2 February 1965. On substance combinations, see also Chapter 3, 98.
91 StATG, 9'40, 5.0.3/0, Kuhn to Stoll, Geigy, 6 July 1965.
92 StATG, 9'40, 5.0.3/32, Kuhn's assessment to Geigy, 4 August 1965, 61.
93 *Ibid.*, 2, 8.
94 *Ibid.*, 23, 55, 75.
95 *Ibid.*, 41–42, 75.
96 Also for adjustments for patients that were difficult to treat; StATG, 9'40, 5.0.3./32, Kuhn to Geigy, 10 November 1965.
97 *Ibid.*, Kuhn's report to Geigy, 10 June 1966, 3–4.
98 See, for example, StATG, ZA KAa 21566; ZA KAa 18485 (with an assessment by Verena Kuhn).

99 StATG, 9'40, 21.3.1/4 preliminary files (publication is missing); located in 9'40, 8.2/52 is the lecture of the same title that was held on 29 May 1965; one cannot clearly determine from the files which of them gave the lecture.
100 StATG, 9'40, 5.0.3/32, Kuhn's report to Geigy, 10 June 1966, 3–4.
101 StATG, 9'40, 3.0.2/7, Kuhn to a doctor, 19 June 1965.
102 For example, StATG, ZA KAa 20549; ZA KAa 18485.
103 See, for example, the three visits to the outpatient facility for underachievement 1969–1972, where Keto and later Ciba 34276 were administered. StATG, ZA KAa 23412. For a similar approach, see ZA KAa 12753.
104 StATG, 9'40, 5.0.3/32, Kuhn to Geigy, 10 June 1966, 2; Kuhn to Geigy, 29 April 1969. On quantities and dispensing, see Chapter 5, 169–176.
105 *Ibid.*, Kuhn to Geigy, 11 July 1970; Geigy to Kuhn, 15 July 1970.
106 *Ibid.*, Kuhn to Geigy, 29 January 1968; Kuhn to Geigy, 29 April 1969.
107 *Ibid.*, Geigy to Kuhn, 15 July 1970; Geigy to Kuhn, 4 August 1970.
108 On the merger, see Chapter 6, 197–199.
109 StATG, 9'40, 5.0.3/32, Kuhn to Bein, Ciba, 1 September 1970; *ibid.*, Oberholzer, Geigy, to Kuhn, 28 September 1970; *ibid.*, Kuhn to Bein, Ciba, 2 October 1970.
110 *Ibid.*, Geigy to Kuhn, 6 October 1970; CA Novartis, Ciba-Geigy, PH 4.00.2, 2 December 1970; StATG, 9'40, 5.0.4/4, Bein, Ciba, to Kuhn, 24 December 1970. Geigy had reported problems with chronic toxicity testing in the United States as early as the third-quarter report of 1968. An expansion of the trial seemed inadvisable for the moment; CA Novartis, Geigy, PP 36, quarterly report, pharma research department, 3/68, 14. In 1967, the Keto trials were temporarily halted in England by the Committee on Safety of Drugs; the authority had requested additional reports on toxicity and effects on fertility; see StATG, 9'40, 5.0.3/32, Geigy to Kuhn, 7 July 1967. After the merger, Ludiomil took the place of Keto; see Chapter 6, 197–198.
111 StATG, 9'40, 5.0.4/4, Kuhn to Bein, 4 January 1971.
112 StATG, ZA KAa 32419 I, female patient to Verena Kuhn, 27 June 1979. On this case, see Chapter 5, 176.
113 StATG, 9'40, 8.3/13, *Über die antidepressive Wirkung von Ketimipramin*, unpublished manuscript, undated (ca. 1970).
114 StATG, 9'40, 5.0.3/32, Kuhn to Geigy, 18 April 1966.
115 The distinction between non-standard therapeutic use and scientific experiments advanced only gradually into the consciousness of the medical community. In Switzerland, it was formalised in 1970 with the guidelines of the SAMS (see Chapter 6, 205–206).
116 StATG, 9'40, 5.0.8/5, Sandoz to Kuhn, 8 August 1962.

117 *Ibid.*, Sandoz to Kuhn, 8 August 1962; Kuhn to Sandoz, 24 October 1962.
118 See Angst and Pöldinger, 'Klinische Erfahrungen'. By then both Janssen and Cilag belonged to the American corporation Johnson & Johnson.
119 StATG, 9'40, 5.0.4/10, Kuhn to Grüter, Ciba-Geigy, 11 December 1972.
120 StATG, 9'40, 5.0.8/2, Kuhn to Jucker, Deputy Director Sandoz, 14 February 1964.
121 A stupor refers to a physical torpor.
122 StATG, 9'10, 10.3/6, day report Ward U, entry of 4 January 1965 on three patients. In the corresponding medical files, there are no entries on FR 33 for 1965.
123 StATG, 9'40, 5.0.8/5, 'Nebenwirkungen', typescript, undated (ca. April 1964).
124 *Ibid.*, 'Einige klinische Versuche mit FR 33/Sandoz', undated typescript (ca. April 1964).
125 Angst and Pöldinger, 'Klinische Erfahrungen', 3–4.
126 Kuhn et al., 'Pharmakologische und klinische Eigenschaften', 358.
127 StATG, 9'40, 5.0.8/5, 'Einige klinische Versuche mit FR 33/Sandoz', undated typescript (ca. April 1964).
128 StATG, 9'40, 3.0.3/5, Kuhn to Hofmann, Neurology Clinic of Vienna, 16 May 1963.
129 StATG, 9'40, 5.0.8/5, Sandoz to Kuhn, 13 February 1963.
130 StATG, 9'40, 3.0.3/5, Kuhn to Hofmann, Neurology Clinic of Vienna, 16 May 1963.
131 StATG, 9'40, 5.0.8/5, Sandoz to Kuhn, 6 March 1963; Sandoz to Kuhn, 13 February 1963.
132 *Ibid.*, Kuhn to Sandoz, 27 April 1963. The patient was treated with FR 33 from September 1962 to February 1963.
133 *Ibid.*
134 StATG, 9'10, 5.4/7345, 21 February 1964.
135 StATG, 9'10, 5.4/10327; no information regarding the collapse.
136 StATG, ZA KAs 21925.
137 StATG, 9'40, 5.0.8/5, Kuhn to Sandoz, 27 April 1963.
138 StATG, ZA KAs 21925, nurse report, 23 February 1963.
139 *Ibid.*, Lier to Cantonal Hospital Münsterlingen, 6 February 1963.
140 *Ibid.*, 15 May 1963; nurse report, 27 April 1963; 9'40, 5.0.8/5, Kuhn to Sandoz, 27 April 1963. The patient was later admitted again as an inpatient.
141 StATG, 9'40, 5.0.8/5, Kuhn to Sandoz, 27 April 1963.
142 StATG, 9'40, 3.0.3/5, Kuhn to Hofmann, Neurology Clinic of Vienna, 16 May 1963.

143 StATG, 9'10, 9.5/3, Sandoz to Kuhn, 11 October 1963.
144 *Ibid.*, Kuhn to Sandoz, 12 October 1963.
145 StATG, 9'40, 5.0.8/5, 'Nebenwirkungen', undated typescript (ca. April 1964), 3–4; ZA KAs 15568.
146 StATG, 9'10, 5.4/13569, 14 February 1964.
147 StATG, 9'10, 5.4/13569. The patient had previously also received Geigy White, Serpasil, Geigy Red, Yellow, Blue, Ciba 24160, Geigy Yellow II, and Metabolite III. That she did not eat enough was already occasionally mentioned earlier in the medical file.
148 *Ibid.*, 4 November 1963. Marantic endocarditis: heart failure due to undernourishment.
149 *Ibid.*, 14 February 1964.
150 StATG, 9'40, 8.1/146, preliminary files for 'Pharmakologische und klinische Eigenschaften eines neuen Butyrophenon-Derivates (FR 33)', undated typescript, published 1966.
151 StATG, 9'10, 5.4/8875, 20 August 1963, 2 October 1963, and 4 January 1964; 9'10, 5.4/9525, extra report; 9'10, 5.4/8678; 9'10, 5.4/10888 and 9'40, 5.0.8/5, extra report; ZA KAs 15844, 27 March 1964; 9'10, 5.4/8678.
152 StATG, 9'40, 8.1/146, Kuhn to Sandoz, 28 September 1964.
153 *Ibid.*, appendix to a letter by Ernst Rothlin (in his capacity as co-editor of the journal *Psychopharmacologia*) to Kuhn, 6 March 1965, written by an anonymous reviewer for the journal *Psychopharmacologia*. The inquiry about the publication by Sandoz had been made in October 1963; see StATG, 9'10, 9.5/3, Sandoz to Kuhn, 9 October 1963.
154 StATG, 9'40, 8.1/146, Kuhn to Rothlin (private), 31 July 1965; Kuhn to Rothlin (private), 15 April 1965.
155 *Ibid.*, Kuhn to Rothlin (private), 29 November 1965,
156 StATG, 9'40, 5.0.8/5, Neff to Kuhn, 16 December 1965. In addition, there were daily allowances for meetings in Basel.
157 Kuhn et al., 'Pharmakologische und klinische Eigenschaften'.
158 CA Novartis, Sandoz, H 121'000, pharmaceutical department, minutes of the management board, 30 May 1967 (resolution on 18 May 1967).
159 RA Novartis, AW 143076 & HF 1854, letters Kuhn and Wander remarks, file note Ringwald, 9 September 1968, 'Besuch bei Herrn Prof. Dr med. R. Kuhn, Psychiatrische Klinik, Münsterlingen, am 3. September 1968 (AW 151129; HF 1854; AW 14306)'.
160 RA Novartis, AW 143076, meeting with Wander Switzerland on 24 and 28 January 1969; *ibid.*, excerpt from the annual report, April 1968–April 1969, undated, 68; *ibid.*, sheet related to HUF 3076, undated.

161 CA Novartis, Wander, subsidiaries folder 1969/I, medical discussions with Wander Switzerland, Bern, 18 June 1969, on the clinical testing of new substances. Wander belonged to Sandoz as of 1967; see Chapter 6, 198.

162 CA Novartis, Sandoz, H 209.005, minutes of the meetings of the clinical research department, appendix to the minutes 42/67, 13 November 1967; ibid., minutes 13/68, 25 March 1968.

163 StATG, 9'40, 5.0.13/0, Wyeth, 'Preliminary Data on WY-3263', October 1961.

164 Pertofran: Metabolite III/G 35030. *Ibid.*, Rothweiler, Geigy, to Kuhn, 8 February 1962.

165 *Ibid.*, Rothweiler, Geigy, to Kuhn, 8 February 1962; Rothweiler to Kuhn, 21 December 1961; Kuhn to Rothweiler, 13 February 1962.

166 *Ibid.*, Rothweiler, Geigy, to Kuhn, 23 February 1962.

167 *Ibid.*, Agathe Christ, directorate secretary, to Rothweiler, Geigy, 13 February 1962 (first form); Kuhn to Geigy, 29 March 1962 (second form), as well as 9'40, 5.1.1/0.3, documentation on Tofranil, undated, two filled-out questionnaires for each of ten cases with G 35020.

168 Kuhn, 'Vorwort', vi.

169 CA Novartis, Geigy, PP 12/5, pharma production, medical department, minutes, psychopharmaceuticals subject-area conference, 6 July 1966, 3–4.

170 CA Novartis, Geigy, PP 1a, pharma production, Geigy pharmaceuticals, annual report 1964, 9.

171 CA Novartis, Geigy, PP 12/4, pharma production, research and distribution meeting, 25 May 1956. See Chapter 3, 99–100.

172 CA Novartis, Geigy, FB 4/4, correspondence, file notes regarding pharma research 1956, discussion on the status of the pharma research work areas on 28 June 1956, 12.

173 See Pignarre, *Psychotrope Kräfte*; Balz, *Zwischen Wirkung*, 334; Tornay, *Zugriffe*, 171–215; Germann, *Medikamentenprüfungen*, 24–25.

174 Quoted in Tornay, *Zugriffe*, 183.

175 AMP, later called AMDP. See Angst et al., 'Über das gemeinsame Vorgehen'; 'Das Dokumentations-System'; Germann, *Medikamentenprüfungen*, 32–36; Tornay, *Zugriffe*, chapter 5.

176 For the Psychiatric University Clinic of Basel, see Germann, *Medikamentenprüfungen*, 24, 43.

177 Germann, *Medikamentenprüfungen*, 24; Rietmann et al., '"Wenn Ihr Medikament"'. The IKS did not declare control studies to be a norm until 1977; see Chapter 6, 204.

178 See Angst, 'Leerpräparate', 9; 'Doppelblindversuch'.

179 Marks, 'What Does Evidence Do?', 89.

180 StATG, 9'40, 5.1.2/2, Benzenhöfer to Kuhn, 21 June 1989; Kuhn to Benzenhöfer, 29 June 1989; 9'10, 0.4/2, Kuhn to Page, Wyeth, 13 November 1961: 'I do not need matching placebos because I never worked with placebos and I have found the antidepressiv [sic] action of imipramine without placebo studies.'
181 StATG, 9'40, 5.0.8/6, Kuhn to Sandoz, 16 November 1965.
182 Healy, *Psychopharmacologists*, vol. 2, interview Kuhn, 99.
183 On this practice, see Chapter 3, 106.
184 StATG, 9'40, 5.0.4/23, Kuhn to Hans R. Vauthier, Astra, Sweden, 5 May 1993.
185 In his daseinsanalysis, Kuhn essentially followed Ludwig Binswanger. Daseinsanalysis distinguishes itself from psychoanalysis and psychopathology and seeks to exclude value judgements and to read and understand the expressions of ill persons as 'psychiatric texts'. Kuhn, *Psychiatrie mit Zukunft*, 21; Kuhn, 'Roland Kuhn', 240, 246.
186 In the 1960s, Kuhn published ten articles on daseinsanalysis (including obituaries for Binswanger), twelve on psychopharmaceuticals (particularly on issues related to depression), four on the Rorschach test, and eleven on psychiatry in general. In 1970, he would also write about the addiction.
187 See Chapter 8, 253.
188 It would be the Zurich psychiatrist Jules Angst, together with the Geigy pharmacologist Walter Theobald, who would publish a monograph on Tofranil, for which Kuhn would provide a preface; Angst and Theobald, *Tofranil*. In addition, the 1960s saw the publication of various psychopharmacological works by Swiss university psychiatrists, who were now researching in cooperation. Here, too, Kuhn remained an outsider.
189 StATG, 9'40, 2.3/0, correspondence and notes on a discussion with Heidegger, 1966; 9'40, 2.3/2, correspondence with Bachelard, 1947–1957; 9'40, 3.1.1951, correspondence with Maldiney, 1947–2014.
190 Kuhn, 'Roland Kuhn', 246.
191 This applied in particular to hermeneutics in the tradition of Hans-Georg Gadamer, whose texts Kuhn read in detail and used for lectures; see StATG, 9'40, 1.0.3/2; 9'40, 10.0/43–47, 50, 71.
192 See Kuhn, 'Roland Kuhn', 246.
193 StATG, 9'40, 2.3/0, transcript of a conversation with Heidegger on 11 March 1966 in Freiburg/Breisgau.
194 Dammann, 'Zur Einführung', 13.
195 On the other hand, he was interested in heritable connections and mental disorders in the family. Noteworthy here is that a

comprehensive lineage archive was set up at Münsterlingen under Zolliker's leadership.
196 StATG, 9'40, 2.3/0, transcript of a conversation with Heidegger on 11 March 1966 in Freiburg/Breisgau.
197 Healy, *Psychopharmacologists*, vol. 2, interview Kuhn, 99.
198 When looking at the medical files, we got the impression that, especially for chronic patients, hardly anything else was noted, which casts doubt on the claim of close supervision. But this does not stand out – one also finds gaps lasting years in the medical files of other clinics.
199 These special reports are sometimes included with the medical files, but they are often missing; a few are also found in the trial dossiers. Most of them probably no longer exist.
200 For outpatients, this is shown by the fact that functionality at school – for example, better grades or passed exams – or in the workplace were weighted highly.
201 CA Novartis, Geigy, PH 7.04, pharma division, copy of a letter from Kuhn to Grüter, Ciba-Geigy, 25 October 1971.
202 See also the effort to create an international psychiatric vocabulary, or the growing importance of the *Diagnostic and Statistical Manual of Mental Disorders* (DSM); Mayer-Gross, 'The Idea', 269.
203 Tornay, *Zugriffe*, 184, 190, 196.
204 See Marks, *The Progress*; Healy, *The Antidepressant Era*.
205 CA Novartis, Geigy, PP 3, pharma production, pharmaceutical department, pharma dossier, packaging file note by Weis, undated.
206 CA Novartis, Sandoz, H 209.005, minutes of the clinical research department, minutes 18, 13 June 1962.
207 StATG, 9'40, 2.3/0, Kuhn to Heidegger, 29 September 1974.

# 5

# Substance logistics, information streams, and money flows

On 17 February 1966, Sister Klara accepted two packages from Basel at the clinic pharmacy. Next, she noted their receipt on a separate sheet of A5 graph paper. She sent the typewritten note – that two lots of 50,000 25-mg ketimipramine tablets had arrived – to Kuhn.[1] Over the last ten years, the nurse had written many notes that informed Kuhn about the inventory, consumption, or delivery of test substances, initially by hand and later with the typewriter. But never before had a shipment arrived with so many units of the same preparation.[2]

As Sister Klara's note shows, produced and distributed within the framework of clinical trials were not only substances but also information. Those who tested substances, thereby creating knowledge, which they reported to the pharmaceutical companies, received free preparations and money. Since the various substances, information, and funds went very different ways, a widely ramified network of flows emerged, which continuously changed. But if we try to take stock, what balance can we strike from all of the flows of substances, information, and money?

This chapter discusses logistics, the tangible and intangible infrastructure of substance testing, which is often backgrounded and remains invisible.[3] It shows the different types of people who administered and received the drugs, analyses the complexities of income and tax accounting, and asks how widely and how well the trials at Münsterlingen were known inside and outside the clinic. Thus the chapter brings together three characteristic fields of pharmaceuticals: materiality, economics, and epistemology.[4] In the process, it clearly shows that boxes filled with test substances, remittances, and data transfers are important subjects of the history of knowledge.[5]

## Supply lines: Dragees, tablets, and ampoules

Packages from Basel were part of the clinic pharmacy's routine. Nurse Klara, who helped Kuhn with logistics, continually received deliveries. Between 1954 and 1980, hundreds of packages with test substances made their way to Münsterlingen. Some came by mail; others were brought by pharmaceutical company employees who regularly visited Kuhn. Some of these preparations were forwarded to others, but most were used in the wards or the outpatient department of the psychiatric clinic. Thus apart from registered medications, the clinic pharmacy also always stored test substances, some of which would never be used up.

By means of the countless inventory surveys, orders, inquiries, delivery slips, confirmation notices, and thank-you letters found in Kuhn's private archive, one can estimate the quantities of test substances that arrived at Münsterlingen throughout the entire period. That Kuhn retained so much logistical information is remarkable. But there are also gaps; if one assumes that each shipment was ordered, delivered, noted in the clinic pharmacy, and finally gratefully acknowledged, it becomes clear that many steps occurred orally and that Kuhn's private archive contains nowhere near all of the letters and notices that might have been able to provide information about the delivery of test substances.

For instance, with respect to the delivery noted by Sister Klara on a slip of paper in February 1966, we have neither a written order nor a thank-you letter that explicitly refers to this shipment. In October 1965, Kuhn had reported to Basel that the

> supplies of G 35259 are already running short again. ... It appears that, at the moment, we are completely using up the ten thousand tablets per month. If the resupply does not then arrive exactly on the day, we will have problems. I would therefore be happy if, as arranged, you could once send me twice as much so that we have a little more freedom of movement.

In November, he ordered another 10,000 dragees of Keto, this time with a 10-mg dosage, which he needed for treating children and for the 'adjustment of difficult-to-handle patients'.[6] As per internal clinic memos, 8,000 10-mg dragees arrived at the end of the year and the aforementioned 100,000 25-mg tablets arrived in February 1966.[7] On 10 March 1966, Kuhn placed a new order for 10-mg tablets.

At the same time, he requested ampoules for injections because for 'severe clinical cases' he 'actually liked [starting the treatment] with ampoules'. As confirmed by a note dated 21 March 1966, 10,000 10-mg tablets and 600 25-mg ampoules in fact arrived at the clinic ten days later.[8]

Thus various types of ketimipramine arrived at Münsterlingen: Keto in the form of tablets, dragees, and injections, 10-mg and 25-mg doses, packages that contained a few hundred, 1,000, and at one point 100,000 units. But how much Keto did the clinic receive in total? To avoid double-counts, one can limit the calculation to those deliveries that are mentioned either in letters from pharmaceutical companies or in thank-you letters or confirmations of receipt. Based on this conservative calculation, almost 950,000 units of ketimipramine arrived at the clinic between 1959 and 1970.[9] That it must have been far more than this is shown by details noted by Kuhn himself. In January 1968, he referred to an 'annual consumption of approximately 300,000 tablets' and added that a large number of patients were now on Keto. In April, he wrote that 'ca. 30,000 dragees' were being used each month at Münsterlingen.[10] One year later, consumption had increased again. Now Kuhn reported to Geigy that they currently had 'a turnover in the magnitude of 4–500,000 tablets per year'. He explained,

> We need plenty of ketimipramine, both clinically but also especially in the outpatient department. Lately, we have also gone over to using relatively large doses in more cases. We are having good experiences with this, disruptive side-effects are not occurring. This way the effect can actually be increased. But if a single patient needs twelve tablets or more per day, then one can easily calculate how quickly the supplies melt away then, even if they are sizeable.[11]

In the case of ketimipramine – the substance used in the clinic's largest, longest, and most comprehensive trial series – Münsterlingen's substance logistics can be very accurately reconstructed. The preparation therefore is well-suited as a central thread to lead us through the jungle of substance and information flows. Supplying the clinic with medications was a challenging undertaking. Test substances were usually manufactured in several dosages and dosage forms, and the spectrum often progressively widened. At the same time, the

## Logistics

demand could strongly change in the course of months or years. This development was not just contingent on the number of patients who received the preparation. Depending on the test phase, substances were also administered in various doses and combined. A medication could be quite varied even when patients received one and the same substance. Some patients were given injections; others swallowed tablets. Many took the preparation once per day, while others took it several times daily. But dosages and dosage forms also varied in individual cases. For 'serious cases', for example, Kuhn usually began with injections and later switched to tablets; for less severe disorders, he started with a relatively low dose, which was gradually increased if the hoped-for improvement did not materialise.

As the delivery quantities and the number of trials grew in the 1960s, Kuhn started keeping a reserve of psychotropic drugs. Sometimes he even ordered fresh supplies when a trial was over. For ongoing trials, he always tried to avoid having to switch patients to other substances. Nurse Klara's painstaking work therefore focused on maintaining an overview, regularly informing Kuhn on the inventory of test substances, and letting him know when supplies were dwindling so he could place new orders in time.

In April 1968, for instance, Kuhn received an 'alert' from the clinic pharmacy that the 25-mg Keto tablets had run out; a 'resupply' had not yet occurred. When Kuhn was unable to reach the director of Geigy's medical department by telephone (he always placed his orders with senior management personnel of the pharmaceutical companies), he expressed his irritation in writing.

> I then tried to connect with you by telephone. You were unreachable. But then your secretary very courteously informed me and arranged for me to be provided with 30,000 dragees, which then also arrived by express. May I remind you of my letter of January this year, in which I drew your attention to the situation? ... The supply I received from the last shipment is only just enough for the month of April, and I am therefore hastening to make you aware that I need resupply at the end of this month.[12]

Despite all efforts, however, bottlenecks cropped up repeatedly at Münsterlingen, whether because the pharmaceutical companies were struggling with problems in the production of a dosage form, because deliveries were delayed for other reasons, or because the demand was greater than anticipated. Since the number of probands, the duration of the trials, and the dosages were not fixed from the start at Münsterlingen, one sometimes lost track of the logistics. Thus medical files frequently note that a test substance had to be temporarily discontinued, or another substance needed to be used because the preparation was no longer in stock. In the case of one patient who received Geigy Red, for example, the latter was replaced by Geigy Green for a week because, as noted in a special report, 'G 22355 [had] run out'.[13]

Notwithstanding such complications, enormous quantities of test substances came to be used at Münsterlingen. In the period under investigation, a total of almost 3 million dragees, tablets, ampoules, and suppositories of various test substances arrived at the clinic.[14] Kuhn received a further 325,000 units of medication for free for a while after they were registered because he had tested the substances prior to their approval. These sums do not include documented deliveries that lack details on quantities[15] and commercially available medications that were tested for new indications.[16] Since the surviving sources are incomplete, the results of these calculations must be treated with caution. Even so, they offer a vivid insight into the quantitative dimensions of the trials, all the more so because they are minimum values.

If delivery quantities are organised according to time or substance, then the numbers strongly vary. The largest quantities of preparations were delivered between 1957 and 1965, back when Münsterlingen had an average of 700 inpatients and just under 1,400 outpatients per year.[17] The year with the highest number of verifiably delivered units was 1965 (just under 460,000); however, similar quantities of test substances had previously arrived in 1955 and 1958.[18] The largest documented delivery contained 300,000 25-mg dragees of Keto;[19] the smallest shipments generally included 100 units. The three surviving metal boxes with various test substances arrived at Münsterlingen at the end of the 1960s (Figure 5.1). Shipments totalling 10,000 units or fewer are documented for two-thirds of the preparations – almost all of them medications that were tested for no longer than one year. One third of all substances were only delivered once; as far as can be determined, these were exclusively substances used for rapid testing or mini-trials that involved very few patients.[20]

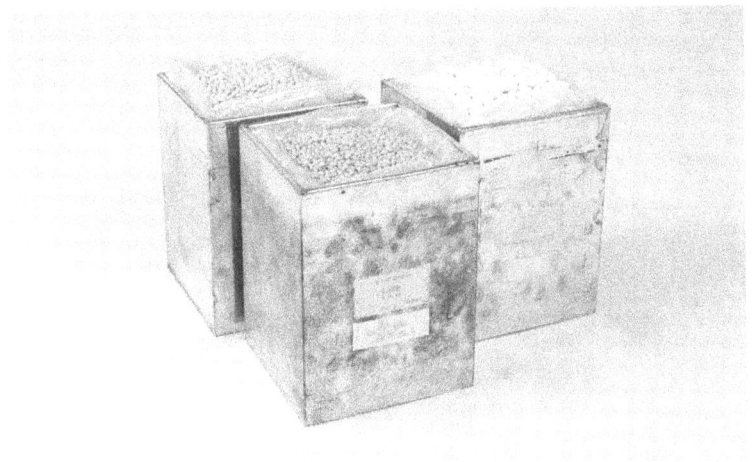

Figure 5.1 Metal boxes with three different test substances, late 1960s

The enormous deliveries of ketimipramine show that vast quantities were used not only of those substances that later came onto the market (Figure 5.2), but even of substances that were never launched. Thus even though Geigy Red (later Tofranil) and Ciba 34276 (later Ludiomil) are in second and third place in terms of quantity,[21] in first place is Keto – the clinic probably received twice as many units of Keto than Ludiomil.[22] While approximately the same number of units of Geigy Red were delivered to the clinic before and after its registration, there is no evidence of free deliveries of Ciba 34276 after its approval. With respect to Geigy Yellow (later Insidon), however, 88,000 units were delivered prior to registration, thus slightly more than two-thirds of a total just shy of 130,000 units.[23]

A quantitative analysis can therefore not only enhance and confirm the perspective on clinical trials and individual test preparations; it can also change it. Compared to other Geigy substances of the 1950s that never came to market, the 88,000 units of Geigy Yellow seem almost paltry. Thus from 1950 to 1956, at least 100,000 units of Geigy White were delivered and from 1957 to 1959, more than 140,000 units of Geigy Pink (G 31406). Almost 60,000 tablets and ampoules of Geigy Black (G 28364), which was only tested for one year, reached Münsterlingen in

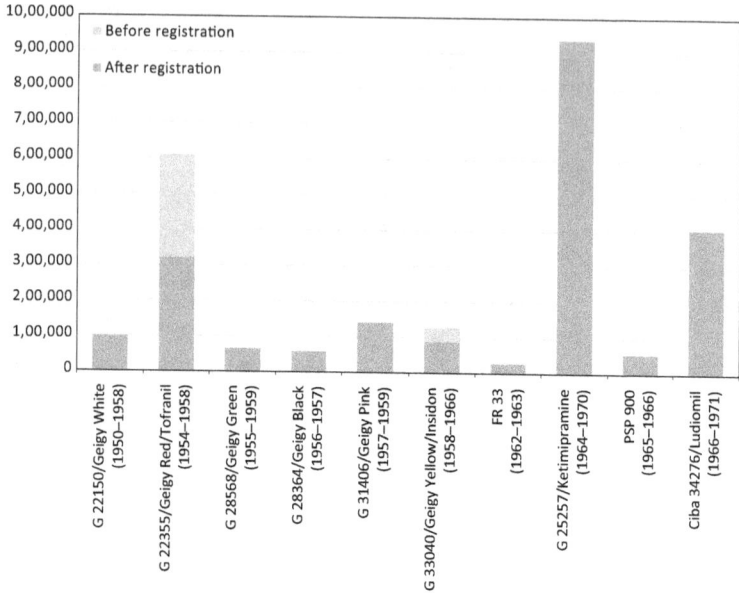

Figure 5.2 Test substances with at least 25,000 delivered units, 1946–1980

1957/1958, corresponding to an average monthly consumption of 5,000 units. Even the neuroleptic FR 33 from Sandoz, which was considered dangerous, was administered in large quantities, with a total of 27,500 units arriving at Münsterlingen between August 1962 and December 1963.[24] Two years later, the company then sent 55,000 dragees and ampoules of the neuroleptic PSP 900 to the clinic. Among the substances used for large-scale trials, however, Geigy products clearly dominated. Two – FR 33 and PSP 900 – came from the Sandoz company, while Ciba was represented by Ludiomil.

As the amounts and trials multiplied in the 1960s, Münsterlingen also became a distribution hub, dispatching test substances to doctors, former patients, even relatives of patients and employees who never had direct contact with the clinic. Anyone who ordered a preparation that was in stock probably received it. That said, however, the medications were distributed free of charge – Kuhn did not actually engage in trade in the proper sense.

Ketimipramine in particular was quite broadly dispersed. In 1965, Kuhn learned from Geigy that a doctor from St Gallen was interested in Keto 'samples'. Even though the company wanted to 'involve no more investigators in the present stage', it agreed to having Kuhn provide the doctor with the substance so that he could continue with 'cases [he had] started treating'. Kuhn then wrote to the doctor, 'If you have another particularly suitable case, then you will probably also be permitted to do another test with the tablets provided to you.'[25] Further letters show that he arranged for Keto to be supplied to various professional colleagues within and outside the Canton of Thurgau in the following years.[26] These doctors had various functions; some wanted to be actively involved in the trial, others did Kuhn a favour, and yet others were treating former clinic patients who had received Keto at Münsterlingen and evidently responded well to the substance. Together with the tablets, the doctors also received a request to tell Kuhn about their experiences with the substance. Such external treatments could last from several months to years. One psychiatrist from the Canton of Zurich, for example, asked Kuhn to send him 'ca. 300 G 35259' for a female patient who had been receiving ketimipramine for ten months. The action, according to the doctor, 'seems not to be unfavourable', but for the moment one had to wait to see whether the 'stabilising effect' persists.[27]

As with many other registered and non-registered medications, Keto was given to patients to take home or sent to them without further ado – even to those who never came to Münsterlingen for treatment.[28] In 1969, a long-term female patient was given Keto to take along while on leave, and it was noted in her medical history: 'The lodger should tend to the regular ingestion.' Since the elderly woman lived on her own without nearby relatives, her lodger took on the tasks of a nurse's aide. He administered the tablets to his landlady and obtained new supplies from the family doctor or the clinic. In summer 1970, for instance, he asked at Münsterlingen for 200 film-coated dragees Ciba 34276-Ba 25 mg V3124 37/877/3' (later Ludiomil); evidently, he had copied down all of the information that he found on the package. At the same time, he expressed thanks for 'the good treatment of his landlady' and reported that 'nothing mentally abnormal [had] become apparent' since he had been giving her the pills.[29]

Even though the man administered ketimipramine to his landlady, neither of their names appear on the clinic's internal 'Keto list' of 1969/1970. The list contains the names of a few dozen people and institutions who were also sent Keto at the time – above all patients, physicians in private practice, and clinics.[30] None of those who ultimately swallowed the dragees were monitored at Münsterlingen, nor were the dosages or the effect of the substance. Even when Geigy decided in late 1970 not to pursue the substance any further,[31] Kuhn did not stop distributing the preparation. Evidently, people elsewhere had become accustomed to the substance too. Jules Angst, who ran the research department of the Psychiatric University Clinic Zurich, asked twice – in late 1972 and early 1973 – whether Münsterlingen 'still [had] ketimipramine in stock', for he had 'a patient who urgently depends on it'. Kuhn arranged for him to receive a total of 2,000 tablets.[32] An older woman to whom Verena Kuhn regularly sent Keto in the 1970s confirmed that she received 500 30-mg tablets as late as 1979. The last reference to ketimipramine found in her file dates from June 1980; some ten years after the Keto trial officially ended, the patient wrote to the doctor, 'Here I still have 3 × 100 G 35259, which I already should have sent back to you long ago, since I have been taking Anafranil (unfortunately, this also does not work against the many feelings of guilt).'[33]

## Hardly a secret: The knowledge of trainee nurses, family physicians, and mothers

Among the Münsterlingen test substances, Keto was in various respects the biggest chunk, that is, in terms of delivered quantities, the extent to which the substance was distributed to other doctors and institutions, and the number of persons to whom it was administered. But what these few examples have illustrated here with regard to ketimipramine also holds true for other test preparations. At Münsterlingen, substances with numbers and colour designations were administered or circulated for more than three decades. As the number of test substances and delivered units burgeoned in the late 1950s and early 1960s, and as the outpatient department became more strongly involved in the trials, the group of people who knew about the non-registered substances continuously grew. Apart from clinic employees, family doctors, independently practising psychiatrists, asylums, and hospitals, the ever-expanding drug supply network now also included the relatives, neighbours, and bosses of patients. Therefore, many people must have known that test substances were being used in Münsterlingen.

In the clinic itself, test preparations were in any event part of everyday life, at least from the mid-1950s to the mid-1970s. One woman who completed her training as a psychiatric nurse at Münsterlingen in 1966/1969 said that during her time nearly all of the inpatients received 'number preparations'. She already knew, as a trainee nurse, that Kuhn was 'developing medications' with various pharmaceutical companies, and that the so-called number preparations were related to these trials.[34] Nursing and administrative staff of the 1970s and 1980s also reported that Kuhn's research activity was known.[35]

People were similarly informed in other psychiatric and somatic clinics.[36] The mother of a boy who was examined in the urology department of the neighbouring cantonal hospital in the second half of the 1970s recounted how she was told, after the examination, that physically everything was fine, and, without further information, was given a small white bag with tablets that were supposed to work against bed-wetting. Under this substance, her son became completely apathetic; he now just lounged around, and he staggered when he walked. Upon learning about the case, an acquaintance working as an oncology nurse in the cantonal hospital immediately responded and declared that the boy in the urology department had received the antidepressants 'from Prof. Kuhn' and that they were being 'tested there'.[37]

Thus many people knew that 'number preparations' were being administered at and distributed from the Münsterlingen Psychiatric Clinic. Another question is: who knew what these substances were all about and what consequences their use could entail? Many people were likely unaware of the interconnections between test preparations, research, possible risks, and financial gains because nobody informed them about such matters. The more anyone knew about medications, clinical research, and the therapeutic state of the art, the more clearly they probably understood how to judge the administration of test substances and their risks. In the sources we examined, however, there are no voices critical of the trials, not even from medical circles.

Closely tied to the question of the state of knowledge is the question of a specific person's position, duties, and rights. If physicians administered test substances to patients, they took on a very different type of responsibility than when a trainee nurse knew that test preparations were being dispensed in her ward, or when a lodger administered substances to his landlady that could only be obtained from Münsterlingen. But what about the responsibility of the cantonal authorities? What was known by those persons and bodies that presided over the Münsterlingen Psychiatric Clinic and were supposed to monitor it?

## Condoning the practices: The clinic director, supervisory authorities, and government

The fact that substances were being tested in Münsterlingen could already be gleaned from the clinic's public annual reports. They repeatedly referred to a collaboration with the pharmaceutical industry, but almost exclusively in less prominent places – for example, when mentioning expert evaluations for pharmaceutical companies or referring to publications on test preparations.[38] But there is at least one prominent passage that unambiguously indicates clinical trials. The 1972 annual report states as follows.

> A preparation that one has been able to use in the clinic for years has now been introduced to Switzerland and is proving very successful. It was a great advantage that we were long able to provide this outstanding medication to the patients of our clinic and the outpatient department.[39]

In light of these sentences, one might have asked how a substance that was only recently available in Switzerland could have been used in Münsterlingen long before.

In contrast to the public, Kuhn's superiors – the cantonal physician and the state supervisory bodies of the Münsterlingen Psychiatric Clinic – had far more opportunities to learn about the trials. Clinic Director Zolliker and Kuhn regularly referred to the collaboration with the pharmaceutical industry. The testing was discussed above all in the financial context, for the supervisory commission and government council were repeatedly being told that Kuhn's pharmacological research immensely benefited the canton. The minutes of a supervisory commission meeting in 1957, for example, state as follows.

> Dr Kuhn notes that the medications for 35,000.00 francs under 'medical needs' are being used very frugally. At the moment, the Geigy company is providing 20,000 tablets and 1,000 ampoules per month to the asylum free of charge for testing purposes. Should the trials be concluded, then the expenditures under this heading could easily increase to double the amount.[40]

With regard to the cost of medication, both Kuhn and Zolliker emphasised that the expenditures for drugs would be much higher if the clinic did not conduct any trials. This applied to ongoing and completed trials, they noted, because even after certain substances were brought to market, clinics that had helped with testing would still receive certain substances gratis for a while. In 1960, for instance, Zolliker remarked in a meeting of the supervisory commission that they were getting Tofranil 'for free at present, but the medications of the Largactil series must now be purchased'.[41]

In 1964, conflict arose between Kuhn and the canton's personnel office. The office had evidently proposed raising the rent for Kuhn's official flat, recommending an increase of 50 francs per month for each child. Kuhn was indignant. In his response, he not only described his working and living conditions but also made it clear that the canton benefited greatly from him without appropriately remunerating his commitment and services. Among other things, he wrote the following.

> Another factor is that I work intensely in science during my free time. The result is that I personally am provided with large quantities of medications for free by chemical factories. I have always provided these medications to the asylum not at some sort of reduced price but for free. In just the last ten years, the asylum has drawn from this a benefit of at least 100,000 francs in the sector of the pharmacy.[42]

Thus from Kuhn's perspective, the trials assisted the canton financially because he generously let the clinic have the test substances for free – substances that he received at no expense. Meanwhile, he never mentions the patients, staff, and clinic infrastructure that he relied on for his research.

Medication costs were never a very consequential part of the clinic's entire budget. Around 1970, the total expenditures amounted to slightly more than 6 million francs, around one quarter of which was borne by the canton.[43] Even so, Kuhn repeatedly used the drug testing as a way to apply pressure. As per his recurring argument as director, the clinic's costs were relatively low because of the trials. If he abandoned them, the budget would soar. 'As you know', Kuhn wrote to the cantonal physician in 1972, 'the clinic has been doing trials of new medications for the chemical industry for years. In exchange, it has the salary of a laboratory technician and draws gratis medications for enormous sums. The savings that can be achieved as a result of this have often amounted to an estimated 100,000 francs a year.'[44] At the same time, Kuhn also emphasised that the collaboration with the chemical industry was 'completely unpredictable'. Thus according to his subliminal warning of the early 1970s, his superiors needed to be prepared for his research activity to stop at any moment and for medication costs to drastically increase.[45] Since the canton was struggling with a growing deficit at the time,[46] this message probably fell on fertile soil in the government.

The clinic and Canton of Thurgau clearly benefited financially from the free drugs – but to what degree is difficult to assess. Kuhn's calculations fail to add up if only because the trials themselves generated costs that were covered by the clinic. Yet if one nonetheless takes him at his word, then, without the gratis preparations, the medication costs for 1954–1963 would have increased by slightly less than 20 per cent, and by slightly more than 80 per cent in the late 1960s.[47] These estimates are so high that, from today's perspective, it would have been advisable to look at the scope of the trials and to ask whether the clinic would have needed that many psychotropic drugs if free substances had been unavailable. The sources, however, contain no indications that Zolliker, the supervisory commission, the cantonal physician,[48] or the government ever scrutinised Kuhn's information or took it as a reason to examine the trials more closely. The supervisory authorities and Kuhn's immediate superior thus knew about the trials throughout the entire investigation period, but they had no further interest in them. The only subject ever discussed was the economic benefits to the canton.

### Remunerations: From rivulet to river

In spring 1951, prior to the intensive collaboration with Geigy, Kuhn received mail from the tax authorities. The Office of the Scherzingen Municipal Council informed him that the tax commissariat was asking him whether it 'would not be possible to obtain a verification document for the 3,000 francs listed as supplemental income for the tax declaration'. Kuhn answered the query just two days later. He explained that 'this declared secondary income is proceeds from various scientific activities and expert evaluations'; however, they could 'not all be calculated as earnings' but were to be understood 'more as sales than as income'. His scientific activities were namely associated with high expenditures. Were he to take these into account, 'nothing at all would remain of the 3,000 francs in question'. Kuhn thus claimed that he was declaring more than necessary; he did not submit any documentation for his secondary income and the associated expenses.[49]

Kuhn's statement, that he had not actually achieved the declared secondary income, had an offended undertone that heightened as the letter went on. 'In the event that there are any doubts at the canton's tax commissariat, whether I have honestly stated my secondary income', Kuhn continued, then it might 'also serve this authority ... as orientation' to learn that, 'for the benefit of the asylum', he had turned down a research contract in the amount of 2,000 francs. Instead, at his request, the sponsor had transferred 3,000 francs to the clinic for the acquisition of an electroencephalography (EEG) device. He had personally paid for all of the costs incurred during the selection of the device and for his training in clinical electroencephalography. Kuhn's conclusion: 'If I wanted to defraud the state of its entitled tax revenue, I would certainly not gift it 2,000 francs that would be owed to me.' To buttress his honesty once more, he finally referred to further merits, but at the same time insisted that he was a modest person: 'I do not like to put on airs with such things. But I hope that the tax commissariat can see from this that it does not need to meet my tax declaration with mistrust.'[50] The tax authority was evidently satisfied with his response – at least, Kuhn's private archive holds no further documents on this matter.

The letter to the Office of the Scherzingen Municipal Council exhibits traits that generally inform Kuhn's correspondence. Even as a senior physician, Kuhn tended to understand questions or statements as criticism, to respond with resentment or concealed aggression, and to turn the tables. On such occasions, adopting a tone that combined arrogance with an ostensible modesty, he also accused authorities of not appreciating his accomplishments, failing to trust him, or basically treating him unjustly. However, the logic of his arguments was astonishingly simple; it was impossible that someone who accomplished so much – for the clinic, the patients, the canton, and science – could make mistakes, be self-serving, or engage in fraud. From this Kuhn concluded that one was not allowed to call him into question, monitor, or even just criticize him – and this also applied to his tax declaration.

The correspondence related to Kuhn's tax declaration is also a key document in another respect. It shows, namely, that the clinical trials in Münsterlingen paid off not only for the clinic and the canton but also for Kuhn personally. The said research contract marked the start. In 1950, Geigy admittedly provided a contribution for the clinic to acquire its own EEG device, but the company also paid Kuhn a fee of 400 francs for the expert evaluation on Parpanit.[51]

The information we have on the secondary income that Kuhn obtained from the clinical trials comes almost exclusively from his private archive and the holdings at Novartis. Thus far, very few files that provide insights into such remunerations have been found in other holdings of the Thurgau State Archives. The tax documents Kuhn submitted were destroyed in due time. Other files – namely, Kuhn's social insurance data and his private accounting records – were inaccessible to us. The totals that actually amounted from Kuhn's income from the trials must remain unresolved, as does the question of whether the pharmaceutical companies arranged for the payment of similar amounts to other investigators who likewise emerged as 'one-man operations'.

If one adds up all of the known remunerations, the result is slightly more than 3.5 million Swiss francs. However, this sum must be noted with caution, just like our calculations for the quantities of substances. For one, the sources have gaps; thus this too is a minimum value. For another, the value of money changes over time. If one uses the consumer price index to adjust Kuhn's annual income to the price level for 2015, then his clinical trials earned him the equivalent of around 8 million Swiss francs.[52] If one measures these remunerations against income from the highest wage level of federal government personnel, then Kuhn's secondary earnings for 1970 matched the annual wages of one high-level federal employee, and for 1975 and 1989 those of two high-level federal employees. A comparison of his income from 1975 and 1980 with the annual wages of a pharmacist shows that the trials brought him around three and half times as much as a pharmacist earned per year.[53]

The pharmaceutical industry arranged for Kuhn to receive various types of remuneration: one-time and recurring, rather low and extremely high, checks and money transfers, amounts that honoured Kuhn's testing in general, and those that were linked to specific trials. The large majority of the remunerations, however, can be assigned to two groups. One included all forms of profit-sharing; the other included fees that accrued during the trials. If one assumes a monetary sum of 3.5 million and adds up the amounts under each heading, then Kuhn received more than 200,000 francs in fees for his 'scientific collaboration'; profit-sharing consisted of slightly more than 3 million.[54]

The largest part of the income that Kuhn obtained from the trials was thus from profit-sharing. Among the numerous medications tested at Münsterlingen were two antidepressants that reached market readiness and were developed with substantial support from Kuhn: Tofranil (G 22355) and Ludiomil (Ciba 34276), which respectively came on the market in 1958 and 1972. Since both products sold like hot cakes, Kuhn profited as well. Starting in 1959, Geigy paid him an annual 'Tofranil bonus' of 30,000 francs. Five years later, the amount was increased to 50,000 francs, with the last money transfer documented in 1976. Income for Ludiomil was added for the first time in 1972. In this case, Kuhn had agreed to a twelve-year profit-sharing arrangement at 0.5 per cent, which would fetch him substantially more than the 'Tofranil bonus'. Whereas the first payment for Ludiomil was slightly less than 500 francs, by as early as 1973 it reached 8,000 francs, and one year later over 30,000 francs. When Ludiomil achieved sales of 25 million francs in 1975, Kuhn received his first six-figure profit-sharing payout. Then in 1980, Ludiomil yielded 200,000 francs for Kuhn; by the next year it was 300,000; and just under 500,000 francs in 1984.

Profit-sharing could admittedly bring in large amounts, but only in the case of successful products. Fees for 'scientific collaboration', on the other hand, did not depend on whether a test preparation was further pursued or ever made it to market. The spectrum of paid-for research endeavours was therefore broad. Alongside fees for reports and expert evaluations, activities such as lectures, participation in conferences, or assistance in the editing of newspaper reports were also compensated. The pharmaceutical industry paid Kuhn sizeable fees, even for short-term, tightly limited services. In 1963, Sandoz paid out a 'daily allowance' of 500 francs; Kuhn received the same amount three years later when he paid the company a one-day visit.[55] In addition, payments were made for otherwise undefined scientific endeavours, in part by money transfers and in part through regular, contractually agreed contributions.

The first such agreement was made in summer 1954. It initially pertained to the testing of Geigy White – it provided for a monthly compensation of 300 francs and was temporally limited, although it was extended twice. In 1956, the company then proposed expanding the contract: 'In light of the notable work that you carry out for us with the testing of our mental drugs, we would like to increase the monthly fee given to you for your personal use ... to 600 francs.'[56] With the continuously extended agreement of 1954, Kuhn began receiving ongoing compensation for his testing work, a type of basic salary that initially amounted to 3,600 francs and then doubled to 7,200 francs in 1956. With the addition of an annual 'research amount' from Ciba as of 1966, it finally reached more than 22,000 Swiss francs per year.[57]

In contrast to clinical trials in the German Democratic Republic (GDR) and at the Burghölzli in Zurich,[58] the money transfers mostly went to Kuhn personally. To be sure, the clinic itself also received funds from the pharmaceutical industry, totalling around 200,000 francs. But this amount consisted almost exclusively of payments for laboratory services accrued as part of testing. Moreover, the sum was based on the assumption that ultimately all compensation for laboratory expenses – salaries and materials – went to the psychiatric clinic.[59] However, at least two 'laboratory payments' (jointly more than 20,000 francs) were transferred to Kuhn personally – whether he forwarded the money is unclear.[60] If one ignores compensations for laboratory costs, the pharmaceutical companies only made three payments to the clinic between 1954 and 1980. Along with the aforementioned payment for the acquisition of the clinic's own EEG device, Zolliker received a sum of 12,000 francs in 1967 for 'the clinical investigations by Dr Kuhn'. The money flowed into a 'scientific fund of the clinic', for which no further information is available.[61] The third payment came from Ciba-Geigy. In 1973, the clinic had sent the company an invoice for 451 francs for three patients who were given a test preparation – who ultimately received this money must also remain unresolved, as does the question of why the clinic suddenly issued such invoices.[62]

The possibility of directing at least some of the revenue from Kuhn's testing into a clinic fund was evidently never up for debate. Such considerations were probably foreign to Kuhn. As early as 1959, he asked Geigy in a privately written note to rewrite a letter about a payment for 30,000 francs and 'in doing so, above all in the address only write: "Senior Physician of the Münsterlingen Sanatorium and Nursing Facility", since mixing up the directorate of the institution with this private matter should absolutely be avoided'.[63] The sources do not in fact clearly show what Zolliker knew about Kuhn's income from the trials and what he thought about it – presumably he did nothing to impede him in this respect either. In any case, Kuhn himself obviously felt that the trials were his personal work and that he was solely entitled to any earnings. For one, he insisted that he performed his research activity exclusively in his free time – an oft-repeated phrase.[64] But this claim seems completely implausible, given that the entire clinic operation was involved in the trials and the amount of work was huge. In addition, the questions arise as to whether Kuhn even separated his work and private life, and what free time actually meant in his situation. Even so, there are no indications that Kuhn's superiors and the competent authorities had any doubts about his assertion.

Second, Kuhn found that his work was not sufficiently rewarded – not only, but especially in Thurgau. 'The prophet counts for nothing in his own country' was the position he more or less explicitly maintained.⁶⁵ In his opinion, however, not only did the canton underappreciate him; it paid him poorly to boot. Hence, he evidently felt he had the right to improve his income; according to Kuhn, even the cantonal physician, who also worked for the government after all, had repeatedly asked for Kuhn's salary to be increased.⁶⁶

What was Kuhn earning as a clinic doctor? His income situation at the clinic, its legal basis, and the cantonal practices cannot be addressed in detail here; they are complex, in part, and also confused.⁶⁷ In addition, most of the files on financial matters found in Kuhn's private archive and in the clinic archives date from the 1970s. Nonetheless, it seems important to compare the amounts Kuhn received from the pharmaceutical industry with his other income sources. In doing so, one should at least also clarify whether Kuhn's income differed from that of other clinic doctors.

In Thurgau, the salary of senior and head physicians consisted of a basic salary and secondary income. Whether a head doctor worked at the psychiatric clinic or at the cantonal hospitals in Frauenfeld or Münsterlingen did not factor into determining the basic salary; individual variations occurred for other reasons.⁶⁸ For supplemental income, however, there were differences. In the somatic hospitals, such income was primarily achieved through the treatment of patients under private insurance schemes. But since no such options existed at the Münsterlingen Psychiatric Clinic,⁶⁹ here physicians improved their income differently. Treating outpatients no doubt brought in the most money; also important were reports, expert evaluations, and Rorschach tests. Until the early 1970s, the revenue from such services probably went directly to the relevant doctor; a pool was then set up in late 1971. Henceforth, all secondary proceeds were supposed to be handed over to the administration. The latter always put half of the proceeds into the pool and distributed the rest to the participating doctors, using a specific distribution key stipulated by the clinic director.⁷⁰ However, compensation for additional services, for example, teaching at the school for psychiatric care, were paid separately even after the pool was established.⁷¹

More extensive legal regulations for secondary income at the psychiatric clinic were not created until 1973. Now the director and the leading physicians were formally issued permission 'to hold consulting hours on their own account, issue expert evaluations, and treat private patients in hospital'. But the 'scope of this secondary activity' had to be approved by the government council, as did other types of secondary activity. Where possible, however, the government avoided discussing the previous practise – such is the impression conveyed by the files we inspected.[72] Thus all in all, the new regulations worked out very well for the doctors. In addition, the government evidently also abstained from closely monitoring the secondary activities at the psychiatric clinic. Neither the pool nor the subsequent legislation could prevent certain doctors from profiting immensely while others had to be content with their basic salary.[73]

The levels of the basic salary and secondary income that Kuhn obtained as part of his clinic activity cannot be completely ascertained from the inspected sources. Basic salaries in Thurgau were relatively low, but no lower than in other cantons.[74] In the mid-1950s, Kuhn's gross annual wages totalled around 17,000 francs, and then 73,000 francs in the late 1970s. Verena Kuhn's gross annual wages in the early 1960s amounted to 26,000 francs, and then almost 65,000 francs twenty years later.[75] The secondary income that the two of them earned in the context of their positions at the clinic had grown prior to 1970, but when Kuhn became director it grew substantially more in just a few years. In 1971, he was paid 16,000 francs from the pool; his wife, who worked chiefly in the outpatient department, received 27,000 francs. Between 1976 and 1979, Kuhn then obtained 100,000 francs each year from the pool, and his wife almost 60,000.[76] The couple's secondary earnings at the clinic therefore increased over time much more strongly than their basic salary; in the mid-1970s, they were ultimately just as high or – in Roland Kuhn's case – higher than the basic salary. If one now adds to this the compensation from the pharmaceutical companies, it becomes clear that, as of the mid-1950s, Kuhn achieved a sizeable income. When the trials in Münsterlingen were expanded and the first 'Tofranil bonus' accrued, the earnings increased more and more. Kuhn's salary peaked in the 1970s during his tenure as clinical director. In this decade, he probably achieved an average gross annual income of over 230,000 francs (around 130,000 from the canton, and approximately 102,000 francs from the pharmaceutical industry).

In 1977, the administrative director of the clinic confirmed to the Thurgau audit office that 'all monies obtained from the pool [were] ... declared on the personal salary statements'.[77] But what about secondary income earned within the framework of the clinic before the pool was set up? And what about the compensation from the pharmaceutical industry? That the government knew about Kuhn's income from his research activities is beyond question.[78] But apart from the letter from the Office of the Scherzingen Municipal Council in 1954, there are no indications that the canton worried any further about Kuhn's income from the trials.

In 1957, Geigy asked Kuhn for 'a brief report ... [as to] who declared our monthly contributions to you to the Federal AHV [Old-Age and Survivors' Insurance], respectively, to which compensation office are the AHV amounts on these allocations being paid'. Kuhn responded that he had paid taxes on the fees from the company as secondary income, but he had not yet paid the AHV contribution, for he assumed this was the company's responsibility as the client. In the event that Geigy had not yet paid the social insurance contributions, he offered to look after the matter himself. The response from the company was brief: 'We have not declared our remunerations to you to our compensation office and therefore also have not paid the amount. We would be very grateful to you if, as mentioned in your letter, you were to handle this from your side.'[79] Kuhn always claimed to have paid the social contributions for the income from his research activities and paid taxes on all income.[80] Whether this statement was reviewed and whether it is actually true must remain unresolved for now.

## Notes

1 StATG, 9'40, 5.0.3/32, note of a nurse for the attention of Kuhn, 17 February 1966.
2 *Ibid.*, Geigy to Kuhn, 20 March 1967.
3 On the subject of infrastructure, see Landecker, *Culturing Life*; Radin, *Life on Ice*; on logistics, Dommann, 'Handling, Flowcharts, Logistik'; Scheidegger, 'Der Lauf der Dinge'.
4 See Appadurai, 'Introduction'; Jasanoff, 'The Idiom'.
5 For the material cultural of psychiatry, see Ankele and Majerus, *Material Cultures*.

6 StATG, 9'40, 5.0.3/32, Kuhn to Kunz, Geigy, 8 October 1965; 10 November 1965.
7 StATG, 9'40, 5.0.3/31, notes by an employee for the attention of Kuhn, 27 December 1965; 17 February 1966.
8 *Ibid.*, 31 March 1966; StATG, 9'40, 5.0.3/32, Kuhn to Kunz, Geigy, 10 March 1966.
9 This sum (938,100) includes all dosage forms and dosages. If it was unclear whether we were dealing with the same delivery (large time interval between the pharmaceutical company's letter and the thank-you letter or the clinic's internal confirmation of receipt), then we only used the number of delivered units specified in the pharmaceutical company's letter.
10 StATG, 9'40, 5.0.3/32, Kuhn to Harwerth, medical director, Geigy, 29 January and 3 April 1968.
11 *Ibid.*, Kuhn to Meissner, Geigy, 29 April 1969. The enormous quantities once more make it clear that ketimipramine was given to far more people than would be suggested by the number of 346 Keto patients who are referred to by name in the psychopharmacological holdings of Kuhn's private archive (StATG, 9'40,5).
12 StATG, 9'40, 5.0.3/32, Kuhn to Harwerth, Geigy, 3 April 1968.
13 StATG, ZA KAs 12360, special report Geigy 22355, 10 April 1956.
14 At least sixty-seven substances were tested at Münsterlingen; there are documented deliveries for sixty-two substances. The sum of almost 3 million (2,994,287) was calculated in the same way as the sum for ketimipramine and is therefore a minimum value.
15 For eight substances, a delivery is documented but without any reference to the number of units delivered.
16 On trials with registered medications, see Chapter 6, 216–220.
17 StATG, 9'10, 1.1.0/60, ARM 1957–1965. Since the annual reports do not list the number of inpatient treatments, the calculation is based on the figures regarding the patient population, which were always determined at the end of the year.
18 458,000 units are documented for 1965, around 451,000 for 1958, and 422,500 for 1955. These peaks are no doubt the result of the testing of Keto, Tofranil, and Geigy White.
19 StATG, 9'40, 5.0.3/32, Geigy to Kuhn, 20 March 1967.
20 In May 1966, Roche, for example, sent a small package with 1,000 tablets of the antidepressant Ro 4–9661 to Münsterlingen. The trial was quickly aborted due to lack of success.
21 The ranking does not change even if those units delivered after the approval are ignored.

22 The surviving documentation for the deliveries of both substances has major gaps.
23 Prior to the drug's registration, 88,350 of a total of 127,350 units were delivered; 39,000 units were delivered after registration.
24 These calculations of the consumption of Geigy Black and FR 33 are based on the assumption that all deliveries of the two substances during this period are documented and that all delivered doses were administered.
25 StATG, 9'40, 3.0.2/7, Kuhn to a doctor in St Gallen, 27 August 1965.
26 Thus for example, Kuhn sent a doctor in Thurgau, 'as requested', 500 10-mg and 500 25-mg tablets of ketimipramine, StATG, 9'10, 1.2.1/3, 9 September 1969.
27 StATG, 9'40, 3.0.2/7, doctor from the Canton of Zurich to Kuhn, 16 May 1966.
28 For a case of 'remote treatment' with Keto, see StATG, 9'40, 3.1.70/0.1, Kuhn to a woman who suffered from depression, 4 December 1968. The woman received 400 25-mg tablets of G 35259.
29 StATG, 9'10 ZA KAs 21827, 6 September 1969; letter of the lodger to the Münsterlingen Psychiatric Clinic, 28 July 1970.
30 StATG, 9'10, 1.2.11/6.3, list 'Notierte Bezüge von G 35259, 1969–70', undated. Most of the patients identified by name had earlier been treated in Münsterlingen.
31 On the discontinuation of the trial with G 35259, see Chapter 4, 138–139.
32 StATG, 9'40, 5.0.3/32, Angst to Kuhn, 23 October 1972 (quote); 9'40, 3.0.2/8, Angst to Kuhn, 15 February 1973. On 26 October 1972, Kuhn sent Angst 1,200 tablets and, on 21 February 1973, 800 tablets. StATG, 9'40, 5.0.3/32, Kuhn to Angst, 26 October 1972; Angst to Kuhn, 15 February 1973.
33 StATG, ZA KAa 32419 I, letters of the patient to Verena Kuhn, 27 June 1979, 1 June 1980.
34 Interview with a former trainee nurse, 13 February 2017.
35 Interview with Jürg Grundlehner, who in 1971–1974 completed his apprenticeship as a psychiatric nurse in the Münsterlingen Psychiatric Clinic, 23 August 2017. Conversation with a former administrative employee of the clinic, 28 November 2016. These accounts contradict many publicly expressed claims of ignorance of the research.
36 See, for example, StATG, 9'10, 1.2.9/3, Kuhn to Hans Binder, director of the Rheinau Clinic in the Canton of Zurich, 16 June 1961.
37 Interview with a mother, 28 November 2016.
38 See, for example, StATG, 9'10, 1.1.0/60, ARM 1949, 9; 1955, 11; 1956, 11; 1957, 12; 1958, 12; 1959, 12; 1973, 20; 1979, 38.

39 *Ibid.*, ARM 1972, 6–7. The corresponding section of the annual report came from Kuhn's pen. The passage referred to Ciba 34276, which came onto the market in 1972 as Ludiomil.
40 StATG, 9'40, 3.0.0/4, minutes of the meeting of the supervisory commission of the Münsterlingen Psychiatric Clinic, 19 July 1957.
41 StATG, 9'40, 1.3/1, minutes of the meeting of the supervisory commission of the Münsterlingen Psychiatric Clinic, 29 June 1960.
42 StATG, 9'40, 3.0.0/6, Kuhn to the cantonal personnel office, undated.
43 StATG, 9'10, 1.1.0/60, ARM 1970. The clinic itself covered the other 75 per cent of the expenditures. The study on the Psychiatric University Hospital Zurich likewise concludes that the institutional incentives for conducting clinical trials should not be overestimated; see Rietmann et al., 'Medikamentenversuche', 241–242.
44 StATG, 9'10. 1.2.8/6, Kuhn to the cantonal physician, Julius Bütler, 18 December 1972. Further evidence is found, for example, in StATG, 9'10, 1.2.8/6, Kuhn to Government Councillor Rudolf Schümperli, 19 May 1972, as well as in connection with Kuhn's basic salary as clinical physician, which is discussed in the next section.
45 StATG, 9'10, 1.2.8/6, Kuhn to Government Councillor Rudolf Schümperli, 19 May 1972.
46 See Chapter 6, 208.
47 StATG, 9'10, 1.1.0/60, ARM 1945–1980. There is no information on the costs of medication in the annual reports of 1969–1971. Between 1954 and 1963, an average of approximately 53,900 francs was spent on medications. If the clinic had actually saved at least 100,000 francs during these ten years, then the cost without the test preparations would have risen an average of 62,900 francs per year, which is equivalent to a budget increase of around 19 per cent. Medications administered in the outpatient department are not included in the budget because they were charged to the patient. Thus Kuhn's estimates pertain only to the savings that could be achieved in the inpatient clinic.
48 The cantonal physician was responsible for the health-regulatory supervision of all medical personnel in the outpatient and inpatient areas. He advised the government council in matters of the healthcare system, prepared the related affairs of the department, and had a very powerful position.
49 StATG, 9'40, 3.0.0/3, Office of the Scherzingen Municipal Council to Kuhn, 31 March 1951; Kuhn to the Office of the Scherzingen Municipal Council, 2 April 1951.
50 *Ibid.*, Kuhn to the Office of the Scherzingen Municipal Council, 2 April 1951.

51 StATG, 9'40, 5.1.0/0.1, Geigy to Kuhn, 26 October 1950. On the testing of Parpanit, see Chapter 1, 37–42.
52 Between 1950 and 1990, prices increased by a factor of 3.63; thus they increased more than threefold during this period. Historical statistics of Switzerland, national index of monthly consumer prices 1921–1995, https://hsso.ch/2012/h/23. The consumer price index gives an approximation of how high to assess Kuhn's income from clinical trials.
53 The figures cannot be compared one-to-one because they are differently defined, but they can serve as approximate values. 'Gesetzliche Besoldungsansätze des Bundespersonals', in *Statistisches Jahrbuch der Schweiz* 89, 1981, p. 379; *Die Volkswirtschaft* (special edition) 86, 1976, pp. 321, 334, and 91; 1981, pp. 380, 396. The calculations were done by the economic historians Joanna Haupt and Florian Müller.
54 Because the pharmaceutical company almost always included expense allowances with fees for meetings or lectures and did not separately list individual items, numerically quantifiable expense payments proved to be negligible (1,200 francs).
55 StATG, 9'40, 5.0.8/5, Sandoz to Kuhn, 9 August 1963; 9'40, 5.0.8/6, Sandoz to Kuhn, 31 January 1966.
56 StATG, 9'40, 5.1.0/0.1, Geigy to Kuhn, 12 August 1954. CA Novartis, Geigy, G_JU/V, ZF Recht, Geigy contracts, Agreement No. 2214, Dr Kuhn, 2 March 1956.
57 For the ongoing compensations from the Geigy company, see StATG, 9'40, 5.0.3/2; for Ciba's 'research contributions', see 9'40, 5.0.2/1. The first fee from Ciba was for 1965 and amounted to 10,000 francs, but it was probably not envisaged as continuous compensation; see *ibid.*, Ciba to Kuhn, 29 September 1965.
58 In the GDR, as of 1964 there was an office responsible for the coordination and financial oversight of clinical studies. Half of the foreign-currency revenue obtained from clinical trials for Western companies went to the Berliner-Import-Export-GmbH, a foreign-trade establishment of the GDR; the other half went to the healthcare system; see Hess et al., *Testen*, 48–49, 91–92. Nor is there any indication that monies flowed directly to individual employees with regard to clinical trials at the Psychiatric University Hospital Zurich; see Rietmann et al., 'Medikamentenversuche', 240–242.
59 As of the 1970s, a portion of the 'laboratory payments' went to the cantonal hospital because it took over certain laboratory tests.
60 In 1977, Ciba-Geigy wanted to transfer 13,200 francs to the clinic for a laboratory technician and 7,200 francs for laboratory costs. Kuhn then asked that the laboratory costs be transferred to his personal

*Logistics* 193

account; StATG, 9'10, 1.2.11/6.5, Ciba-Geigy to Kuhn, 21 April 1977; Kuhn to Ciba-Geigy, 20 June 1977. CA Novartis, Geigy, G_JU/V, ZF Recht, Geigy contracts, no. 2214, 10 March 1980.
61 StATG, 9'10, 9.5/2, Ciba to Zolliker, 19 December 1967.
62 The substance is the antidepressant Ciba 21024. CA Novartis, Geigy, G_JU/V, ZF Recht, Geigy contracts, no. 2214, 18 April 1973.
63 StATG, 9'40, 5.0.3/2, Kuhn to Director Krebser, Geigy, 16 February 1959, 3.
64 See, for example, StATG, 9'40, 1.0.1/0, Kuhn to Government Councillor Rudolf Schümperli, 10 February 1971; 4'802'139, Sanitätsdepartement, Allgemeine Akten, § 251, correspondence with Bruno Stadelmann, Stadelmann to Government Councillor Alfred Abegg, 28 October 1972, quote from a letter from Kuhn dated 17 June 1972.
65 StATG, 6'11'** 1989, S 48, files on the Schenker case, pleading of Hans Schenker's defence attorney before the court of appeal, 1 September 1989.
66 See, for example, StATG, 9'10, 1.2.8/6, file note on a discussion between Kuhn and the cantonal physician Julius Bütler, 26 June 1971; 9'40, 1.0.5/5, Kuhn's statement for the attention of the court of appeals, 17 July 1989, 4. See also Chapter 8, 266–267.
67 Kuhn's salary as a clinic doctor consisted of a basic salary, various supplements, and secondary income. Using the files we inspected, it is not possible to precisely reconstruct the individual salary components.
68 This information must be clarified for clinical directors. The directors of the cantonal hospitals and the Münsterlingen Psychiatric Clinic had the same basic salary, but the basic salary of the director of the Cantonal Hospital Frauenfeld had been lower until 1980.
69 Although officially two insurance benefit classes were recognised at the Münsterlingen Psychiatric Clinic, a corresponding differentiation of services was not on offer. The clinic therefore had only one or two private patients per year; StATG, 9'40, 3.0.1/3, Kuhn's interview in the *Thurgauer Volksfreund*, 2 June 1973.
70 StATG, 9'10, 1.2.11/6.5, Regulations for the organisation of a pool for the secondary income, undated (early 1972); 9'40, 1.0.5/2, establishment of a fee pool for doctors, ca. 1971–1974.
71 StATG, 9'40, 1.0.5/3, accounting statements from the fee pool for doctors, 1972–1979.
72 StATG, 4'802'147/201, RRB No. 73/1080, 21 May 1973; 3'00'564, RRB No. 73/1083, 21 May 1973. Unambiguously illegal prior to 21 May 1973 were secondary activities by the director. Verordnung des Grossen Rates über die Besoldungen der kantonalen Beamten und

Angestellten (11 May 1959), in *Neue Gesetzessammlung für den Kanton Thurgau*, vol. 23 (Frauenfeld: 1963), 3; StATG, 9'40,1.00/0, Reglement für die Kantonale Heil- und Pflegeanstalt Münsterlingen von 1951, § 39.2.

73 The decision on which doctor could pursue what and how many secondary activities was made by the director. The question of which doctors could participate in the pool led to conflicts, as did the distribution key. Kuhn only allowed 'experienced' physicians to work in the outpatient department. See, for example, interview with René Bloch, 14 March 2018; StATG, 9'10, 1.4/6.1, Kuhn to Dr Wyss, director of the Münsingen Psychiatric Clinic, 9 August 1968; 9'40, 1.0.3/0, 97, 14 July 1972.

74 StATG, 9'10, 2.1/3, comparison of the salaries in the psychiatric clinics of Münsterlingen, Breitenau (Canton of Schaffhausen), Wil (Canton of St Gallen), Waldhaus (Canton of Graubünden), Königsfelden (Canton of Aargau), Hasenbühl (Canton of Basel-Landschaft), and Herisau (Canton of Appenzell Ausserrhoden), 1957.

75 StATG, 9'40, 3.0.0/3, pay computation for Roland Kuhn, 25 January 1956; 9'40, 3.0.0/5, pay computation for Roland and Verena Kuhn, 1962 (autumn); 9'10, 2.1/5, pay receipts of Münsterlingen Psychiatric Clinic 1971, pay receipts for Roland and Verena Kuhn; 9'10, 4.4.0/213, Roland Kuhn personal dossier.

76 StATG, 9'40, 1.0.5/3, accounting statements from the fee pool for doctors, 1972–1979.

77 StATG, 9'40, 1.0.5/4, Administrative Director Rohner to Financial Audit Department of the Canton of Thurgau, 18 March 1977; original emphasis.

78 In a clinic invoice from 1976 that went to the tax authorities, Kuhn's total earnings were footnoted with the comment, 'Without direct payments from the chemical industry'; see StATG, 4'802'207, § M46/528, audit report Münsterlingen Psychiatric Clinic, shares of doctors' fees for 1975 and 1976, appendix 1, earnings of clinical physicians for 1976, 19 January 1977.

79 StATG, 9'40, 3.0.0/4, correspondence between the staff pension fund of the Geigy company and Kuhn, 29 January–9 February 1957. See also StATG, 9'40, 5.0.7/6, Roche to Kuhn, 29 October 1969.

80 For further agreements in this regard between Kuhn and the Ciba and Geigy companies, see StATG, 9'40, 5.0.2/1, Ciba to Kuhn, 30 January und 20 February 1968; 9'40, 5.0.3/2, Geigy to Kuhn, 18 September 1968; Kuhn to Geigy, 8 October 1968.

# 6

# The 1970s: Between doldrums and success

Like it did every year, in February 1979, the Münsterlingen Psychiatric Clinic celebrated Carnival, a festival where roles are exchanged and boundaries transgressed. Along with more or less elaborately costumed patients and clinical employees, attending the Carnival ball that year were two clowns, a man and a woman, who as per the writing on the backs of their costumes were named Ludio and Mili (Figure 6.1). Together they represented a medication: Ludiomil. The round laughing faces on their costumes point to the fact that Ludiomil tablets are supposed to create a good mood – after all, the medication was an antidepressant.

On a different photo, Ludio and Mili each hold a marmalade jar in their hands, filled with colourful sweets, which they are evidently distributing to the crowd. Ludiomil had in fact been dispensed in Münsterlingen for years – as generously as candies, the clowns seem to suggest. Known by the company's abbreviation Ciba 34276, the substance began being tested in Münsterlingen in 1966. In the late 1960s, Ciba delivered thousands of tablets to Thurgau, at least 150,000 tablets in 1970, according to records of the orders and deliveries, and then almost 400,000 in 1971.[1] Initially just one test substance among many, Ciba 34276 quickly showed a lot of promise and was pursued for years until finally being approved in 1972. In this case, too, there was a seamless transition from testing to therapeutic application.

The Carnival photos of 1979 were made after the long period of economic growth that had paralleled the boom in psychotropic drugs.[2] In the 1950s and 1960s, Western countries had achieved substantial affluence. The clowns are wallowing in excess, which they are simultaneously parodying with their handouts. An

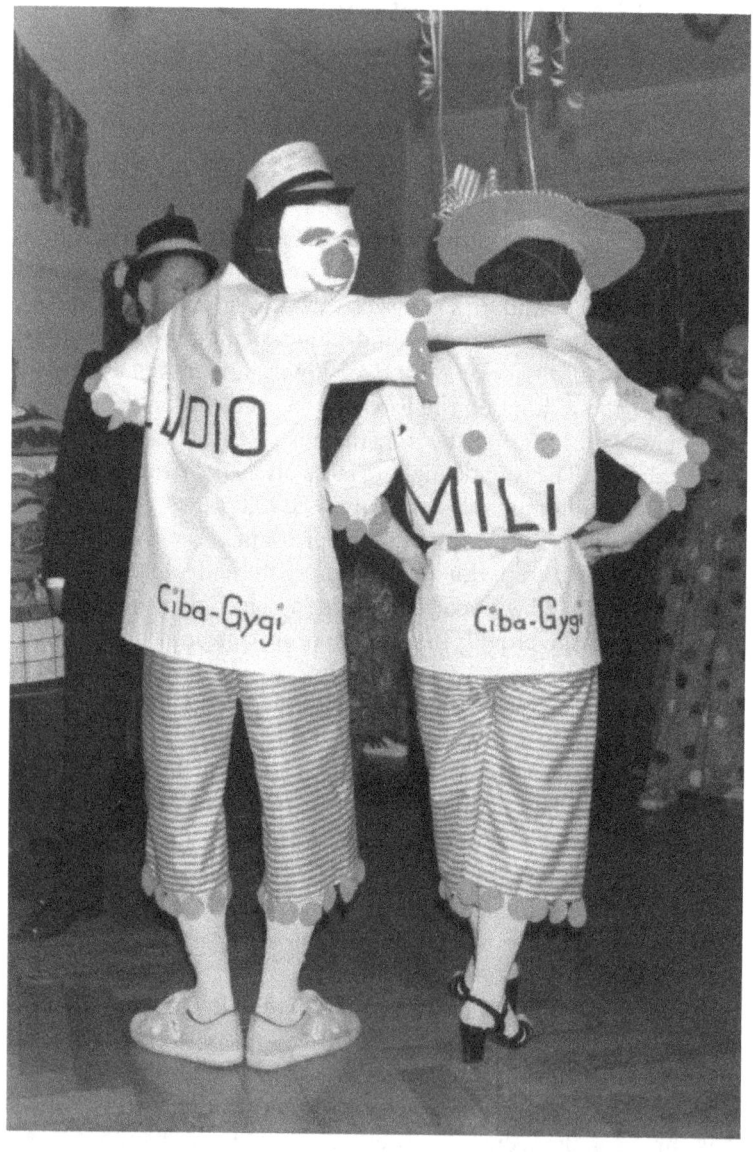

**Figure 6.1** Ludio and Mili, Carnival 1979

overabundance of antidepressants had namely been achieved in the meantime as well. Since the 1950s, a plethora of substances had been tested, some of which had proven successful. But the coveted magical drug had still not been found. Hence, every promising innovation had given rise to new hope. But then, after the large number of trials that Kuhn had conducted in the 1960s, in the 1970s drug innovation seemed to have actually run into a wall. Important breakthroughs never materialised, new regulations complicated quick registration, and approved medications were being tested for additional indications. Ludio and Milli embodied a substance that had already been used in Münsterlingen for thirteen years, and seven years had passed since its approval. 'Will there be nothing new anymore?', Kuhn might have thought when he saw the clowns.

The same question also troubled the pharmaceutical industry. But if we shift our gaze away from the lack of breakthroughs, it quickly becomes clear that the 1970s did indeed feature new developments. In the history of knowledge and science, it is now generally agreed that actors, practices, and objects that fail to prevail or do so only briefly must be given at least as much attention as the 'discoverers', 'innovations', and 'therapeutic revolutions' that have been the focal point of early histories of medicine.[3] Success stories run the risk of obscuring all those things that have led to dead ends but that nonetheless – as this chapter shows – contributed to creating knowledge.

## The Basel pharmaceutical companies: Strategies against stagnation

Ludiomil was originally called Ciba 34276. Thus the preparation came from the Ciba company and was often called 'Ciba' or the 'Ciba remedy' in Münsterlingen. However, when the drug was approved in 1972, the company no longer existed in this form. It had merged with Geigy in 1970, so the place of origin indicated on the costumes of the clowns at the Münsterlingen Carnival of 1979 was not 'Ciba' but rather 'Ciba-Gygi'. Much had changed with the merger, including in the area of psychotropic drugs. To avoid overlapping product lines, hard choices had needed to be made. With regard to test substances, Ciba-Geigy had to decide between the

Geigy product G 35259, Kuhn's beloved ketimipramine, or the Ciba product 34276. The company chose to continue with Ludiomil.[4]

Ciba and Geigy merged just as twenty-odd years of economic growth were winding down. In the 1960s, it had become increasingly difficult to manufacture new drugs of commercial interest. The pharmaceutical advances seemed to have run dry and fears of a certain stagnation took hold. The confrontations over drug prices between the pharmaceutical companies, health insurance funds, and state health authorities intensified. The companies were worried about their returns and, citing research costs, were already defending their prices in advance; at the same time, they deliberated on how they could reinvigorate the innovation process and reinvest their profits.[5]

During this last phase of prosperous growth, the Basel companies decided to diversify. They expanded their product lines in the fields of agro- and photochemicals, plastics and adhesives, and cosmetics and medical equipment, among others. Since they did not clearly prioritise any product group, pharmaceuticals became less important for the companies for the time being.[6] The trend to build strong positions in as many sectors as possible also included mergers. In 1967 Sandoz took over Wander, and in 1970 Ciba and Geigy merged.[7] In both cases, the newly reconfigured companies expected the merger to substantially strengthen their pharmaceutical sector, especially since it seemed that drug approval policies would tighten up.[8] However, this hope was not entirely realised. Although companies still made profits, they then ran into problems as a result of the oil crisis, the recession, and the collapse of the international monetary system. From 1974 to 1975, sales declined a few percentage points, for the first time in decades. The strongest declines occurred with older and mass-produced products, that is, with dyes, chemicals, and plastics. Agrochemicals and pharmaceuticals, on the other hand, held up well.[9]

For Ciba-Geigy, the concrete implementation of the merger was not a simple matter. It led to tensions and uncertainties, for one had to decide, among other things, who would take over which positions and functions, and how to design wage policies, employment conditions, and employee-benefit provisions. Speaking to subordinates in 1970, the medical doctor Hugo Bein, who had directed Ciba's biological research department since 1965 and who took over the management of pharmaceutical research after the merger, tried to allay people's fears, but without sugarcoating anything.

> On the part of the product line, few overlaps and frictions apparently arise. The situation is different when we consider the areas of preparations in development and the position of individual employees in the company. We do not want to deceive ourselves: the merger prearrangements have created tension, areas that are filled with anxious and aggressive tension.[10]

In fact, not only were employees made redundant; there was also resistance and friction, especially among academically trained staff. The Ciba and Geigy merger resulted in a collision between very different corporate cultures. The medical doctor Alexandra Delini-Stula, for example, who worked in research for Geigy from 1966 to 1970 and then for Ciba-Geigy, experienced the merger as a severe crisis – 'a major drama'. As she recalled, even though the merger was officially between two equal partners, Geigy had actually been taken over by Ciba. Afterwards, parallel structures continued to exist at first, until the company was gradually reorganised. Two colleagues, she noted, had committed suicide because of the merger.[11] According to Paul Erni, who wrote a history about 'the Basel marriage' in 1979, the 'strong will to draw the greatest possible utility from the synergy of the merger', and the strict pursuit of this goal, could 'simply not always be harmonised with the personal expectations of many affected persons'.[12] The merger was also a major topic for the public and the media, and certainly for Kuhn. He collected newspaper and magazine articles related to his field of expertise, and now he also saved texts about the Basel merger: carefully clipped articles from the business section of the *Neue Zürcher Zeitung*, an organisational chart of Ciba-Geigy's corporate structure, a so-called *Schnitzelbank* (humorous song) from the Basel Carnival, and a poem from a satirical magazine.[13]

## Ludiomil: A long-time trial

How did this substance, which prevailed over Keto, found approval in 1972, and seven years later took centre stage at the Münsterlingen

Carnival, come about? In February 1965, Ciba's pharmaceutical research committee decided to subject the psychoactive substance 34276, which according to the committee's minutes had been produced at a clinician's request, to toxicity studies.[14] However, the toxicity tests dragged on. In September 1966, the committee decided to press ahead with the production of the preparation as quickly as possible so that the toxicity studies could be concluded and it could start the clinical trials. The pharmacological report on the conducted animal experiments was sent out in November. In the cover letter, the company assured, 'As soon as we have larger quantities of the preparation available, we will first and foremost endeavour to precisely clarify tolerability in the case of repeated application, also on a dog.'[15] By this time, Kuhn had already been using the substance for almost a year, having started the first patients on 'Ciba' by no later than December 1965.[16]

The clinician who proposed the synthesis of Ciba 34276 was not named in the committee's minutes, but he was none other than Roland Kuhn. As noted earlier, in the 1960s, Kuhn had developed into a hobby pharmacologist, and he always later emphasised that Ciba 34276 had been synthesised at his initiative.[17] In fact, Kuhn was promised a commission 'on the future sales';[18] he was the first, and until the autumn of 1966 also the only, clinician who tested Ciba 34276. The company had granted him an exclusivity right, which shows the strength of Kuhn's position back then. Other physicians could only carry out trials and publish about the substance with his consent. When articles nonetheless appeared in spring 1966, Kuhn expressed his disappointment and reminded the company of his prerogative. Ciba explained by return mail that the publications in Germany had occurred without the company's knowledge and that the trial would only be expanded with his consent: 'The preparation has thus far not been given to any other investigator and it remains reserved for you.'[19]

After the first preliminary test in late 1965, the number of Münsterlingen patients who were given Ciba 34276 persistently grew. In late 1966, it stood at thirty-four; in March 1967, there were eighty-two cases.[20] A Ciba file note written after a visit to Münsterlingen states that the preparation had thus far only been tested by Kuhn and his wife. However, as of June 1967 – one and a half years after the trial began – the substance was now being used as 'routine therapy' throughout the entire clinic.[21] As the testing gradually evolved into therapy, the numbers quickly climbed. According to Kuhn, 225 patients were treated with Ciba 34276 in 1968, and in 1970 he spoke about 400, and in 1971 about 617 cases. Of these 617 patients, around one quarter were children; as was already the case in 1967, more than half of the subjects had been treated as outpatients.[22]

A few months after expanding the trial internally, Kuhn began involving other clinics and doctors. His long-term partner was the private clinic in Münchenbuchsee in the Canton of Bern. In November 1967, Kuhn sent 1,000 tablets of Ciba 34276 to the head doctor, whom he probably knew from his time as an assistant physician at Waldau. He asked him 'not to say anything about the preparation anywhere', told him about his impressions thus far, and explained how to proceed with the trial of the substance.

> I ask you not to use the medication in a big way, but rather only for selected cases, and for each case to let me know: sex, age, brief description of the illness with the duration of the illness, the course thus far, the therapy thus far, therapeutic effect, dosage, side-effects. The dosage is similar to that of a standard antidepressant of the imipramine series.

The trials at Münchenbuchsee continued until 1971, and Kuhn incorporated at least some their findings in his assessments.[23] Ciba evidently knew that Kuhn had passed the preparation on. In 1969, a company employee told a doctor at the Cantonal Hospital St Gallen 'that various patients with other psychiatrists were receiving preparation 34276 through Prof. Kuhn'.[24]

However, the trial was not limited to Kuhn and his confidants. After Kuhn had agreed to the expansion of the trial in summer 1967, the company decided to make Ciba 34276 'available for targeted testing' starting in the autumn.[25] At first, the trial's expansion was limited to German-speaking regions. Then in late 1968, the executive management decided to test the substance internationally. In February 1970, the first report arrived from Milan, which by October 1971 was followed by reports from other parts of the globe – for example, from Australia, Scandinavia, and the United States.[26]

The goal of having Ciba 34276 registered in various countries drew nearer. Although by then Kuhn had repeatedly told Ciba about his impressions of the preparation, an actual test report had still not been written. Thus in April 1971, the company asked him for a comprehensive report, which was also supposed to include the number of patients treated with Ciba 34276.[27] This request was difficult for Kuhn to fulfil. Apart from the lack of time, the evaluation of the long-term trial confronted him with various methodological problems. How many patients had actually been treated with the substance since late 1965? Was it even possible to numerically quantify the findings and to review them statistically? And how was one to deal with the fact that Ciba 34276 had long been used almost exclusively in combination with other substances, above all to counteract its worrisome side-effects, namely, weight gain and vertigo? After five years, Kuhn was sure he knew a lot about the Ciba substance, but compiling a quantitative overview confronted him with major challenges.[28]

In January 1972 the time had finally come: at the annual symposium that Ciba had been holding in St Moritz since 1970, Kuhn reported on 'clinical experiences with a new antidepressant', and his wife spoke about the administration of Ciba 34276 to children. Many of the other lectures also dealt with Ludiomil – in the meantime, the substance had been given a brand name. Ciba-Geigy published the articles after the symposium, while also no doubt including them in the approval applications.[29]

Kuhn's article differs sharply from previous ones; it contains quantitative information and even features two tables. Nonetheless, it can hardly be compared with the other clinical conference reports, all of which were based on double-blind studies. Even though Kuhn concluded in 1971 that he had treated more than 600 patients with Ciba 34276, for methodological reasons only 320 cases could be included in the assessment. More than half – 181 – had taken Ciba 34276 merely as a 'main medication'. And although the other 139 patients had received only Ludiomil, they had various diagnoses.[30] It was no wonder that Kuhn and the company had decided not to statistically review the significance of the values.

## Increased drug regulation

Before Ciba-Geigy could put Ludiomil on the market, the company needed to apply to the Intercantonal Office for the Control of Medicines (IKS) to register the substance. Viewed from an international perspective, Switzerland was an exception when it came to the approval of drugs insofar as the cantons were responsible for the supervision of medications until 2002, when the first Therapeutic Products Act was enacted at the federal level.[31] The regulation of therapeutic products had been part of the cantonal legal systems since the mid-nineteenth century. But it soon became clear that this responsibility could be better met within the framework of an intercantonal association. After the failure of initial attempts to create a concordat in the second half of the nineteenth century, the first five cantons entered into an agreement in 1900, which was gradually joined by other cantons. Although the jointly operated Intercantonal Office for the Control of Medicines reviewed and registered new medications, it did not issue marketing approvals. Since the regulatory amendments of 1942, however, new drugs had to be reviewed and registered by the IKS before the cantons could approve them as medications. With the agreement of 1954, the testing and review of medications was finally completely handed over to the IKS,[32] which over the following decades acquired more and more competencies.[33]

This standardisation served not only the cantons but also the pharmaceutical industry and the retail sector, for it substantially simplified their work. As a member of the World Health Organization (WHO) and the Council of Europe,[34] Switzerland was furthermore obliged to cooperate in the elaboration and realisation of international recommendations in the area of drug monitoring. The international development of the drug market and government health policies also greatly contributed to ensuring the gradually increasing coordination and regulation of registration requirements in Switzerland in the second half of the twentieth century.[35] In 1963, the IKS expanded the documentation obligation after other countries had tightened their approval regulations in the wake of the thalidomide scandal.[36] Apart from pharmacological documents, manufacturers now had to submit precise information on the clinical effect, the character of the effect, and any side-effects. The IKS thus actually introduced clinical effect verification for new preparations.[37] In 1971, the cantons again transferred competencies to the IKS, which was now also supposed to monitor the manufacturing of new medications. As the director at the time wrote in 1975, this did not yet mean the IKS had legislative authority, but it had established a 'bindingness exercised in daily practice'.[38] In 1977, the registration guidelines of 1963 were reworked, which led to a further clarification and tightening of documentation obligations. Clinical studies on humans were now basically to be conducted as controlled clinical studies, which needed to be checked against trials with either a placebo or a known medication. The new guidelines were based, for the first time, on the four-phase model for clinical trials,[39] which at the same time was also being mandated in the United States.[40] Originally set up to combat so-called patent medicines (medications of unknown composition), the IKS was gradually expanded into a 'comprehensive system for monitoring safety and effectiveness'.[41]

The ever-greater tightening of registration requirements and their adaptation to international standards is also reflected in the IKS annual reports. A survey of rejected medications shows that until the mid-twentieth century most of these substances were denied registration because of dishonest marketing – unproven indications and gimmicky advertising. After that, the reports increasingly cite the inadequate documentation of the pharmacological effect and toxicity. With the thalidomide scandal, the international perspective began gaining more priority; as of 1965, statements are regularly made on injury reports of the WHO.[42] Starting in 1977, the reports are dominated by commentary on the development of guidelines for 'good laboratory practice' (GLP), which were issued in 1982 by the OECD (Organisation for Economic Co-operation and Development) and established the organisational procedures and the conditions according to which laboratory trials were to be planned, conducted, and supervised.[43] However, the cantons remained responsible for the regulation of clinical trials. The IKS itself did not issue regulations on medications in clinical trials until 1992, which entered into force in 1995.[44]

The increasing requirements that numerous countries established in the 1960s and 1970s for the approval of new medications were primarily directed at the pharmaceutical industry. However, insofar as they established the conditions that determined the market launch of new medications, these requirements also inevitably influenced the standards of clinical research. Thus in its annual report of 1969, for example, the IKS emphasised that, for a registration request, indications had to be 'verified not only by open but also by controlled trials with reference substances or placebos' and the submitted documents had to 'meet the international methodological standard'.[45] For the clinical testing of psychoactive substances, however, the statistical turn seems to have gained acceptance only gradually. Thus in the 1970s, the IKS annual reports still state that a large share of newly registered psychotropic drugs were rejected because the clinical trials had not fulfilled the 'strict standards'.[46]

The stronger regulation of the approval of medications therefore also resulted in the gradual, irreversible transformation of the clinical trial. If pharmaceutical companies wanted to obtain the approval of a new medication, then as of the late 1960s they had to submit clinical studies that satisfied the heightened requirements with regard to trial design, standardisation, and documentation.[47] This not only led to a standardisation of clinical research, but also contributed to a general standardisation of psychiatry, which increasingly aimed for consistent diagnoses and comparable findings related to the course of diseases and therapies.[48]

Furthermore, the stricter regulation of medication monitoring and clinical research went hand in hand with growing professional self-regulation in medicine and psychiatry. In 1964, the World Medical Association established research ethics guidelines for clinical trials with the Declaration of Helsinki.[49] Building on this declaration, six years later the Swiss Academy of Medical Sciences (SAMS) issued its own 'guidelines for research studies on humans'. As stated in the guidelines' introduction, the SAMS wanted them to 'make doctors and their employees who conduct research studies on humans aware of the fundamental issues that arise'. At the same time, however, it stressed that the guidelines did not absolve anyone of their 'personal professional, civil, or criminal responsibility'. The guidelines distinguished between 'research studies in the interest of the person to be studied' and other 'research studies'. With the first type of study, the doctor could combine testing with treatment only insofar 'as it is justified by the diagnostic, therapeutic, or prophylactic value for the patient' and entails 'no considerable risk'. The 'consent declaration of the person to be studied or his legal representative' was defined as an 'essential precondition' for both types of study. Consent could be provided orally or in writing, but it was supposed to be recorded. The same applied to the 'research studies' themselves; they had to be noted in the patient's medical history and recorded and stored in a separate study protocol.[50]

From the Swiss perspective, the 1970 SAMS guidelines are a milestone.[51] As with recommendations at the international level, they admittedly had no direct legally binding force,[52] but they launched discussions among Swiss doctors about ethical guidelines and the design of clinical trials. That said, this debate evidently took time to get going. Along with two copies of the guidelines, which contain neither markings nor comments, Kuhn's private archive also includes two letters from the SAMS that served as a reminder of those guidelines. A letter of February 1975 states that a head doctor from Zurich reported being asked on a TV show whether provisions on the regulation and supervision of research studies on humans existed in Switzerland. In his response, according the letter, the professor had referred to the SAMS guidelines of 1970 and mentioned two clinics with corresponding advisory committees, but he did not know 'whether and in what way the guidelines [were] applied in practice elsewhere'. The board and senate of the SAMS took this information as a reason to once more point to the guidelines and make it clear that the academy had no monitoring responsibilities. Since 'the problem could become the subject of a public discussion', however, it seemed worthwhile to ask the medical faculties and forty-five large hospitals of Switzerland whether they had commissions that monitored research studies on humans.[53] There is no response enclosed with the letter, which, although unusual because Kuhn generally responded quickly and reliably to incoming correspondence, is also not surprising since he did not otherwise partake in the debate about research guidelines.

In the mid-1970s, the number of publications in which clinicians spoke about ethical guidelines and the design of clinical trials started to grow. For example, Brigitte Woggon and Jules Angst from the Psychiatric University Hospital Zurich published a three-page text that presented the 'perspective of the clinical investigator' on the 'fundamentals and guidelines for the initial testing of psychotropic drugs'. In the introduction, the authors point out that, as a rule, clinical trials of psychotropic drugs consist of 'clinical research in conjunction with medical care'. Since when transitioning to a trial with sick persons the effect of test substances often cannot be predicted, whether it was a therapeutic trial or 'purely scientific' research could only be determined after the fact. Therefore, Woggon and Angst not only called for pilot studies but also brought up for discussion whether these 'would have to enlist certain patient groups for ethical reasons, for example, patients with mild symptoms'.[54] Along with administrative regulation under public law, as was implemented, for instance, in Switzerland in the 1970s, requirements were also established in industry and medicine. In the aggregate, these provisions all contributed to a slow but definitive transformation of the practice of clinical testing.

## A late promotion in turbulent times: Kuhn as clinical director

During his entire time at Münsterlingen, Roland Kuhn was a very busy man. In the 1970s, above all in the first half of the decade, however, his workload became especially large. In 1971, Adolf Zolliker retired, whereupon Kuhn, after more than thirty years as a senior physician and deputy director, took over his position at age 59. Kuhn had accomplished much; he was considered the discoverer of the first antidepressant; he was an honorary professor, the author of numerous publications, and now also a clinical director. At the same time, he could count on Ciba 34276 reaching market readiness soon. In short, Kuhn was at the pinnacle of his career.

However, the heavy workload was not just the result of his being chosen as clinical director. As he wrote in his application to take over Zolliker's position, as the latter's deputy Kuhn had already assumed 'numerous ... responsibilities' of the director. He had long been managing the 'everyday work' at the clinic and the training of the doctors, looking after the medical assistants, ergotherapy, and the laboratories, and organising the school for the psychiatric nursing staff.[55] In his thank-you letter after his appointment, he then also assured the government that 'not much [would] change in the management of the clinic' after he took office.[56] But this prophesy would turn out to be false. In his last ten years of work at Münsterlingen, Kuhn brought about quite a bit of change – probably more than he originally planned.

That Kuhn's tenure as clinical director occurred in a new era can also be discerned from the Carnival photos of 1979. Thus while Mili wears open shoes with heels, as was appropriate back then for festive occasions, Ludio's feet are in running shoes. A different picture shows a costumed woman with a green wig. She is obviously impersonating a female psychologist, for she is holding two issues of the journal *Psychologie heute* in her hands; the cover picture of one issue displays the headline, 'The Rebel in Us'.[57] Standing next to the female psychologist is a younger man in a dressing gown and pyjamas. As shown by a sign, he represents 'teaching personnel today' and is also wearing running shoes. The man has a large clinical thermometer in his hand, which indicates a life-threatening body temperature of forty-two degrees. The prescription furnished with Kuhn's signature, however, merely orders 'three days' bed rest'.

A female psychologist, running shoes, and a nurse who points to a catastrophic situation – signs of a transformation in psychiatry and society that had also made its way to Thurgau. Kuhn's tenure as director took place during a period when previously unchallenged authorities were confronted with harsh criticism and new actors. Admittedly, some of the problems Kuhn struggled with in the 1970s had already been familiar to his predecessor, such as a lack of staff and dilapidated buildings. But as the ripples from the broad criticism of psychiatry in the 1960s reached Thurgau and he himself was publicly attacked in 1972/1973, other questions arose as well. The new director found himself under immense pressure, both within and outside the clinic.

In July 1971, Kuhn took over an institution in dire need of reform. At the same time, since the 1960s, the Canton of Thurgau had been recording sharply increasing expenditures, which were tied to a growing deficit. To be sure, Thurgau was no worse off financially than other cantons. The clinic's structural renovations were primarily covered by its own higher revenues, and by the end of the 1970s the canton was in the black again.[58] But even so, the economic situation was not especially conducive for capital investments in psychiatry. Nonetheless, even Kuhn believed that certain reforms were indispensable. Thus in his second annual report, he felt obliged to make it clear that he did not deny there were problems at Münsterlingen.

> In the course of the reporting year, one has criticised the director, his annual report for 1971 constitutes whitewashing and does not correspond to the factual circumstances. Therefore it is again expressly put on record that the lack of staff and the building conditions of the clinic make it difficult to treat the sick.[59]

The renovation of the clinic was already long overdue. Even though individual renovation projects had been carried out in the 1950s and 1960s, urgent construction measures were waiting to be dealt with after Zolliker's resignation. As Kuhn wrote in a historical survey in 1990, 'one of his first official acts' consisted of inviting the canton's architect to the clinic for an inspection. The latter came to the conclusion that while a few of the newer buildings met 1920s standards, most had far greater deficiencies.[60] Planning now began for a total renovation of the clinic, which would continue throughout the 1970s. Much of the renovation and new construction work would not be completed until the 1980s, which meant that the situation remained unsatisfactory for quite some time.[61]

Parallel to the planning work, Kuhn brought in innovations that many other psychiatric clinics had also introduced since the late 1950s; the clinic management was divided into a medical directorate and an administrative directorate that no longer answered to the head doctor. Ergotherapists, music therapists, and movement therapists began working alongside psychologists; in the late 1970s, a dance therapist offered a three-week course at Münsterlingen each year. After a four-year experiment in a smaller, newly established ward, the separation of the sexes was eliminated in two further wards. In 1979, a psychologist regularly conducted a group discussion in Ward F, in which patients could voice their concerns.[62]

Beyond the realm of psychiatry, the range of therapies expanded too. Chronic and geriatric patients could be transferred to newly opened nursing and old-age homes. As a result of this institutional differentiation, the number of outpatient treatments continued to increase at the Münsterlingen Psychiatric Clinic, while the number of inpatients steadily declined in the 1970s. Just prior to Kuhn's retirement from the clinic, a rehabilitation facility was set up in the former Ittingen Charterhouse as an 'outstation', and the External Psychiatric Service and the outpatient centre in Romanshorn were founded during the tenure of Kuhn's successor.[63]

At least as serious as the building situation in 1971 was the lack of staff. Kuhn had already pointed out the impending problems to the government council before taking office. 'We must be clearly aware', he warned, 'that substantial difficulties are ahead for us'. Even now already, the 'medical staff' was incomplete, and the existing shortage of not only doctors but also nurses would continue to grow. In addition, ergotherapy was understaffed and the same would likely soon apply to the laboratory.[64] The 1972 annual report then addressed the 'early termination of various employment agreements' with assistant physicians, which was why in late 1972, along with two senior physician posts, one third of the assistant physician positions were also unoccupied. The staffing situation had also deteriorated in the nursing area. The large number of unfilled positions led to persistent overburdening, and difficulties were further aggravated by the huge fluctuation of staff.[65]

In 1972, the lack of nurses was so severe that it became necessary to reduce the number of beds on the 'women's side' and to introduce a 'block on the admission of women with geriatric illnesses'. In mid-1973, the clinic faced a shortfall of eleven 'male nursing students', thirty-three 'female nursing students', as well as seventeen male and thirty-one female fully trained nurses.[66] Female residents of the region were urged on radio and television to assist the clinic. Married former nurses took night watches. Women's associations recruited housewives who were supposed give the nurses a hand, helping with spring cleaning, for example, and airing out beds. In 1974, at least the number of nursing trainees began to increase again. At the same time, patients were entrusted with nursing tasks,[67] and unqualified assistants were hired, who often came from abroad and spoke no German. In the second half of the 1970s, the staff shortage was therefore limited to 'fully trained, well-qualified nursing personnel'. Even Kuhn's last annual report states that the clinic still lacked more than thirty certified male and female nurses.[68]

It was long-known that psychiatric clinics had to struggle with a shortage of staff, especially female nurses; Kuhn himself blamed the staff shortage in Münsterlingen on, among other things, the 'very difficult working conditions with the many agitated and unsettled sick persons' and the 'inadequate pay in comparison with other analogous institutions'.[69] During the first years of his tenure as director, however, the staff shortage was particularly severe and also affected the medical personnel, which raised the question of whether the problem might perhaps also be traced back to the clinical director. In fact, former nurses and assistant physicians consistently report that Kuhn had been very hard-working and present, but also 'very strict' – 'a patriarch'. They say he cultivated an authoritarian leadership style, which was viewed positively or negatively depending on one's attitude, and that he brooked neither criticism nor dissent.[70]

In 1972/1973, criticism was voiced in public. Appearing in Thurgau newspapers were articles and letters to the editor that referred to the conditions in the psychiatric clinic.[71] Kuhn took it as a deep personal offense. In correspondence and in the diary he kept at the beginning and end of his term as director, he spoke about 'witch hunts', 'press campaigns', and 'sleepless nights'.[72] Bruno Stadelmann, a young Social Democratic teacher, submitted to Kuhn a list of questions, which later also appeared in the newspaper.[73] In February 1973, there was finally an interpellation in the canton parliament, which, apart from the staff shortage, the building situation, and other grievances, also discussed Kuhn's leadership style. Clinical testing was never mentioned anywhere; the only point of criticism pertaining to medications was the accusation that patients were being kept subdued and quiet with sedatives because of the lack of personnel.[74]

In August 1973, Kuhn submitted a forty-four-page position paper to the government council and a handful of published letters to the editor that backed him up. Kuhn rejected all of the criticisms except for the building situation and the staff shortage. Regarding the psychotropic drugs, he wrote that the new medications worked 'on the illness itself', whereas before only anaesthetics, sleep, and sedative medications had been available. In addition, because of his own scientific work the clinic was well acquainted with 'modern psychopharmacological treatment'. As he explained, 'for me it is troubling to encounter the accusation that, in the clinic I lead, the patients are being numbed in a way that is harmful to them, since decisive discoveries were made at Münsterlingen precisely in the elaboration of non-numbing psychotropic drugs'.[75]

The nurse shortage, which Kuhn described as 'catastrophic', was caused neither by a 'restrictive personnel policy' nor by a 'rigorous hierarchy in the operation'. Referring to his launching of an employee newsletter as an example,[76] Kuhn insisted that he had always endeavoured to meet the requirements of 'modern leadership principles'. For that matter, the director of a psychiatric clinic could by no means simply do as he pleased, for he was 'bound to the objectively given possibilities, the good intention to cooperate, and the enthusiasm of his staff'.[77]

Finally, Kuhn pointed out that the interpellation mixed up 'sociopolitical and social-psychiatric problems of a general nature with a specific critique' of the Münsterlingen Psychiatric Clinic. In his opinion, the interpellation contained many antipsychiatric motives, which he repeatedly addressed in his position paper.[78] An appended reader's letter by a doctor also refers to the antipsychiatric attitude, stating that the 'attacks from the camp of leftist intellectual sociologists against clinical psychiatry are very much to be understood in the context of revolutionary activity'.[79]

Looking back, however, Uwe Moor, a Thurgau resident who witnessed the parliamentary interpellation on the psychiatric clinic, fully rejected the notion of a Marxist conspiracy. He noted that the Great Council viewed the young parliamentary members behind the interpellation as 'revolutionary' and 'mutinous' just because they were members of the Social Democratic Party and intellectuals, but Moor described them simply as 'a group of young people ... against this establishment' who were prepared to 'pose questions that the society actually wanted to render taboo'.[80] Thus by the early 1970s, the harbingers of the new social movement had also reached Thurgau. Previously unchallenged authorities now had to deal with 'draft-dodgers' and long-haired 'hashish youngsters' while at the same time being generally confronted with a critical attitude – an attitude that assistant physicians or nurses of a psychiatric clinic could also display.[81]

## The end of the Münsterlingen trials?

The 1972/1973 'press campaign' also brought up the question of whether it would be better for the clinical director to fulfil his extensive responsibilities instead of doing scientific work. However, Kuhn unequivocally rejected the allegation that he was overburdened and neglecting other tasks for the benefit of science, noting he had always pursued scientific interests in his free time. Moreover, for a head physician, scientific activity was key 'in order to keep up the clinic'. However, in this case Kuhn probably understood scientific work to mean activities such as participating in conferences or reading technical articles; clinical trials were no longer mentioned.[82]

Apart from his heavy workload, there are also other factors that suggest Kuhn was rarely involved in testing anymore during the 1970s. First, apart from documents on Ludiomil, his private archive contains relatively few sources regarding trials. In his diary, too, Kuhn rarely speaks about research. Second, he found that there was 'more of a stagnation ... in the development of new [psychopharmacological] medications'.[83] Because he rejected the benzodiazepines Librium and Valium, he never became involved in this branch of research, and there did not appear to be any new antidepressants in sight after the approval of Ludiomil. Third, the increasing regulations in the drug sector had a negative impact on Kuhn's work as a clinical investigator. This also undoubtedly applied not only to his willingness to collaborate on the testing of substances but also to the interest of pharmaceutical companies to recruit him.

Kuhn was sceptical about the new testing methods from very beginning. Over the 1970s, as more and more colleagues fell in line with the statistical turn, his criticism grew. When looking back, he usually complained about the downfall of research, which in his opinion was linked to the rise of modern testing methods. At first, he was still rather cautious and even conceded that questionnaires, double-blind testing, and statistical evaluations could be fruitful,[84] but by the by the late 1970s he was loudly complaining about 'so-called controlled studies'. If well planned and analysed, they could admittedly 'serve as valuable confirmations of open trials', but they were not suitable for identifying the mood-brightening effect of new, unknown substances. In addition, he felt that psychology had been permeated with popular, ambiguous terms and concepts while rating scales disregarded the main symptom of daily fluctuation. Therefore, it came as no surprise when this produced 'completely distorted results'.[85] In a speech Kuhn gave to the medical community of the Canton of Thurgau shortly before leaving the clinic, he prophesied that psychopharmacology would 'still make substantial advances ... but only with intelligent, targeted research in combination with very good psychopathological-clinical observation'.[86]

Kuhn's aversion to the new research methods is also reflected by sources that were not meant for publication. In 1975, upon being asked by the Byk Gulden company to test a new substance,

Kuhn made it clear that he would only accept such an offer under certain conditions.

> I must tell you ... from the outset that I am not prepared to do double-blind studies and to agree to complicated provisions on the execution of such trials. My successes in the testing and discovery of psychopharmacological substances came about only by means of simple clinical methods, and I have no reason to deviate from these methods.[87]

And how did the pharmaceutical industry view this position? Whereas in the late 1960s Kuhn increasingly developed into a preliminary investigator because of his rejection of standardised methods, he was now pushed even further towards the margins. Although still being asked to conduct trials,[88] he no longer had the same importance, even for companies with which he had closely worked for a long time. This is illustrated by the documents that Ciba-Geigy submitted in 1972 with the registration application for Ludiomil. Along with referring to open trials, the company now also referred to controlled double-blind trials that had compared Ludiomil with two other antidepressants. Kuhn, however, was never mentioned, despite having been crucially involved in the preparation's development.[89]

How contemporary psychiatrists perceived Kuhn's psychopharmacological research is difficult to assess. Jules Angst, who directed the research department of the Burghölzli in Zurich, reported that Kuhn observed how patients changed under a medication and wrote up case histories of individual patients – 'perhaps on half a page'. His results, however, were based neither on checklists nor measurements. Kuhn was considered the 'discoverer of Tofranil' and a daseinsanalyst, and he had engaged in 'psychopharmacology for a certain length of time', but he 'never [became] an actual psychopharmacologist'.[90] Two former assistant physicians at the Münsterlingen Psychiatric Clinic strongly criticised Kuhn's research methods. Whereas one felt that his former boss 'did science according to his own taste' without worrying about scientific standards, the other wondered why specialists did not question Kuhn's results – it was simply impossible to closely investigate groups of several hundred patients in a clinic such as Münsterlingen in the way Kuhn claimed in his publications.[91]

One would need to see whether other such voices exist, and in what context they were heard. But in contemporary specialised publications, we have thus far only stumbled across one statement that criticises Kuhn's methodology. In 1972 in St Moritz, when Kuhn lectured on his experiences with Ludiomil, Karl Rickels, a professor at the University of Pennsylvania, piped up during the subsequent discussion. Originally from Germany, the psychiatrist began by confirming the importance of conducting open tests 'at the start of the "career" of a new preparation in order to discover possible ... indications, which can then be reviewed as hypotheses in controlled studies'. But he then criticised Kuhn's long-term trial.

> Yet I doubt that one needs hundreds of patients for this. I believe, on the contrary, that one could have already investigated several of the patients treated by Herr Kuhn in a controlled study, whereby more valid information would probably have resulted. I find somewhat unfortunate above all the combination of a test preparation with one or several already known medications within a clinical trial.[92]

Compared to other commentary, these were harsh words; the specialists who participated in the Ciba-Geigy seminars in the 1970s otherwise always voted for their own methodological approach, but without criticising other ones.[93]

## Or further testing under new auspices?

In his response to the Byk Gulden company, Kuhn plainly stated what he would not do. At the same time, however, he still made it clear that he was basically interested in testing substances. In trials, he explained, he sought to 'find something new, to work out new indications and to observe the individuality, so to speak, of a certain active substance, its particular indications and the course of its effect over a longer time'.[94] But under the changed conditions of the 1970s, was it still even possible for Kuhn to conduct such trials?

While the portents were different, more trials actually took place in the Münsterlingen Psychiatric Clinic in the 1970s than one would suspect from the psychopharmacological holdings in Kuhn's private archive. For one thing, eighteen test preparations were trialled that left few traces – either because the trials were barely documented or because the sources have not survived. For another, trials were carried out that are not immediately recognisable as such in the medical files. These were trials with substances that had already been approved, and they were supposed to clarify whether the drug also worked for other indications or patient groups. In contrast to substances with test numbers, which can be immediately identified in the sources, medications such as Tegretol (an antiepileptic), Lioresal (an antispasmodic), and Trasicor (a medication against cardiac arrhythmia) do not stand out in medical files and other clinical records.

Among the clinic's many thousands of outpatient medical files, for example, is that of Rita Suter, an 11-year-old girl who was referred to Verena Kuhn in late 1974. According to the treating psychiatrist, the child's mother had long suffered from endogenous depression. She was undergoing treatment and had recently brought along her daughter, who was not sleeping and was very passive, especially at school, and sometimes also became aggressive against her younger sister. An examination by the paediatrician produced no findings; the treating psychiatrist suspected a depression, but he did not want to treat Rita Suter without a thorough examination. Verena Kuhn considered the girl to be 'rather of a somewhat below-average intelligence' and 'strongly retarded'. She prescribed two antidepressants and at the next appointment added Tegretol, since she found that the EEG curve could 'possibly indicate a slight organic affection after all'.[95] Tegretol had been launched in 1963 as an antiepileptic. Because in the case of some epileptics it also showed a psychotropic effect, individual clinics, including Münsterlingen, began using the medication for depression and behavioural disorders. As Roland and Verena Kuhn reported at a symposium in 1975, they 'often [obtained] excellent results' with Tegretol, especially with patients with abnormal EEG findings.[96]

At the next check-up, however, Verena Kuhn concluded that Rita Suter's medication could be even better adjusted. She recommended a trial with Trasicor, adding that she would be 'above all interested, whether one [could] see an effect of Trasicor in such a case'. Sometime later, Roland Kuhn inquired with the treating psychiatrist; in a handwritten phone memo, he noted that the patient's condition was 'very much better' under Trasicor. In 1977, the doctor asked whether the medication could perhaps be reduced, for

Rita Suter was doing well. Two years later, he wrote that the girl was refusing the medication. Even so, she was still required to take Tegretol, Trasicor, and antidepressants every day.[97]

Where did Verena Kuhn get the idea to prescribe Trasicor for Rita Suter? Trasicor had been approved in Switzerland in 1968 as a drug for the treatment of heart disorders. Between 1975 and 1982, other application possibilities were gradually added. The package leaflets, which back then were meant for doctors,[98] described Trasicor as a medication that, among other things, worked against stress and could also be used in the event of functional cardiovascular disorders. Under this indication in the leaflet of 1982, 'psychogenic, e.g., anxiety-related cardiovascular disorders' are finally mentioned for the first time.[99]

That Ciba-Geigy was testing Trasicor for new indications in the 1970s is shown by technical publications from this time.[100] For example, in 1976, the international symposium held by the company each year was dedicated to the topic 'Betablockers and the Central Nervous System'. Fifty-eight people from twelve countries participated in the symposium, reporting on their experiences. Roland and Verena Kuhn attended as well. The symposium was chaired by Paul Kielholz, the director of the Psychiatric University Hospital Basel, who opened proceedings with a short retrospective on the state of research.

> Since the introduction of betablockers ... doctors and patients have repeatedly observed that the pharmacons also have an anxiolytic or stress-inhibiting effect. In recent years they were therefore also increasingly used in psychiatry: for the treatment of anxious and phobic states, to combat anxiety in the case of depressions with an anxious character, to attenuate stress reactions, and for the treatment of stage fright, opening-night, exam, and public-speaking fears.[101]

Ciba-Geigy had invited Roland and Verena Kuhn to join in the discussions. Their contributions suggest that at Münsterlingen betablockers were primarily combined with antidepressants to combat anxious states; the scope of the trials remains unresolved.[102] Kuhn's private archive contains the names of thirty-five patients who received Trasicor. But given that we came across seven additional Trasicor patients in a different context, the substance must have been prescribed more often. Most of the forty-two known Trasicor patients underwent treatment for a long time and also received other medications. Almost all were outpatients, around one fifth were women, and more than a third were children and youth.

Roland and Verena Kuhn worked closely together. This is shown by documents that they jointly processed, as well as by entries in Kuhn's diary: 'In the evening as usual, discussions with my wife about cases.'[103] Verena Kuhn played a key role in the Trasicor trials; she treated almost all of the participating patients from our sample. She also wrote a handwritten list with the heading 'Trasicor', compiled on a calendar page from 1974. Evidently, the list was also used by her husband, for he inserted addenda for certain names.[104] The medical files of the Trasicor cases verify that Verena Kuhn was very interested in the drug's effect and expressly asked patients, family doctors, and treating psychiatrists for their input.[105] Responding to the implicit question as to why she was prescribing such a preparation, she explained to the doctor of an 18-year-old on Trasicor that at Münsterlingen they had been trying for some time to treat states of anxiety with the drug and 'often [had] really good success'.[106] At the symposium in St Moritz, she also made the case that betablockers could render 'great service' for children.[107]

One cannot clearly say at whose initiative the trials took place at Münsterlingen. Kuhn's private archive admittedly holds an excerpt from the company's own test plan of 1971, according to which Trasicor was supposed to be tested for the treatment of agitated psychoses, thus for a different indication. But Kuhn did not receive the plan until 1976; therefore, it probably served him more as background information. Since the enclosed letter refers to prior oral discussions and announces the 'consignment of sufficient quantities of Trasicor', he must at least have informed the company that he wanted to try the substance for mental disorders.[108] The delivery of gratis preparations also suggests a test.

In the case of Lioresal, an antispasmodic, the impulse came from Ciba-Geigy. When the pharmaceutical research committee learned that Lioresal might possibly also work against schizophrenia, it decided, 'in view of the considerable commercial importance of this indication', to search for prospective cooperation partners at the St Moritz symposium.[109] 'Interesting lectures on Tegretol and many interesting discussions with various colleagues', Kuhn noted in his diary, 'above all suggestions ... on the Lioresal treatment of chronic schizophrenics'. After returning from St Moritz, Kuhn informed his employees and immediately began to administer Lioresal to the first schizophrenic patients.[110] At the same time, Ciba-Geigy arranged for him to receive the unpublished article of the Swedish doctor who had made 'the discovery' of the new indication for Lioresal.[111]

In summer 1975, Kuhn compiled a handwritten list with notes on all of the patients who had thus far been involved in the trial. In doing so, he relied on notes that had been written by assistant physicians or nursing personnel.[112] Regarding one patient, for example, a report and file note have survived in which the deputy head nurse summarised observations on the effect of Lioresal. Attached to the note is a slip of paper dated mid-August with the remark, 'Please give to Herr Prof. Kuhn'.[113] The medical file of a different man states, 'a temporary test with <u>Lioresal</u>, which is supposed to have a favourable effect for defect schizophrenics, completely miscarried, the lad simply fell <u>asleep where he stood and sat</u>. To not further reduce the work capacity, this test was aborted.' Kuhn read the remarks that the treating doctor had made in late February 1975, corrected the misspelled name of the medication, underlined individual words, and included the case in his list.[114]

At the end of August, seven months after the last entry on Lioresal, Kuhn spoke about the preparation again in his diary: 'The company has written to fifteen clinics and requested, one should do tests. Nine have responded, telephone reports are available from five on altogether just a few cases, in which one saw nothing.' The remaining four clinics were invited to a conference where the said doctor from Sweden also participated. Kuhn travelled to Basel as well, but he was very disappointed by the presentations: 'one again sees above all how one should not investigate new medications, and how inadequate are the skills of people and the absent understanding for major problems'.[115]

Kuhn had therefore created the list in light of the meeting in Basel. The conclusion that he drew at the end of document does not seem particularly positive: '21 chronic schizophrenics: → 3–4 improvements. 12 unchanged. 4 worse. – 3 neurological cases. perhaps somewhat better 1, unchanged 1, worse 1'.[116] Yet, Kuhn nonetheless believed to have identified 'a certain effect' with his patients, and he continued the trial. Three months later, he participated in a conference in Nuremberg, where he spoke about 'Lioresal for psychoses'.[117] Following the presentation, Kuhn noted in another diary entry, 'an interesting discussion developed', one had 'ascertained similar effects elsewhere'. In the end, he concluded, 'There seems to be something to it'.[118] The trial was continued for a few more months, but then was evidently abandoned after all in 1976.[119] As with other trials, Kuhn's persistent optimism also came to bear in the case of Lioresal. Even when facing less-than-encouraging results, he tended to see a 'certain' effect and to suggest that colleagues who reported negative results were making methodological mistakes.

Trasicor, Tegretol, and Lioresal, and perhaps other preparations as well, were used at Münsterlingen outside the approved applications area (off-label use). These were not cases where the medications were administered for therapeutic reasons only. In the 1970s, the impetus for these trials no doubt usually came from outside. Kuhn perhaps received a suggestion or query from the pharmaceutical industry, or picked up on something while reading technical literature or at a conference. And then started trying things out himself.

His role for the pharmaceutical industry changed during this decade. The 1970s were dominated by the economic crisis and increased regulation in the area of medications, while larger breakthroughs in psychotropic drugs failed to materialise for the pharmaceutical companies. Clinical trials were therefore confronted with new challenges.[120] The signs were particularly bad for Münsterlingen; Kuhn, who had always rejected quantitative methods, definitively lost his prominent position as an investigator. Having taken over the clinical directorate, he had to focus on other urgent tasks, for he was faced with a major personnel shortage, buildings in need of renovation, and public criticism. Nevertheless, Kuhn's career as a clinical researcher did not come to an end completely after the success with Ludiomil.

## Notes

1 StATG, 9'10, 1.2.11/6.3; 9'40, 5.0.2/2; 9'40, 5.0.2/4; 9'40, 5.0.4/4, orders and deliveries of Ludiomil, 1966–1971.
2 On the period after the boom, see Doering-Manteuffel and Raphael, *Nach dem Boom*; Rodgers, *Age of Fracture*.

3 For the field of pharmaceutical history, see Rosenberg, 'The Therapeutic Revolution'; Greene et al., *Therapeutic Revolutions*; Majerus, 'Making Sense'; Henckes, 'Magic Bullet'.
4 See Chapter 4, 138–139.
5 König, 'Besichtigung einer Weltindustrie', 214–215.
6 For Ciba and Ciba-Geigy, for example, pharmaceuticals made up 46 per cent of their manufactured products in 1961, but only 27 per cent in 1980; see König, 'Besichtigung einer Weltindustrie', 227–229.
7 *Ibid.*, 194–195, 210.
8 Erni, *Die Basler Heirat*, 145. See also CA Novartis, PE 4.01(Hugo Bein, Ciba), manuscript of a speech to subordinates of the merged companies, undated (1970).
9 König, 'Besichtigung einer Weltindustrie', 234.
10 CA Novartis, PE 4.01(Hugo Bein, Ciba), manuscript of a speech to the subordinates of the merged companies, undated (1970), 17.
11 Interview with Alexandra Delini-Stula, 19 June 2017. On the 'equal value' of Ciba and Geigy, see Erni, *Die Basler Heirat*, 140; on the 'sometimes tragic individual fates' of employees, *ibid.*, 167.
12 König, 'Besichtigung einer Weltindustrie', 227, 233–234; Erni, *Die Basler Heirat*, 159–160 (quote).
13 StATG, 9'40, 5.0.4/25.
14 CA Novartis, Ciba, FO 5.03 Forschung, Zweckforschung, chemische Protokolle, pharma research committee (PFA) no. 39/65, 17 February 1965. On the new toxicological requirements during this time, see Chapter 4, 119–125.
15 StATG, 9'40, 5.0.2/2, information on preparation Ciba 34276-Ba (maprotiline), 31 October 1960; Hugo Bein, Ciba, to Kuhn, 11 November 1966. The impression that Kuhn started testing Ciba 34276 before the company sent him written information about the substance is confirmed by a file note from October 1966; Novartis clinical archive, BSM00002218, box 470, file note, visit, 31 October 1966.
16 CA Novartis, Ciba, FO 5.03 Forschung, Zweckforschung, chemische Protokolle, pharma research committee (PFA) no. 78/66, 13 September 1966.
17 StATG, 9'40, 8.3/20, Kuhn's file note, 14 August 2000.
18 StATG, 9'40, 5.0.2/1, Bein to Kuhn, 15 October 1968. See Chapter 5, 183.
19 StATG, 9'40, 5.0.2/4, Kuhn to Kaufmann, Ciba, 31 May 1966; Kaufmann, to Kuhn, 2 June 1966.
20 *Ibid.*, Kuhn to Kaufmann, Ciba, 31 May 1966; Novartis clinical archive, BSM00002218, box 468, view card/green folder, preparation 34276-Ba (antidepressant), chronological listing of appointments with investigators, visit report, 1 July 1966. StATG, 9'40, 8.1/174,

Über eine neue psychopharmakologische Stoffgruppe, undated manuscript by Kuhn, Bein and Wilhelm (the parts by Bein and Wilhelm are missing), cover letter, 17 March 1967.

21 Novartis clinical archive, BSM00002218, box 470, file note on a visit in Münsterlingen, 23 June 1967.

22 StATG, 9'40, 5.0.2/4, Kuhn to Bein, Ciba, 21 December 1968; 9'40, 3.0.3/7, Kuhn to doctor from Bonneval, 8 June 1970; 9'40, 5.0.4/4, trial 34276, Kuhn to Prof. Grütter, 27 July 1971.

23 StATG, 9'40, 5.0.2/4, Kuhn to Dr Plattner, Münchenbuchsee Private Clinic, 2 November 1967; overview of previous trials, 8 November and 12 December 1968; 9'40, 5.0.2/5, additional correspondence with various doctors at the Münchenbuchsee Private Clinic, 1967–1971.

24 Novartis clinical archive, BSM00002218, box 470, file note Hugo Bein, Ciba, 9 January 1969.

25 Novartis clinical archive, BSM00002218, box 468, view card/green folder, preparation 34276-Ba (antidepressant), chronological listing of appointments with investigators, visit report, 1 July 1966; CA Novartis, Ciba, file note, visit 1 July 1966, decision.

26 StATG, 9'40, 5.0.2/4, Bein, Ciba, to Kuhn, 23 December 1968; Novartis clinical archive, BSM00002218, box 468, view card/green folder, preparation 34276-Ba (antidepressant), list.

27 StATG, 9'40, 5.0.2/4, Bein, Ciba, to Kuhn, 2 April 1971.

28 *Ibid.*, Kuhn to Kaufmann, Ciba, 31 May 1966; 9'40, 8.1/174, Über eine neue psychopharmakologische Stoffgruppe, undated manuscript by Kuhn, Bein and Wilhelm (the parts by Bein und Wilhelm are missing), cover letter 17 March 1967.

29 Kielholz, *Depressive Zustände*.

30 The 320 cases pertained to 237 outpatients and 83 inpatients; Kuhn, 'Klinische Erfahrungen', 199.

31 There is not much literature on the regulation of clinical research in the German-speaking world, particularly as pertains to the 1950s and 1960s. Isolated writings, usually in support of the pharmaceutical industry, can be found following the thalidomide scandal. More publications began appearing in the 1970s; the closer one gets to the present, the greater the increase in the number of publications. Not all types of regulations have been equally well researched. If one adopts Gaudillière's and Hess's heuristic categorisation into professional, industrial, administrative, and public regulation, then the existing works deal above all with administrative regulation and less often with professional regulation. Historical studies such as Gaudillière and Hess, 'General Introduction' are still lacking for Switzerland.

32 The cantons could now only supervise the manufacturing of medicines.

33 The history of the Intercantonal Office for the Control of Medicines and its successor institution, Swissmedic, which was created in 2002 through the merger of the IKS with the Special Unit for Medicine of the Federal Office of Public Health, has hardly been researched thus far. A brief survey is offered by Ratmoko, *Damit die Chemie*, 105–108; Tornay, *Zugriffe*, 211–212; Germann, *Medikamentenprüfungen*, 30–31. Beyond that, there is a brief overview in a *Festschrift* (Fischer, 'Werdegang') and a dissertation in the field of law (Wüst, *Die Interkantonale Vereinbarung*). See also Wüst, 'Die Arzneimittelkontrolle'. For more information, one primarily needs to rely on the monthly and annual reports, directives, regulations, and Festschrifte of the IKS.

34 Switzerland is a founding member of the World Health Organization (WHO), established in 1948; it joined the Council of Europe in 1963.

35 Wüst, *Die Interkantonale Vereinbarung*, 106–110.

36 See AR IKS 1962, 5; AR IKS 1963, 8–10. On the thalidomide scandal, see Chapter 4, 120–121.

37 Fischer, 'Werdegang', 37, 42; monthly report of the IKS 1963, 2–7; Interkantonale Vereinbarung über die Kontrolle der Heilmittel, 3 June 1971, 812.2. Richtlinien der IKS betreffend Anforderungen an die Dokumentation für die Registrierung von Arzneimitteln der Humanmedizin (Registrierungs-Richtlinien), Bern, 16 December 1977; Germann, *Medikamentenprüfungen*, 30–31.

38 Fischer, 'Werdegang', 46. Hägele even makes the case that IKS decrees were *de facto* binding because the cantons were obliged to comply with intercantonal requirements; Hägele, *Arzneimittelprüfung*, 299.

39 See Chapter 4, 121–122.

40 IKS guidelines regarding requirements for evidence for new active substances, 7 January 1963, in Monatsberichte der IKS, 63 (1963), 2–7; IKS guidelines regarding documentation requirements for the registration of medicinal products for human use (registration guidelines), Bern, 16 December 1977; Germann, *Medikamentenprüfungen*, 31; Brandenberger, *Psychiatrie*, 60.

41 Undritz, *Rechtshandbuch*, 32.

42 See, for example, AR IKS 1965, 12.

43 AR IKS (1950–1995). In contrast to GLP, good clinical practice (GCP), which was declared binding for the United States by the FDA, was not enforced in Switzerland. GCP was discussed above all in the IKS annual reports of the 1990s.

44 The regulations were supposed to ensure the safety of test subjects and the quality of research results. They stipulated that clinical trials had to be supervised by independent ethics commissions.

The provision was included in modified form in the Therapeutic Products Act, which entered into force in 2002. Since then, research on humans must follow the GCP directive. www2.zhlex.zh.ch/appl/zhlex_r.nsf/0/C1256C610039641BC12561AB00455790/$file/812.24_18.11%2093.pdf;www.admin.ch/opc/de/classified-compilation/20002716/index.html (accessed 8 April 2024).
45 AR IKS 1969, 14.
46 See AR IKS 1971, 18; AR IKS 1975, 29; AR IKS 1976, 18; AR IKS 1977, 21.
47 Tornay, *Zugriffe*, 210.
48 Ibid., 184, 190, 196.
49 See Chapter 4, 125.
50 SAMS, *Richtlinien*.
51 See Sprumont, *La Protection*; Schläpfer, *Probandenschutz*; Germann, *Medikamentenprüfungen*.
52 Since the SAMS was and is a private foundation without the powers of a public authority, it cannot stipulate any legally binding norms. For a historical overview of the international ethical code for research on humans, see Tröhler, *Doctors' Ethos*.
53 StATG, 9'40, 5.1.2/0, letter of the SAMS, undated (ca. 1971–1974), 14 February 1975.
54 Woggon and Angst, 'Grundlagen', 1258 (quote).
55 StATG, 9'40, 1.0.1/0, Kuhn to Health Director Rudolf Schümperli, 10 February 1971.
56 Ibid., Kuhn to Health Director Rudolf Schümperli, 5 April 1971.
57 *Psychologie heute*, no. 5 (1978).
58 Ritzmann, *Historische Statistik*, 973.
59 StATG, 9'10, 1.1.0/60, ARM 1972, 11.
60 Kuhn, 'Geschichte', 104.
61 See, for example, StATG, 9'10, 1.1.0/60, ARM 1971–1980; 9'40, 1.0.3/0–3.
62 StATG, 9'10, 1.1.0/60, ARM 1971–1985; 9'40, 1.0.0/0, regulations of 1951 corrected and supplemented by Kuhn, undated (August/September 1971); 9'40, 1.0.11/0, group discussions in Ward F, minutes of 30 August, 6 September, and 13 September 1979. For other Swiss psychiatric clinics and clinical psychiatry in general, see Meier, *Spannungsherde*, 261–296, 314; Meier et al., *Eingeschlossen*, part 3.
63 StATG, 9'10, 1.1.0/60, ARM 1971–1985.
64 StATG, 9'40, 1.0.1/0, Kuhn to Health Director Rudolf Schümperli, 5 April 1971.
65 StATG, 9'10, 1.1.0/60, ARM 1972, 3–6; ARM 1973, 9.

66 StATG, 9'40, 1.0.1/3, Kuhn's statement on parliamentary criticism of the Münsterlingen Psychiatric Clinic, 1 August 1973, 38.
67 That patients helped in nursing and worked was a widespread and previously common practice.
68 StATG, 9'10, 1.1.0/60, ARM 1971–1979; Kuhn, 'Geschichte', 108.
69 See, for example, Kuhn, 'Geschichte', 108. See also StATG, 9'40, 1.0.1/3, Kuhn's statement on the parliamentary criticism of the Münsterlingen Psychiatric Clinic, 1 August 1973, 38.
70 See, for example, interviews with Albert Lingg, 7 September 2016, Colette Grosspietsch and Doris Meili-Nyffenegger, 13 September 2016 (quotes), and Jürg Grundlehner, 23 August 2017.
71 See, for example, StATG, 9'40, 3.0.1/3, *Thurgauer Volksfreund*, 28 June 1973, insert.
72 See, for example, StATG, 9'40, 1.0.3/0, 131–136, 31 January–20 March 1973.
73 StATG, 9'40, 3.0.1/3, *Thurgauer Volksfreund*, 28 June 1973, insert. From the sources we examined, it is not clear how Stadelmann arrived at this information.
74 See, for example, StATG, 9'10, 1.2.8/6 and 9'10, 1.2.8/7, Kuhn to Government Councillor Alfred Abegg and Cantonal Physician Julius Bütler, 19 July 1972, 6 March 1973, 30 April 1973, 1 August 1973, 22 August 1973; 4'802'139, Sanitätsdepartement, Allgemeine Akten, 1972, §251, correspondence with Bruno Stadelmann; 4'802'151, Sanitätsdepartement, Allgemeine Akten, 1973, §475, Interpellation Gross.
75 See also StATG, 9'40, 1.0.1/3, Kuhn's statement on parliamentary criticism of the Münsterlingen Psychiatric Clinic, 1 August 1973, 7, 42.
76 Kuhn created the small employee newsletter – referred to as a *Mitarbeiterbrief* – after taking over the clinical directorate. In the first issue he justified its introduction by noting that 'it is no longer possible for the director to cultivate a personal relationship with every individual assistant'. He was therefore choosing the format of an employee newsletter 'to address all of you from time to time and to inform you about facts and problems of our joint everyday work and to announced certain guidelines'; StATG, 9'40, 1.0.4/0, Mitarbeiterbrief no. 1, 1 July 1971, 1.
77 StATG, 9'40, 1.0.1/3, Kuhn's statement on the parliamentary criticism of the Münsterlingen Psychiatric Clinic, 1 August 1973, 10–17. Also in his survey of the clinic's history, Kuhn wrote retrospectively that he had cultivated a 'fully open leadership style'; Kuhn, 'Geschichte', 110.
78 StATG, 9'40, 1.0.1/3, Kuhn's statement on the parliamentary criticism of the Münsterlingen Psychiatric Clinic, 1 August 1973, 1, 8–9, 36–37.

79 *Ibid.*, appendix.
80 Interview with Uwe Moor, 15 November 2016.
81 See, for example, StATG, 9'40, 1.0.1/3, Kuhn's statement on the parliamentary criticism of the Münsterlingen Psychiatric Clinic, 1 August 1973; 9'40, 1.0.3/0, 22, 42, 98, 130, 132.
82 StATG, 4'802'139, Sanitätsdepartement, Allgemeine Akten, §251, correspondence with Bruno Stadelmann.
83 StATG, 9'10, 1.1.0/60, ARM 1975, 8.
84 Kuhn, 'Beobachtungen', foreword, vi.
85 Kuhn, 'Erkennung', 7–8, 10. On the main symptom of daily fluctuation, see Chapter 2, 80.
86 StATG, 9'10, 1.1.0/60, ARM 1979, 16.
87 StATG, 9'40, 3.0.3/9, Kuhn to Byk-Gulden, 8 March 1975.
88 See, for example, StATG, 9'10, 1.2.11/6.3, query of Cilag Chemie regarding the testing of an otherwise unidentified preparation, 30 May 1973.
89 Swissmedic archive, documentation on Ludiomil.
90 Interview with Jules Angst, 5 September 2016.
91 Interview with a former assistant physician of the Münsterlingen Psychiatric Clinic, 17 January 2018; interview with René Bloch, 14 March 2018.
92 Kielholz, *Depressive Zustände*, 206.
93 Ciba Aktiengesellschaft, *Entspannung*; Ciba Aktiengesellschaft, *Entspannungstherapie*; Kielholz, *Die larvierte Depression*; Birkmayer, *Anfall*; Kielholz, *Betablocker*.
94 StATG, 9'40, 3.0.3/9, Kuhn to Byk-Gulden, 8 March 1975.
95 StATG, ZA KAa 24598, Verena Kuhn to the referring doctor, 31 January 1975.
96 See Kuhn, 'Die psychotrope Wirkung', 268 (quote); Kuhn-Gebhart, 'Die psychotrope Wirkung', 263.
97 StATG, ZA KAa 24598; 9'40, 4.7/3, Kuhn's notes regarding three 'Trasicor patients', undated. As of spring 1980, the girl was evidently being attended to by the child psychiatry service of the Canton of Zurich (as well as by the psychiatrist).
98 For the expansion of approvals, long applications for changes to the text in the package leaflets could evidently be submitted to the IKS; by the late 1970s, they were directed at both patients and doctors. The expansion of indications was not applied for or approved as such. Instead, the company applied for a new package leaflet, which listed the corresponding indication.
99 Swissmedic archive, documentation on Trasicor.

100 See the numerous hits produced by a literature search on the key word Trasicor or Oxprenolol in Pubmed, the database of the US National Library of Medicine and the National Institutes of Health of the United States.
101 Kielholz, ed., *Betablocker*, opening address, 9. Anxiolytic: relieving states of anxiety and tension.
102 Kielholz, *Betablocker*, 139–140, 163–164, 174–175; StATG, 9'40, 7.0/22; 9'40, 8.2/104.
103 StATG, 9'40, 1.0.3/0, 89, 9 May 1972.
104 StATG, 9'40, 4.7/3, handwritten list 'Trasicor', undated (1974).
105 See, for example, StATG, 9'10, 6.2/33754, Verena Kuhn to treating family doctor, 24 March 1975; ZA KAa F 19824, 17765, Verena Kuhn to the treating psychiatrist, 18 August 1975; ZA KAa 34583, Verena Kuhn to the patient, 14 August 1975.
106 StATG, ZA KAa 30460, Verena Kuhn to treating family doctor, 11 November 1975.
107 Kielholz, *Betablocker*, 139–140, 163–164, 174–175. StATG, 9'40, 7.0/22; 9'40, 8.2/104.
108 StATG, 9'40, 5.0.4/17, Ciba-Geigy to Kuhn, 21 January 1976.
109 CA Novartis, Ciba-Geigy, PH 4.00.2, Division Pharma. Forschung: Protokolle. Pharmaceutical research committee (PFA), PFA 12 February 1975, 2.
110 StATG, 9'40, 1.0.3/1, 52–53, 5–11 January 1975, Ciba-Geigy symposium in St Moritz; 21 and 28 January 1975.
111 StATG, 9'40, 8.1/202, Kuhn to Bein, 23 January 1975. The text is by P.K. Frederiksen, bears the title 'Preliminary Report Concerning Lioresal (Baclofen) in the Treatment of Schizophrenia', and has a personal greeting from the author. It appeared in March 1975 in *The Lancet*.
112 StATG, 9'40, 5.0.4/15, Kuhn's handwritten list with the title 'Lioresal', undated (first half of 1975).
113 *Ibid.*, file note on the administration of Lioresal as of 18 February 1975.
114 StATG, ZA KAs 20241, 27 February 1975 (underlining in the original). Defect schizophrenia: schizophrenia with a chronic progression that is accompanied by the irreversible degeneration of mental capabilities.
115 StATG, 9'40, 1.0.3/1, 72, 26 August 1975.
116 StATG, 9'40, 5.0.4/15, Kuhn's handwritten list with the heading 'Lioresal', undated (first half of 1975). The category 'chronic schizophrenia' also included various mixed diagnoses.
117 StATG, 9'40, 8.1/203. See also Kuhn, 'Carbamazepin'.

118 StATG, 9'40, 1.0.3/1, 80, 6–7 November 1975.
119 StATG, 9'40, 5.0.4/15; 9'40, 5.0.4/16.
120 In the 1970s, the number of patients treated by the research department also continuously declined at the Psychiatric University Hospital Zurich. Rietmann et al., 'Medikamentenversuche', 214.

# 7

# Fatal incidents

In the Münsterlingen Psychiatric Clinic, incidents repeatedly occurred that were related to the administration of test substances or medications. Problems could arise if a substance was dangerous, if it led to difficult-to-control reactions or had undesirable effects, if someone could not tolerate a test preparation or combination of substances, if the dosage was too high, or if a substance was administered or ingested inadvertently. Moreover, when it came to test substances, whether they could lead to long-term harm – for example, damaging the liver or affecting the blood count – was mostly unknown.

Both test substances and approved medications can have undesired consequences. The longer and more widely a drug is used, the greater the knowledge about its risks and side-effects, such as when it is combined with other substances. For a drug to be approved, one must verify that the risks and side-effects stay within certain limits as defined by the authorities. Once a medication is on the market, other regulations kick in to continually improve its safety. For test substances it is different. Effects must first be worked out in clinical trials and distinguished from undesired effects, which are then classified as side-effects.

Problems such as weight gain and dry mouth, which occurred both with approved medications as well as test substances, were considered rather minor side-effects, which one accepted or tried to counter with other medications or by varying dosages. But sometimes the side-effects were so strong that the treatment was discontinued. Now and then serious complications arose at Münsterlingen that had longer or permanent consequences or even led to death. For the doctors, however, the causes of these complications mostly seemed unclear or at least inconclusive. They recognised certain symptoms and perhaps clarified one or the other. In addition, an autopsy was performed at the clinic in the case of every fatality. But rarely did these investigations lead to unequivocal conclusions. Complications remained a matter of interpretation and were virtually never linked to test substances.

Along with ignorance that was supposed to be transformed into knowledge, there were also other forms of not-knowing at Münsterlingen. The aforementioned risks[1] associated with the administration of new or largely unfamiliar substances could be described as a structural not-knowing intrinsic to substance trials that cannot be eliminated but only kept in bounds. Beyond that, however, one can also identify wilful not-knowing, as well as inventories of knowledge that were ignored, repressed, hidden, or presented in a distorted manner.[2]

This chapter looks at such phenomena of not-knowing. The focus is on incidents with a fatal outcome, which are taken from the entire investigation period.[3] In most of these cases, it is difficult to assess retroactively why the patients died and whether the test substances played a role. Furthermore, the sources usually do not address the fatalities in great detail. Thus the following does not try to get at the 'actual' causes of death but rather considers whether patterns can be discerned with regard to the fatalities we found. Can the cases be divided into specific groups? Under which circumstances was a connection made to the medication in question? How was information about fatalities reported?

## Numbers and groups

To estimate the fatalities among Münsterlingen test patients, a quantitatively representative sample of medical files needed to be selected and investigated. But in the absence of resources, we only looked into incidents and fatalities that came to light as we worked through the sources: clues can be found in Kuhn's private archive, which, for instance, includes lists of names for specific preparations in which individual patients are marked with the symbol '†' for deceased. Other incidents are mentioned in his correspondence and in reports to the pharmaceutical industry. When one considers that the trials involved well over 1,000 patients and the administration of several million units of test substances, relatively few incidents and fatalities are recorded in Kuhn's private archive. However, we also came across incidents and fatalities in medical and clinic files that do not show up at all in Kuhn's private archive – his documentation therefore features gaps in this respect too.[4] The number of unrecorded cases is difficult to estimate.

All told, when working with the sources we came across thirty-six people who died during or shortly after the administration of test substances. The analysed cases can be divided into three groups. The first consists of eight cases where there are no indications that the doctors asked whether the patient's death might be linked to the test preparation.[5] In 1951, for example, one of the first patients who received Geigy White died. When the physical condition of the long-time schizophrenic patient suddenly deteriorated, the substance was discontinued. But a connection between the problems that arose is not explicitly considered in the patient's medical history; the treating physician assessed the effect of G 22150 positively. Shortly thereafter, an umbilical hernia operation was performed, which resulted in complications that led to a lung infection and ultimately death.[6] Another female patient, who suffered from depression and received test preparations during her third stay at the Münsterlingen clinic, committed suicide in 1968 while on leave. The sources provide no indication that anyone considered whether the suicide could be traced back – even just in part – to the administered substances. The patient had already been taking two drugs – Keto and Ciba 34276, the later Ludiomil – for a year; previously, other drugs had been discontinued because they had triggered severe side-effects.[7]

The second group – half of the cases we investigated – consists of patients whose deaths were likewise not seen as linked to test substances. But in contrast to the first group, these were people who received the test preparations while already on the brink of death.[8] Almost all were elderly, seriously physically ill men who received various Geigy substances in the second half of the 1950s and are included on lists of test patients from Ward U.[9] The fact that we know of more fatalities of men than of women therefore undoubtedly has to do with the surviving records; presumably, there was a comparable number of fatalities among female test patients in the corresponding women's wards (Figure 7.1).

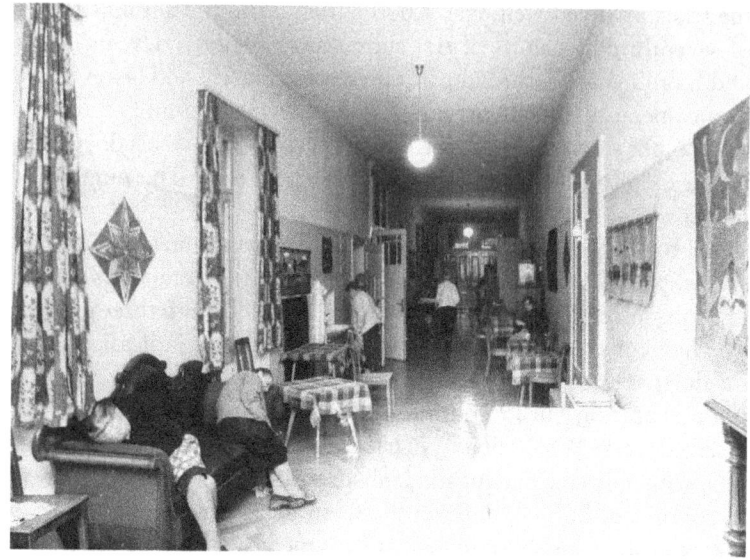

Figure 7.1 Corridor of a ward for chronically ill and disabled women, 1980

Why did Kuhn take the risk of administering test substances to patients in poor general health, and what did he expect to accomplish? Until into the 1970s, the sought-for effect and dosage of a substance when a trial began was far less clear than it is today. Thus in many Münsterlingen trials – all the more so in preliminary testing – the initial goal was to gain knowledge about tolerability, effects, and side-effects. Kuhn's test reports always have a section on side-effects and or case descriptions in which a distinction is made between positive and negative effects. At least into the 1960s, many psychiatric professionals viewed side-effects as a possible sign for a substance's effectiveness.[10] This applied particularly to physical reactions and to neuroleptics; for this substance group, side-effects signalled that something was happening, that a change was being brought about.

Some substances, however, were not associated simply with side-effects but also with major risks. In such cases, the pharmaceutical companies or Kuhn himself weighed whether these risks seemed manageable, appropriate, or too great. Kuhn interpreted risks in much the same way as side-effects. In his eyes, they did not necessarily prevent a preparation from reaching market readiness but rather could very well augur huge potential and great effectiveness.

Chronic patients with poor prognoses were therefore often included at the start of a new trial. In doing so, Kuhn was trying to learn about the substance's tolerability, determine the appropriate dosage, and get a feel for whether the preparation showed any effect that could be discerned with the naked eye. For him, a poor prognosis also precluded any spontaneous recovery, thus ensuring that the progression of the disease could not distort the substance's effect. To observe the effectiveness more precisely, he then searched for other patients, such as those who could provide better information and responded more strongly.[11] At a therapeutic level, in his dealings with patients who were severely ill and difficult to care for, the hope that they could be sedated with the help of a test substance sometimes shines through. But other long-proven medications would also have been available for this purpose. However the motives were weighed in an individual case, Kuhn presumably felt that there was no longer much to be lost here and, in the best-case scenario, the administered test substances would have a positive effect.

The third group consists of ten patients – around 28 per cent of the analysed fatalities – for whom the sources contain remarks on the cause of death and on a possible link with the administration of test substances.[12] Here, a precise analysis can bring to light deeper results, especially since the cases cover the entire investigation period. Our question is whether anyone thought about if the administered test substances were dangerous or, in fact, too dangerous. What did the communications with the outside world look like? Which actors were informed about the fatality, the administered substances, and any deliberations on a possible connection? And is it possible to detect any change through the decades?

## Dangerous test preparations? Kuhn's deliberations

The ten fatalities where a connection to the administration of test substances was considered occurred between 1947 and 1970; thus they span a period of almost twenty-five years. Eight patients were hospitalised in Münsterlingen at the time of their death; two were undergoing outpatient treatment but had already been looked after as inpatients several times. At the time of their death, all of the patients had already been treated at the Münsterlingen Psychiatric Clinic for a long or very long time (between one and thirty-four years) and were very well known there.

Three of the ten fatalities were patients in a poor general health. In their case, deliberations on a possible connection between the test preparation and death are found only in Kuhn's report to the pharmaceutical industry, but not in the medical files. Two of these three patients died in 1947 and 1949, respectively; both were men who, after the trial with Parpanit, continued to be treated with this substance and died in the process. As he wrote in an evaluation on the long-time effect of the preparation, however, Kuhn did not see a connection between the treatment and either patient's death.[13] Regarding the third patient – a man who died of cirrhosis of the liver in 1967 at age 73 – Kuhn pondered vis-à-vis Roche whether the rapidly advancing jaundice was caused by the longstanding administration of Largactil. During the 'trial period', Kuhn reported to the company, the patient had shown initial symptoms of icterus and died within just a few days. But the jaundice falls 'completely beyond consideration with regard to side-effects of your preparation'. According to Kuhn, it was caused by a liver carcinoma. The medical file does not even mention the test preparation Ro 6-5136, which was being given to the patient shortly before his death.[14]

The other seven cases – four women and three men – were people who died very suddenly.[15] That these cases in particular are well documented is hardly surprising, for one must assume that their sudden deaths sparked discussions and deliberations that also found their way into the files. A further reason could be their age. Except for one 70-year-old female patient, they were all relatively young (27 to 52 years). It is also immediately apparent that all of the conclusive remarks in the patient histories are by Kuhn – not by the treating doctor, for example, or by the clinical director. In this context, too, Zolliker is nowhere to be found.

Kuhn usually recorded his deliberations in the medical history several months or years after a patient's death. Josef Wenger, for instance, was admitted to the clinic in 1953. He suffered from schizophrenia and in 1956 initially received Geigy Green for five weeks, and then Geigy Red – the later Tofranil – for several days. As the cure started with Geigy Green, the nursing report and medical history both similarly noted that the patient was refusing the new drug.[16] Shortly thereafter, the man stopped eating and drinking, and then he fell into a catatonic stupor, an akinesia that 'the Geigy medications no longer addressed'.[17] Ten days later, Josef Wenger suffered a circulatory collapse and died. The pathological institute that performed the autopsy was not told about the medications, and nor was Geigy.

Josef Wenger's death evidently still occupied Kuhn seven years later. Reflecting back on the case in 1962, he concluded that the circulatory collapse was presumably not due to the administered medications but rather to the catatonic stupor. Although not categorically ruling out the possibility that Geigy Red and Green had negatively impacted the patient's condition, he emphasised, however, that there were 'no severe toxic brain changes'. In his opinion, this finding spoke against the idea that the death could be linked to the medication.[18]

In a few cases, Kuhn made his entries shortly after the patient's death. In 1966, for example, Regina Gerber was admitted by her family physician to the Cantonal Hospital Frauenfeld because of a high fever, respiratory distress, and oedemata. One week later she died, 35 years old, of severe liver damage that caused inner bleeding. Ever since 1952, she had repeatedly been under psychiatric treatment as an inpatient or outpatient, with a diagnosis that read 'depression in a hysterical, infantile psychopath'. At Münsterlingen, she had received numerous psychotropic drugs, including three test substances; most recently, however, she had also ingested, as self-medication, high doses of a laxative.[19]

Soon after her death, Kuhn wrote as follows in her medical history.

> On the basis of the knowledge of the entire case, one can consider whether the massive use of laxatives ... could have led to a cirrhosis of the liver. Then one must naturally also ask whether the many psychotropic drugs could have brought about liver damage. But it must be noted that, to our knowledge, the patient never had icterus [a medical term for jaundice].

Although the autopsy record – a post-mortem was performed on Regina Gerber in Winterthur – refers to the patient's high consumption of medications, it only mentions approved substances. The changes to the liver could not be more closely determined because the postmortem decomposition was too advanced and no tissue sample had been taken after her death. Aetiological conclusions were therefore impossible; but from the medical examiner's perspective, there were 'nonetheless ... certain indications for a medicamentous-toxic' cause. In short, a drug may have caused her death.[20] No comments were made about these results in the psychiatric medical history.[21]

Kuhn's conclusion – that it was admittedly possible but unlikely that the administered psychotropic drugs caused or at least contributed to the patient's death – is also found in the other five cases. The sources we examined therefore give the impression that Kuhn basically did not, or did not want to, link fatalities to psychotropic drugs. In most of the cases (twenty-six out of thirty-six fatalities), there is no sign that he even took such a connection into consideration. In the files that contain the corresponding deliberations, Kuhn admittedly sometimes tacked back and forth, but he always came to a negative conclusion. This attitude was condensed into a linguistic pattern that Kuhn repeatedly used: 'one must naturally ask' whether the administered drug is related to the fatality, 'but' one can immediately deny this in the next sentence. There are no indications that Kuhn's assessment was any more cautious when dealing with test substances than with approved medications. At the very least, he felt that the deaths of patients who additionally suffered from physical diseases or who took more than one preparation were unclear. Cases that Kuhn himself would have found straightforward are thus no doubt hard to find, if only because combining several substances was the norm at Münsterlingen.

## Explaining fatalities: Information practices

When patients die, this not only raises the question of the cause of death. It is also necessary to inform relatives, authorities, and perhaps also other doctors or the pharmaceutical industry. Since the pharmaceutical companies were working towards developing and selling drugs with the fewest possible risks, they were interested in learning about severe incidents or fatalities if there was any possibility they could be traced back to an administrated drug. This applied both to test substances and to approved medicines. In Switzerland, as of 1965 such cases had to be reported to the Swiss Academy of Medical Sciences (SAMS), which conducted investigations and then issued recommendations to the relevant companies, the Intercantonal Office for the Control of Medicines, and the Swiss Medical Association (FMH).[22] How did Münsterlingen communicate to the outside world about fatalities? Who informed whom about what?

Deborah Lang's death was discussed with many actors. The patient died in 1958 at age 27. She had been injected with Trilafon, an antipsychotic drug approved since 1957, which led to an acute cardiac arrest.[23] The patient had been admitted to the clinic in 1950; her diagnoses ranged from depression through psychopathy to schizophrenia. During her eight-year stay at the clinic, she had been given a wide array of substances over a long period of time – including the test substances Geigy White, Red, and Pink. Deborah Lang's relatives were told that the reason for the 'sudden cardiac arrest' was an unknown heart condition. The immediate cause had been an 'additional stress', like that which arises during a more acute phase of such a mental disorder or in the case of physical exertion.[24] In communications with the family, therefore, the test substances were no more mentioned than were the Trilafon injections she had been given just before she died.

Writing to Geigy, however, Kuhn noted that the patient had 'for years at times [received] large quantities of Tofranil'. 'In the last months before her death, she almost continuously had ca. 25 mg of Tofranil a day, but aside from that 25 mg G 31406 [Geigy Pink] and also aside from that all kinds of sleep medications and sedatives.' Despite this mention of test substances and approved psychotropic drugs, Kuhn nonetheless linked Deborah Lang's sudden death to heart damage. The reason Geigy learned about the patient's death was related to a query from the company that arrived at Münsterlingen shortly after the fatality. Kuhn was asked whether it was possible and worthwhile to examine the brain 'of a patient treated over a longer time with Tofranil'. He responded that her case would admittedly be suitable for such an examination, 'but [would] probably be too ambiguous for one to be able to declare anything'.[25]

Deborah Lang's death strongly preoccupied Kuhn. At the clinic, people were deeply moved by the sudden death of the young, long-time patient. Even the supervisory commission was informed (no such corresponding documentation exists for other cases), but it evidently made no inquiries.[26] According to Kuhn, the death was 'very unpleasant' for the clinic.[27] Deliberations on the cause of death are not only found in the patient's medical history and in the correspondence with Geigy and the patient's relatives; Kuhn also questioned specialists at other institutions. He informed Manfred Bleuler, the director of the Burghölzli in Zurich, who likewise knew the patient; he contacted the director of a German university hospital where someone had died of a 'Trilafon complication', and he discussed possible causes of death with Ernst Grünthal in Bern, a cardiologist in Geneva, and the pathologist at the Cantonal Hospital St Gallen.[28]

The last entry in the medical history was made three years after Deborah Lang's death. After brain-related findings were established in early 1962 by the Brain Anatomy Institute in Bern, Kuhn believed he could finally answer in the negative to the question of whether the administered psychotropic drugs could be linked to the death. He suspected, according to his conclusion, that the organic cardiac injury and the small area of infarction in the brain 'probably most likely might be linked to the insulin treatment that was carried out in another institution'.[29]

The case of Christine Räber, a patient who died from severe liver damage in 1970, was not discussed nearly as long. At the time of her death, she was 42 years old and for several years had suffered from Huntington's disease, an incurable, inherited affliction of the brain that is indicated externally by emotional and muscle-control disorders. She stayed at Münsterlingen for just under a year. Three months after being admitted to the clinic, the patient began being treated with SUM 3170, a preparation from the Wander company that between 1966 and 1968 was tested for psychoses and then for Huntington's. Even though Christine Räber's condition initially seemed to improve somewhat, no clear success could be identified over a longer period. The substance was replaced by an approved medication. When the patient appeared to be doing poorly again, she was put back on SUM 3170. Shortly thereafter, her physical condition quickly deteriorated and she died within a few days.[30]

The treating physician wrote a long entry in her medical history, which ended with the conclusion that the high fever was 'most likely' caused by the Huntington's disease, while 'the dystrophic exacerbation of the liver [was] no doubt most likely [caused] by the necessary high dosage of medications'.[31]

Christine Räber was actually a patient of Zolliker, who was researching the heritability of Huntington's disease. But because Zolliker was away on holiday, Wander learned about the fatality from Kuhn. Here, too, he raised the question about the cause of death.

> Naturally, the question is whether any of the administered medications could be to blame for the liver disease and thus for the death. We cannot simply determine this. ... The Huntington's chorea itself would no doubt surely have led to death in the near future, even without the liver disease. ... Overall, one can say that the preparation did in fact bring a certain improvement to the patient for months, that the discontinuation evoked a deterioration, and the resumption of the treatment brought an improvement again, even though the patient found herself in a terminal stage.

As in the case of Deborah Lang, Kuhn emphasised to Wander that Christine Räber would have died from her disease sooner or later anyway.[32]

Despite the lack of clarity over the cause of the patient's death, SUM 3170 evidently continued to be used at Münsterlingen – at any rate, another 3,000 tablets were ordered in December 1970.[33] The fatality seems to have bothered Kuhn less than Wander, for the company actually analysed the case in detail, albeit not until one year after the patient's death. But it also brought in results from other clinical trials with SUM 3170. In November 1971, the company finally produced a five-page report. If one or more medications had contributed to the patient's death, it stated, this was probably an individual intolerance, not a liver toxicity caused by 'the chemical structure' of the preparation. Among the administered preparations, Largactil, Phenergan, and SUM 3170 were considered. The fact that Christine Räber had received high doses of the test substance over nine months even though the instructions originally envisaged a treatment period of twelve weeks was never mentioned. The final conclusion, however, reads: 'Since SUM-3170 cannot be absolved with certainty, any possible relationship of SUM-3170 to liver damage should be carefully considered in the next trials.'[34]

As in the case of Deborah Lang, nothing in Christine Räber's file suggests that the family was informed about the administration of the test preparation and the possible connection with the patient's death. Although the clinic had informed relatives that the patient's condition had severely deteriorated, it linked the change to Huntington's disease: 'Very high fevers have arisen, which are connected with her nervous disorder, and her condition is not good, such that one must reckon with a fatal development.'[35]

Anna Tuchschmid suddenly came down with leukaemia in 1961 at 70 years of age, which led to her death a few days later. She suffered from endogenous depression and had been hospitalised six times between 1955 and 1961, and at the time of her death she had been taking high doses of imipramine for more than six years, first as a test substance and later as an approved medication. According to Kuhn, she was one of the first patients who was given Geigy Red, the later Tofranil; she had responded well to the treatment and had spoken about 'miracle tablets'. During her last clinic stay, she was tested for three months on Geigy Yellow, the later Insidon, but she was then put back on Tofranil because Geigy Yellow failed to show a positive effect. Since the patient had exhibited fluctuating blood counts for a long time, after her death Kuhn looked into whether a new blood count had been taken during her last hospitalisation.

> It is clear that this did not happen, which no doubt probably related to the fact that during the time in question ... there was a change of laboratory technicians and, apart from that, the move to the new medical centre took place. Apart from that, we have thought the situation over very carefully. Cf. letter to Geigy.[36]

On the same day Kuhn that made this entry in the medical history, he also told Geigy about the death. He wrote that the patient suddenly became severely ill and died of leukaemia within a few days. Then he considered whether the leukaemia could be traced back to the longstanding administration of Tofranil. 'Even though it is, of course, not very likely', he continued, 'the question arises whether the medication and especially its very long use could be connected with the illness'. Therefore, he would be interested to know whether similar observations had been reported.[37] Kuhn was evidently concerned that changes to the patient's blood count could have been linked to the ingestion of Tofranil. This fear was related to experiences with other substances that had been made at Münsterlingen and other clinics. After a test substance had led to blindness in the case of two patients at the Friedmatt in Basel, there were concerns that Geigy White could likewise lead to eye damage; later, attention focused on liver damage and blood-count changes. The testing with Geigy Yellow, however, was not mentioned to the company. The patient's medical history as recorded by the Cantonal Hospital Münsterlingen, where the patient died, only notes the repeated psychiatric treatments, making no mention of the medication.[38]

One can therefore conclude that when it came to communications with the outside world, Kuhn did not systematically and transparently investigate fatalities. The policy of selective information affected relatives of the deceased patients, the pharmaceutical companies whose substances were used, and other hospitals and doctors who were involved in the respective case. Thus even though autopsies were routinely performed on all patients who died in the clinic, the pathologists were not told if someone had received test substances. Therefore, the autopsy reports do not, as a rule, pursue the question of whether the death could be related to the medication. If for once results nonetheless arose indicating a possible connection – for example, when it was noted that there were certain signs that liver damage might have been caused by drug toxicity – this occurred in a vacuum.

## Leponex: New reactions in the 1970s

If Kuhn felt a preparation was quite promising, incidents and fatalities would not easily frighten him off. Apart from the fact that Kuhn never seemed strongly interested or disturbed by the deaths of patients in poor general health, he also tended to pay less attention to incidents and fatalities in later years compared to earlier in his career. Interestingly, this shift took place even as clinical trials became increasingly regulated over time. This is illustrated quite clearly by two cases from the 1970s, which can unequivocally be traced back to the administration of Leponex, a neuroleptic by the

Wander company that by then had already been approved. While under Leponex, the two patients, a young woman and a 74-year-old man, developed an agranulocytosis, a severe blood formation disorder, from which they soon died. In these cases, too, Kuhn made no effort to track down the causes of the agranulocytosis. But in contrast to earlier, he now found himself confronted with actors who wanted to pursue these cases, even though they did not involve a test preparation.

Sarah Linder died in 1973, just a few months after Leponex had been approved in Switzerland. Her treatment with the neuroleptic only began after the approval, thus she did not receive a test substance. Kuhn is conspicuous in her file primarily because of his absence. To be sure, he was informed about the patient's condition and treatment; she was a very young woman who suddenly became severely psychotic. He himself, however, made no entries in Sarah Linder's medical history, not even after her death, unlike other cases whose medical files contain his thoughts about the respective patient's cause of death.[39] The order for the transfer of the patient to the cantonal hospital, which is on the clinic directorate's letterhead, was written and signed by the treating assistant physician. Moreover, Kuhn, who two years earlier had taken over the management of the clinic, neglected to tell Wander about the fatality. A confidential internal company memo shows that Wander learned about Sarah Linder's death from a former assistant physician at Münsterlingen. When the company then contacted Kuhn, he responded that he had not considered it appropriate to inform Wander. 'He for his part did not report the case because the illness was so complex that any speculation about the cause of the agranulocytosis would be futile.'[40]

The assistant physician who supervised Sarah Linder's ward left Münsterlingen shortly after the patient's death. According to his own account, he had originally planned to stay there for two years but was completely dismayed by conditions at the clinic; he even contemplated suicide or quitting the profession. Kuhn had 'exploited' the patients and staff 'by hook and by crook'. His relationship with Kuhn had been extremely conflictual, which, he noted, was also true for many of the other doctors. Despite Sarah Linder's condition, only by overcoming immense opposition was he able to transfer the patient to the cantonal hospital. Her death broke the camel's back. The assistant physician resigned on the next possible date and found a new job, where he told a Wander employee about the fatality.[41]

In 1975 – two years after Sarah Lindner's death – two more cases of agranulocytosis occurred under Leponex within a short period in Finland. Wander conducted further investigations, informed the IKS, and sent out a circular letter that drew attention to the need to regularly monitor the blood count.[42] In late November, Kuhn hosted a representative of the company, with whom – as he noted in his diary – he discussed the 'problematic harmful effects of Leponex'.[43] By this time at the latest, it was clear that extreme caution was called for when administering the medication.

At Münsterlingen, however, the risks of the drug were assessed differently. Franziska Weiss, for example, left the clinic in December 1975. Her discharge medication consisted of sleeping medication, Leponex, and Trasicor, even though for years she had suffered from leukopenia, a low white blood cell count, and the ingestion of Trasicor had led to bronchitis. After being discharged, the patient continued to be supervised in the outpatient department, where the physician treating her decided during their first consultation to discontinue Trasicor. But because the leukopenia increased the risk of agranulocytosis, he felt the administration of Leponex was problematic as well and soon switched the patient to a different drug.[44]

In 1976, the 74-year-old Ulrich Tanner was admitted to the Münsterlingen Psychiatric Clinic for the first time because of persecutory delusions. He was diagnosed with old-age schizophrenia and right away given Leponex, as well as a second neuroleptic later. After three months, Ulrich Tanner had a high fever, but no infection could be found. A few days later, his white blood cell count was checked, which produced an alarming finding. The patient was immediately transferred to the cantonal hospital, where he died of agranulocytosis, however, after just a few days. Following the death, Kuhn received a report from the medical clinic of the cantonal hospital which considered the possibility of 'medicamentous-toxic agranulocytosis on Leponex' and requested the patient's psychiatric medical history.[45] Ultimately, Wander also learned about Ulrich Tanner's death, but how it did so is unclear. However, since corresponding information cannot be found either in the patient's medical file or in Kuhn's private archive, it seems likely that the company was informed by the medical clinic of the Cantonal Hospital Münsterlingen.[46]

In 1977, the Cantonal Hospital St Gallen conducted a nationwide study on haematological incidents that occurred under Leponex. When Kuhn was asked to participate in the survey, he seemed cagey.

> We had one fatality because of agranulocytosis and isolated cases of more or less asymptomatic leukopenia. We reported these cases to the Wander company. The latter analysed our cases very closely. Answering your questionnaire would be a lot of work for us, in addition our documents are in part insufficient.

Kuhn recommended contacting Wander for further information, adding that Leponex was prescribed to a great many patients at Münsterlingen. It is 'a very excellent medication' and therefore often used, 'which naturally automatically [increases] the number of dangerous complications'.[47]

The results of the study were published in 1977. The impetus for this work, according to the authors, was provided by two of the hospital's own agranulocytosis cases 'as well as the suspicion of a cluster' of cases in eastern Switzerland. The basis for this suspicion is not mentioned. The survey was sent to all of Switzerland's psychiatric clinics and acute care facilities, just under half of which responded. A total of twenty incidents were reported (eight with lethal outcomes), a few of which were unknown to the manufacturing company. The authors concluded that the cluster of cases in eastern Switzerland was 'conspicuous' but did not comment on the results. Elsewhere, however, what they thought about colleagues like Kuhn shimmers through.

> Extremely illuminating were the numerous responses to our survey, which ranged from comments such as 'Leponex was recognised as unsuitable and prohibited for any use', through interested cooperation, to indifference and refusal. In any case, we can state that neither the fact of potential lethal complications of this medication nor the need for regular blood checks are known everywhere.[48]

Thus in the 1970s, severe incidents and fatalities under test substances or medications were no longer a matter exclusively for manufacturing companies and clinical investigators. The awareness within professional circles of the residual risk of clinical trials and medications had grown, and the demand to investigate such cases as closely and systematically as possible and to discuss them was increasing. Kuhn always claimed to be able, by means of his practised gaze, to tell whether a substance was effective or not. However, according to the conclusion one can draw based on the thirty-six cases we analysed, when it came to fatalities he evidently did not look particularly closely.

That the times definitively changed in the 1970s can be seen not only from the fact that Kuhn was increasingly confronted by actors who dealt with fatalities differently than he did. At the time, psychiatry's self-perception and its perception by others was undergoing a fundamental transformation, which also influenced how patients were seen. Kuhn's authoritarian attitude seems to have therefore increasingly alienated the clinic's staff. In late 1978, for example, he ordered that a long-term patient who caused major problems for the staff needed to stay in her room unless at least four male or female nurses were nearby. A few months later, a nurse wrote under Kuhn's directive with a red pen: 'There is no more need to ask about a cancellation of this order. Prof. Kuhn is of the opinion it should remain in place forever because it does the girl good.' How long the directive applied is unclear, but certainly not 'forever'. Kuhn left the clinic in 1980 – long before the patient.[49]

## Notes

1 See, for example, Schlich and Troehler, *The Risks*; Itzen and Müller, 'Risk'; Mohun 'Constructing'.
2 The history of knowledge is increasingly examining the phenomena of ignorance, doubt, or agnotology; see Proctor and Schiebinger, *Agnotology*; Croissant, 'Agnotology'.
3 For a careful historical classification and assessment of the analysed cases, it would also be necessary to investigate deaths of patients who did not receive any test substances. These results then would have to be compared with results from other psychiatric clinics.
4 Whether Kuhn documented incidents and fatalities in his study documents no doubt strongly depended on whether these occurred before or after his reporting to the pharmaceutical industry.
5 StATG, 9'10, 5.4/2951; 9'10, 5.4/12687; 9'10, 5.4/13552; 9'10, 5.4/14539; ZA KAs 17160 (at the same time ZA KAa 18360); ZA KAs

17889; ZA KAs 17952 (at the same time 9'10, 6.2/3306); ZA KAs 17160 (at the same time ZA KAa 18360).
6. StATG, 9'10, 5.4/2951.
7. StATG, ZA KAs 17952. More recently, a correlation has been shown between certain antidepressants and an increased suicidal tendency; hence, according to today's criteria, a link between a test substance and suicide would not be ruled out. However, other factors would also need to be considered.
8. StATG, 9'10, 5.4/10488; 9'10, 5.4/13022; 9'10, 5.4/13599; 9'10, 5.4/13820; 9'10, 5.4/13837; 9'10, 5.4/13840; 9'10, 5.4/13849; 9'10, 5.4/13923 (at the same time 9'10, 6.2/7591); 9'10, 5.4/13953; 9'10, 5.4/14017 (at the same time 9'10, 6.2/3727); 9'10, 5.4/14145; 9'10, 5.4/14187; 9'10, 5.4/14202; 9'10, 5.4/14296; 9'10, 5.4/14631; 9'10, 5.4/14699; 9'10, 5.4/14743 (at the same time 9'10, 6.2/9093); ZA KAs 18879.
9. See Chapter 2, 77–78.
10. See, for example, Schmuhl and Roelcke, 'Heroische Therapien'.
11. On this patient hierarchy, see Chapter 4, 146.
12. StATG, 9'10, 5.4/8168; 9'10, 5.4/10205; 9'10, 5.4/11783; 9'10, 5.4/13569; 9'10, 5.4/14182; 9'10, 5.4/14808; ZA KAs 15568 (at the same time 9'10, 6.2/3891); ZA KAs 15810 (at the same time 9'10, 6.2/139); ZA KAs 17303 (at the same time 9'10, 6.2/5832.1/2); ZA KAs 18871.
13. StATG, 9'10, 5.4/10205; 9'10, 5.4/11783; 9'40, 50.0.3/3, Kuhn's expert evaluation to Geigy, 20 June 1949.
14. StATG, 9'10, 5.4/8168; 9'40, 5.0.7/5, Kuhn to Dr Foglar, 29 September 1967.
15. StATG, 9'10, 5.4/13569; 9'10, 5.4/14182; 9'10, 5.4/14808; ZA KAs 15568; ZA KAs 15810 (at the same time 9'10, 6.2/139); ZA KAs 17303 (at the same time 9'10, 6.2/5832.1/2); ZA KAs 18871.
16. StATG, 9'10, 5.4/14182.
17. *Ibid.*, summary, undated (spring 1956).
18. *Ibid.*, 12 March 1962.
19. StATG, 9'10, 6.2/5832; ZA KAs 17303. It was known that the patient ate little and, when outside the clinic, took high doses of laxatives that led to severe diarrhoea.
20. *Ibid.*, 27 January 1966; discharge report of the Cantonal Hospital Frauenfeld, 14 February 1966; 9'10, 9.1/16, autopsy report of the Pathological Institute of the Cantonal Hospital Winterthur, 24 January 1966.
21. StATG, ZA KAs 17303, 11 January 1966. Jaundice would have suggested damage to the liver. The ingestion of certain substances can

## Fatal incidents

lead to liver damage, especially if the ingestion occurs in high doses and over a long period. For test substances, the risk of liver damage is still unclear or not as clear as for approved medications.

22  CA Novartis, Geigy, PP 12/3, Produktion Pharma, pharma committee minutes 2/65, 2 February 1965, 5. For more detailed information, see Chapter 4, 121–122.
23  StATG, 9'10, 5.4/14808.
24  StATG, 9'10, 5.4/14808.2, Kuhn to the patient's family, 28 March 1959.
25  StATG, 9'40, 5.0.3/11, Kuhn to Oberholzer, Geigy, 24 November 1958.
26  StATG, 4'840'33 Aufsichtskommission, Protokolle 1935–1964, minutes of the two-person supervisory commission delegation of 26 November 1958, 2.
27  StATG, 9'40, 5.0.3/11, Kuhn to M. Bleuler, Zurich Psychiatric Clinic, 27 November 1958; 9'10, 5.4/14808.2, Kuhn to patient's family, 21 November 1958.
28  StATG, 9'40. 5.0.3/11, Kuhn to Prof Flügel, Erlangen Psychiatric Clinic, 27 November 1958; Kuhn to E. Grünthal, Waldau Psychiatric Clinic, Bern, 13 January 1958, 31 May 1960; Kuhn to M. Bleuler, Zurich Psychiatric Clinic, 27 November 1958; Kuhn to G. Pilleri, Waldau Brain Anatomy Institute, Bern, 2 March 1962; Grünthal to Kuhn, 12 January 1959; pathological institute of the cantonal hospital to Zolliker, 23 December 1958. *Ibid.*, 9'10, 5.4/14808.1–2, 21 November 1958–8 March 1962; Kuhn to the patient's family, 28 March 1959.
29  StATG, 9'40. 5.0.3/11, Kuhn to G. Pilleri, Waldau Brain Anatomy Institute, Bern, 2 March 1962.
30  StATG, ZA KAs 18871.
31  *Ibid.*, 12 August 1970.
32  StATG, 9'10, 9.5/4, Kuhn to Wander, 17 September 1970.
33  StATG, 9'10, 1.2.11/6.3, Kuhn to Wander, 19 December 1970.
34  StATG, 9'10, 9.5/4, Wander to Zolliker, 29 and 30 September 1969; Kuhn to Wander, 13 August 1971; Wander to Kuhn, 30 December 1971, including report of 3 November 1971.
35  StATG, ZA KAs 18871, letter to the patient's family, 10 August 1972.
36  StATG, 9'10, 6.2/139; ZA KAs 15810, 27 February 1956 and 2 March 1962 (quotes); 9'40, 5.0.3/10, typescript on G 22355, undated.
37  StATG, 9'40, 5.0.3/15, Kuhn to Rothweiler, Geigy, 2 March 1962.
38  *Ibid.*; 9'40, 5.0.3/10, copy of the patient's medical history of the Cantonal Hospital Münsterlingen, including results of the autopsy.
39  StATG, 9'40, 1.0.3/0, 131, 3 and 4 February 1973.

40 StATG, ZA KAs 20371, copy of a file note of the Wander company, 28 September 1973, that a Wander employee sent to Kuhn as information on 29 September 1973. In the cover letter, the man promises that, apart from the director of Wander's medical office, only the management of the research office for human toxicology of the Sandoz corporation will learn about the case.

41 Interview with a former assistant physician of the Münsterlingen Psychiatric Clinic. In the interview, the man actively recalled the patient's name, age, and date of death, but said he assumed that Kuhn, too, had reported the case to Wander.

42 StATG, 9'40, 5.1.1/7, circular letter of Wander company, 4 September 1975.

43 StATG, 9'40, 1.0.3/1, 82, 28 November 1975.

44 StATG, ZA KAa 34377/II, 4 May 1976.

45 StATG, ZA KAs 21863, report of the medical clinic of the Cantonal Hospital Münsterlingen to the directorate of the Münsterlingen Psychiatric Clinic, 15 September 1976.

46 StATG, 9'10, 9.5/4, medical office of the Wander company to Kuhn, 26 October 1976.

47 *Ibid.*, Kuhn to Dr Senn, Cantonal Hospital St Gallen, 15 February 1977. See also Senn et al., 'Clozapine'. At least for the example mentioned above, Kuhn's statement that the cases were reported to Wander is not true. Our sample does not include any other agranulocytosis cases.

48 Jungi et al., 'Gehäufte durch Clozapin', 1862. See also Senn et al., 'Clozapine'. The two cases of agranulocytosis at St Gallen were observed within a three-month period.

49 StATG, ZA KAs 18288, report decision of 15 December 1978, addendum dated 21 February 1979.

# 8

# The 1980s: A long, restless finale

In February 1980, Kuhn retired from the Münsterlingen clinic, where just a few months earlier he had celebrated his fortieth anniversary of service. He was succeeded by Karl Studer, who came from the Psychiatric University Hospital Basel.[1] 'Unified songs of praise in the press accompanied the farewell', notes a letter to the editor; another points out that, according to the government, Kuhn 'tirelessly devoted himself in word and writing and deed ... to the new pathways in psychiatry'.[2] Signing both as author was Walter Dahinden, an engineer who had refused to perform military service and therefore spent a couple of weeks at Münsterlingen. To set a counterpoint to the many tributes, he reported on his clinic stay in various media, where he criticised not only the conditions there but also Kuhn and the government.[3]

With Kuhn's departure from the Münsterlingen Psychiatric Clinic in 1980, the setting changes for us, too. The clinic recedes into the background, and the focus turns to Kuhn's activities after his retirement, his self-perception and the perception of others, the nascent historicisation of his work and the field of psychopharmacology itself, as well as his personal preoccupation with his own biography (Figure 8.1). This shift also makes it clear that the writing of history, too, is a multilayered process involving a struggle over interpretations. The practices of collecting, storing, and archiving involve including some things and excluding many others.[4] In this respect, they resemble the filtering and translation processes in the textualisation of knowledge.[5] Who gets a chance to speak, and from whom are there surviving traces? Who is allowed to write whose history?[6] Proceeding from such methodological and theoretical considerations, this chapter looks at Kuhn's struggle for

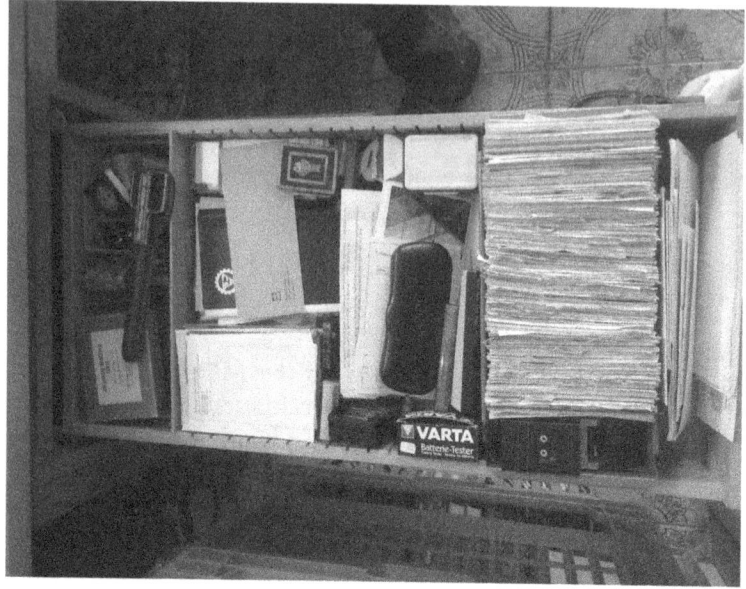

Figure 8.1 Roland Kuhn's desk drawer, 2013

one last pharmacological 'discovery' and his gradual and increasingly controversial historicisation.[7]

After Kuhn retired from the clinic, he would live for another quarter century. It was a life he spent together with his wife, cultivating friendly collegial contacts, and reaping the harvest of his indefatigable activities, and it gave him the opportunity to reflect on a broad field of experiences and accomplishments. But one searches in vain for signs of him taking stock of his life, or that he took satisfaction with what he had accomplished. Much more frequently, Kuhn shifted into a sullen and plaintive tone. His perspective on contemporary psychiatry became increasingly critical, with him portraying an image of decline. He evidently did not notice that this entailed the collective denigration of the younger generation. In his opinion, psychopharmacology was in an equally tragic state. 'Forty years ago, Switzerland was a world leader in this field; today one does nothing for psychopharmacology.'[8] So radically did Kuhn summarise the situation in early 2001. In this case, he was not wrong. Huge changes had taken place in the pharmaceutical industry. The companies he had worked with – Geigy, Ciba, Wander, Sandoz – no longer existed in their old form. Since the merger of Ciba-Geigy and Sandoz in 1996, all that remained of the companies he had worked with most was Novartis,[9] where the 'great strategy' of restructurings and takeovers was what mattered most. Any interest in past accomplishments had disappeared. Apart from Novartis, there was naturally Hoffmann-La Roche, but Kuhn's contact network there had always been modest.

## The busy pensioner

When Kuhn took his pension in 1980, one can hardly say that he stopped working. He continued to pursue a wide range of activities and interests and was often on the go. When he left his job at the clinic, he was 68 years old. The purchase of a detached house in nearby Scherzingen cleared the way for the transition to life as a pensioner. He now had sufficient space to bring his library and extensive documents home, including many files from the clinic, particularly trial documentation and patient medical files (taking the latter was illegal).[10] In 1980, he opened a private practice in his home.

At first, he maintained a close relationship with the clinic, all the more so since his wife continued working there until her own retirement in 1983.[11] It was within walking distance, and Kuhn often came by to ask for copies of articles from specialised journals. Moreover, he needed to use the clinic laboratory, for, with the help of a German doctor, he wanted to complete a biochemical study he had started that dealt with noradrenaline metabolism in depressive patients. To this end, Kuhn set up a freezer in the clinic for urine samples, which, with the knowledge of his successor, he had analysed by a laboratory technician.[12]

Thus many things stayed the same after Kuhn's retirement, including his regular lectures at the University of Zurich, which Kuhn finally ended in July 1998 with a farewell lecture ('Science and Art in Psychiatry: After Forty Years') that harkened back to his inaugural lecture in early 1959.[13] The Wednesday philosophical roundtable of a small circle of faithful, where he also lectured, met for even longer.[14]

Kuhn possessed an extensive archive; he was forever the fastidious documentarian of his own activities. After retiring from the clinic, he privately engaged a secretary to help him set up a new classification system adapted to his current interests.[15] He collected widely according to persons and topics – careful clippings of newspaper articles, technical articles, advertisements, and book announcements. He underlined things he found important, never without a ruler. He started using a computer in 1987 and even learned how to use email.[16] He dutifully answered letters – and resented it when his own letters went unanswered. He repeatedly turned to the cantonal library in Frauenfeld with complicated bibliographical search requests and with copy jobs to expand his own holdings.[17] 'I am naturally collecting statements about me. Of those there are many that I do not all have. Every link in this chain of publications about me is very valuable to me.'[18] Sometimes he nonetheless got lost in his self-constructed labyrinth of files – and this too he documented with a note: 'Somewhere there is even more under this key word. I do not know where to look today! 8.XI.04. R. Kuhn.'[19]

His retirement from the clinic, however, also meant that he had more time, which was something he had hoped for. In late 1980, he wrote that he was now already enjoying 'a little more freedom', but then immediately qualified his statement.

> But I still have a private practice and various obligations, so I am fully occupied and far from being able to do what I would actually like to do, especially scientifically, and what I also believe I should do. But I still hope, as in previous decades, for better times.[20]

The hope remained unfulfilled. His correspondence is replete with repeated references to countless appointments, conferences, and lectures, in conjunction with small journeys that he usually took with his wife. One moment he complained about the permanent stress, and the next he was speaking with a certain pleasure about how he was in great demand.

> I am starting to slowly adapt to my so-called retirement, practice somewhat, but have too many patients, such that not everything takes shape according to the program. I still do not know how I am going to keep doing this, for actually I would finally like to be able to do what I have always wanted to do throughout my life and was unable to do.[21]

He was driven by the desire for intellectually challenging work, not only in daseinsanalysis, which had interested him all along, but now also in the field of psychopharmacology.

The output of publications remained high. They included weighty and labour-intensive essays, now and again also of a historical nature.[22] However, he was unable to realise the dream of a larger publication. For a time, he pursued the idea, which arose in the 1970s, of publishing a text book together with his friend Hugo Bein.[23] But when they simply could not get anywhere with the work, Bein withdrew.[24] Kuhn pursued the project on his own for a while. 'I now already have a manuscript of over one hundred pages', he reported in 1982,

> wherein are recorded my experiences and my theoretical conceptions on psychopharmacology and which in many points are different from everything that one reads. I have therefore decided, a long time ago already, to change my entire project and to publish a text with the title: 'Studies on Psychopharmacology'. The chapter headings are very unusual, and likewise what is in the individual chapters.[25]

But the work was not as far along as this passage suggests – it was never finished.[26] In the end, there was still the hope of publishing an anthology of his most important articles. But for too long he had been busy with other matters, and now he no longer had the strength. When things did not work out with his publishing contacts, he suspected secret enemies and sabotage. 'Evidently some sort of advisors are asked each time, who have an interest in that my unusual publications are no longer distributed', he wrote in 2003.[27] Finally in 2004, with the help of his former psychiatry students, a small volume was published after all. Along with some his own essays, it also contained articles by friends and colleagues in honour of his ninetieth birthday, as well as a useful catalogue of this writings.[28]

The size of the private practice of Roland and Verena Kuhn is unknown. Both started holding consultation sessions at their home immediately after they stopped working at the clinic. At first the practice must have been quite popular, but the number of patients sharply declined in the 1990s, no doubt because of the Kuhns' age. In summer 2002, Kuhn apologised to the cantonal physician, reporting that he and his wife could no longer participate in the survey of general practitioners.

Each week I have one to two consultation hours, Vreni has a few more, but also very little, and so, with the best intentions, we cannot answer the questions posed. In recent weeks I have even received a new patient, the son of a patient whom I have been treating for decades, and have achieved a wonderful success with 10-mg Ludiomil. This gives me the courage to continue working as a doctor even at ninety years of age, even though I am naturally also very reticent.[29]

### Levoprotiline: A final trial

Thanks to crucial suggestions from Kuhn, Ciba-Geigy had achieved a major success with the approval of Ludiomil in 1972, which had immediately led to work on related substances in the hope of finding something even more effective. The period of great optimism had admittedly long since passed. The cost of developing newer substances had continuously increased and the rate of innovation had declined. At the same time, however, it was clear that maintaining Ciba-Geigy's current lead in the field of antidepressants would require a steady stream of new products. A strategic paper by the pharmaceutical division in autumn 1976 noted that, with a market share around 24 per cent, the company was among the frontrunners, just behind Merck and Sharp & Dohme and best placed internationally.[30]

> The commercially available antidepressants (our own and the competition) are moving – since Tofranil and amitriptyline – in the area of me-too [imitation products]. This has made the market so competitive that only genuine innovations can be expected to have larger sales and will be able to jump the ominous barrier of a 5–10 per cent market share.

One of the newly synthesised substances from those years, CGP 12103 A, was first introduced to the pharmaceutical research committee in June 1978.[31] They assumed that they were looking at another potential antidepressant.[32] The testing began in Germany, directed by Ciba Frankfurt, although it is unclear exactly when.[33] The broader clinical trial, which was supposed to reach its goal in five years, probably did not start until 1983. But the process became bogged down as early as 1985, when regulations were abruptly intensified as the result of a drug-related scandal at a West German hospital.³⁴ For the time being, nothing was moving, so Ciba Frankfurt looked into continuing the trials in the GDR and Czechoslovakia. This allowed work to resume by 1986. The reason for the relocation was the desire to resume the trials as quickly as possible, not the hope for lower standards – in fact, the work in the GDR tended to be performed more carefully than in West Germany.³⁵

This was the situation when, starting in summer 1986, Kuhn had another turn as an investigator. The initial contact is poorly documented. Alexandra Delini-Stula, who supervised the trial from Basel, remembers the initiative coming from Kuhn himself.³⁶ However, this raises the question of how he heard about the new substance in the first place (it came to be called levoprotiline in 1987). By this time, his formal connection with Ciba-Geigy had come to an end; the payments for his participating interest in Ludiomil had also contractually expired at the end of 1984.³⁷ But informal contacts still existed. Documented is a visit by Kuhn to Director Max Wilhelm in summer 1986, where they evidently agreed on the delivery of the new substance.³⁸ Ciba-Geigy wanted to resume the collaboration because it wanted to counter the bottleneck that had developed in the clinical trials and because the results thus far had been too ambiguous. Kuhn, for his part, had trouble understanding why the development of new antidepressants should have become so difficult (Max Wilhelm seems to have said something to that effect).

> I cannot quite understand why in your company one has such difficulties with antidepressants. Just today I read again, the World Health Organisation estimated the number of persons suffering from depression to be 3 per cent of the world population. ... Every medication that can help here somewhat surely has very good prospects, and after all, the success of Ludiomil should not be entirely disregarded.³⁹

Thus began for Kuhn the last trial of a potential antidepressant, which would occupy him for many years. Verena Kuhn was involved from the beginning, with one third of the patients coming through her; but, like always, all communications ran exclusively through her husband. Ciba-Geigy described the operation as an 'open, non-comparative, multicentred trial to comprehend the effect profile and tolerability of levoprotiline. A total of seventy to eighty patients is intended. ... The treatment should consist of at least six weeks per patient. The intended treatment period, however, is six months or longer.'[40] The additional time was at Kuhn's request – he had always felt that a trial of only a few weeks was insufficient. Since the Kuhns could not muster all of the expected patients from their private practice, they convinced a friendly colleague in Porrentruy to participate.[41] By the end of 1989, thirty-five of their own patients were taking part in the trial, thirty-one of whom are recorded by name; a large majority (twenty-four) were female. Another fifty, about whom there are no further details, joined the trial through their colleague.[42] Professors Hugo Bein in Oberwil near Basel and Boris Luban-Plozza in Locarno also participated with several patients from their private practices.[43]

Kuhn received the first 300 dragees in November 1986; at the same time, Delini-Stula referred to the inadequacy of the previous trials and what was expected of his participation: 'In all of these studies, the only criteria for therapeutic efficiency was a change of the Hamilton scores [a rating scale on the presence of depression], and you know how little this says about the quality of the effect of antidepressants. Your observations will therefore have a very particular value.'[44] Shortly thereafter, Kuhn announced the start of the trial with three patients, which he followed up in July 1987 with a 'first preliminary report'. He noted that the substance was scientifically very interesting because it encouraged reflection on the mechanism of action. Furthermore, it exhibited several tangible advantages, namely, that it did not trigger weight gain or impair the sexual function for men, as happened above all with Anafranil. Unfortunately, it also raised questions, since

> as with all of the other antidepressants, it is difficult to determine whether or not there is an effect. Sick persons, who no doubt are typically vitally depressed but do not suffer very severely from their condition, are very suggestible, [they] hope a new medication will have an effect, one must educate them about the medication so that [they] are willing to take it, they then have a pronounced expectation and then believe they can feel something that perhaps is not the case in reality. Gradually it then turns out that there are indeed a few doubts as to whether or not the effect really existed.[45]

Patient consent as Kuhn described it could evidently no longer be bypassed in the case of ambulatory patients. But another fundamental aspect had changed as well.[46] The levoprotiline trial marks the first time signed consent declarations appear in Kuhn's private archive.[47] Ciba-Geigy had created a trial protocol for the levoprotiline tests and also insisted that it be observed. 'For this trial, the ethical requirements apply as they are stipulated in the Declaration of Helsinki', it stated. The criterion of voluntary participation had to be ensured; the patients had to be 'adequately informed' about the preparation and the goal of the trial. The information had to orally presented to the patient and 'also orally explained'; the patient was supposed to 'record in writing that he has understood the information and is in agreement with the treatment'. Moreover, he or she was entitled to withdraw from the trial at any time.[48] The company thus substantially restricted the investigator's freedom. Two years later, Ciba-Geigy would further stipulate that the levoprotiline tablets were only provided for the patients individually registered on the forms.[49] The metal boxes with vast quantities of test substances were a thing of the past.

In December 1987, Kuhn gave a lecture at a Ciba-Geigy meeting in Basel, having by this time included twenty patients from his private practice in the trials.[50] 'In seven cases, the new substance could be tested on its own, in the others it was added to an already existing treatment.'[51] Kuhn tried hard to once again give a very nuanced explanation of his qualitative, individualising research method. He explained that one made more headway with this approach than with the 'exact scientific methods' (placebo-controlled, double-blind procedures, etc.), which evidently had thus far delivered very few clear results. Levoprotiline was no doubt an antidepressant 'that has roughly the same effects as other known substances. ... One can repeatedly check, compare, and weigh the available numbers, but one does not really learn anything.'[52] Fascinating, however, was the fact that levoprotiline did not prevent the reuptake of noradrenaline, one of the body's own neurotransmitters – a characteristic that was previously thought to be crucial for antidepressant action.[53] Concerning the effect, Kuhn maintained: 'In our opinion, the most important point, even with regard to a launch of the preparation, is the lack of increased appetite. Here lies one of the biggest problems of therapy with antidepressants, especially for women.'

This was also a problem with Ludiomil, 'since the preparation, as is well known, leads most strongly to weight gain'. Under certain circumstances, there even might be the potential for an application against adipositas (obesity), which would result in 'an enormous field of action'.[54]

And that was as far as it went. The tests dragged on – nothing else was said of 1988 as the originally intended year of completion. Kuhn ploughed ahead, without ever following up on the 'first preliminary report' with a more comprehensive one. Sometimes, however, he brought a few of his old favourite ideas into play again. The effect of levoprotiline, he wrote to Director Max Wilhelm in late 1987, is often not very sustained. 'I think that various tests with modified substances would be worthwhile, whereby I am thinking about making the change of the sidechain not only for Ludiomil but also in the same way for Anafranil and perhaps also for Tofranil.'[55] It was as if time had stood still – Kuhn was making good suggestions and developing commercially promising pharmacological ideas just like he had more than twenty-five years before. Except there was no longer anyone on the other side who could hear his message; the bureaucratised corporate giant no longer functioned like Geigy's earlier pharmaceutical department, where personal contact was key. Director Wilhelm found the proposals interesting, but he confessed in his delayed response that he 'no longer [had] all that much contact with the laboratories anymore' and was absorbed by larger organisational restructurings in the company.[56]

What the restructuring was all about would soon become clear. After a break in communications that lasted months, Kuhn received news in summer 1989 that Alexandra Delini-Stula had been relieved as project manager for CGP 12103. Evidently, numerous Ciba-Geigy people had been replaced, and the language now was English. Delini-Stula said her goodbyes (she went to Roche soon thereafter) and added: 'I also do not know whether the new manager of the project intends to cultivate the good tradition of our collaboration.'[57] To reengage the investigators, in December 1989 the company invited them to a meeting in Basel.[58] The new manager urged Kuhn to deliver the patient reports on the forms provided by the company. Kuhn, however, still dragged his feet. He excused himself by saying he was ill and did not deliver the reports until eight months later, in August 1990. The summarised assessment was still not yet done. According to Kuhn, the work and the necessary studies of the literature were extensive, and he did not know how long it would take him. The report would never materialise – on 26 November 1990, the company told him that the development of levoprotiline had been abandoned, effective immediately. 'The data gained from controlled studies with large numbers of patients do not indicate any statistically ensured difference in effect from placebos and also show that the antidepressant effect of levoprotiline is inferior to that of amitriptyline.' Kuhn was asked to stop treating his patients with levoprotiline.[59]

Kuhn was consternated. For a while, he continued to fight for 'his' drug, and he even won over a few allies at the company who also felt that the decision was misguided.[60] But he gradually had to accept that Basel had lost interest, and again he went through the painful experience of having a company abandon a substance that he fully believed in.[61] He was only able to negotiate a limited additional supply for patients still being treated. One year after the project was terminated, he received another 5,000 tablets. He was repeatedly asked to switch his patients to a normal commercial preparation, which particularly annoyed him because, from his perspective, no such preparation existed. 'It appears to me as if what I say and write is not considered worth taking seriously, and this makes me feel hurt.'[62] He was equally upset when he failed to get a serious response to his request to produce a joint publication to present the opposing positions. At first, the company was apparently prepared to accommodate this request. Other people would also be publishing on levoprotiline, Kuhn said. 'If one wants to prevent me from doing the same, then I feel this is not only disconcerting but also offensive and an insult to me.'[63] His earlier interactions with the company had been different; 'the gentlemen from the research department and the clinical testing came to me frequently, at least once a month, and asked about how the trials were doing'. Now, they 'simply [sat] in the office' and waited 'for results to come that deliver numbers with which one can travel to the competent authorities'.[64]

The experience with levoprotiline once more prompted Kuhn to explain why he felt the testing procedures and documentation required by the official regulations were fatal. They were 'not only worthless but also highly harmful because they virtually suppress new findings'.[65] He pointed out that 'large controlled studies' had also shown 'that imipramine was no different than a placebo', which contradicts 'totally the clinical experience of the action of imipramine on millions of ill people'.[66] In addition, Kuhn accused the current studies of lack of due care.

> If, for example, a main indication consists of the avoidance of the secondary effect of weight gain of typical antidepressants, then it is obvious that one must limit a controlled study to patients who in fact suffer from weight gain when under antidepressant therapy. ... If ... your large trial series were not carried out while taking this criterion into account, then the negative result says nothing and is completely meaningless![67]

Kuhn's criticism shows that he did not fully understand the new procedures and was methodologically confused. The 'main indication' was the use of levoprotiline as an antidepressant. Introducing a second main indication at the same time was impossible; a specific consideration of weight gain would have required a different approach.

Kuhn proposed to Ciba-Geigy that they should form a common front against state regulation and its agencies. 'This would be an outstanding example, which would show that and why the currently common research methods in psychopharmacology are failing, why it is that, for more than two decades, no clinically important progress has been achieved in psychopharmacology, and what measures must be taken to remedy this evil.'[68] Together, one needed to repudiate 'the regulations of the approval authorities that make the development of new preparations impossible, which lies not only in the interest of the sick and that of research, but above all also that of the pharmaceutical industry!'[69] Ciba-Geigy's internal responses to Kuhn's proposal are unavailable. But it easy to imagine what company insiders probably felt about the prospects of such a frontal assault against state agencies, including the powerful US authorities, which had long been decisive.

Kuhn definitely addressed points that were causing problems for the pharmaceutical companies, namely, the complicated approval process and the staggering amount of statistical evidence that was now required to verify the effectiveness of a new substance. But at the same time, his insistence on qualitative exploratory methods seemed positively outmoded. Keto was simply a poor drug, recalled the former Ciba-Geigy employee Alexandra Delini-Stula, who was well-disposed to Kuhn.[70] Laurent Maître, who worked for the same company, felt similarly. 'You show ... a certain longing for older preparations (e.g. ketimipramine, Geigy Pink, and levoprotiline)', he wrote to Kuhn in 2001.

> From my standpoint, that is, from the standpoint of a former industry person, I do not particularly view the suspension of the first two substances – despite [their] incompletely characterised, interesting qualities – with sadness, but I do that of levoprotiline – and how! Now, around ten years after the suspension of levoprotiline, I find even more than back then: that was in many respects a disastrous and not to mention very costly decision by the company.[71]

Alexandra Delini-Stula dated the loss of interest in antidepressant research as early as 1986/1987. 'I have the impression that classical psychiatric indications are slowly losing their importance for big companies because I believe, they are not considered as very profitable.'[72] A new generation of managers, more interested in commerce than in the speciality of medicine and psychiatry, had moved to the fore at Ciba-Geigy. 'There was no further active research in antidepressants. In Roche the same thing is happening in the benzodiazepine field and in Sandoz, I guess, in neuroleptic research.'[73]

Levoprotiline was thus definitively stranded,[74] another annoyance for the ageing Kuhn. 'I see how Swiss research, which in its day stood at the forefront worldwide, has now forfeited all significance', he wrote to Maître in 1996. 'At the big congress in Paris, where the future of antidepressants in the next century was discussed, there was no talk at all about Switzerland. In this regard, our country has sunk into insignificance.'[75] Maître, who was familiar with the decision-making channels at Ciba-Geigy, explained: 'Levoprotiline is a good example of repetitive industrial mistakes.' He himself, however, did not want to make any further public comments on the matter. 'My verdict was recently strengthened by a report according to which the last batch of the pure substance (or the rest of it, and it was a lot of material!) was burned: for a <u>lot</u> of money, but on the other hand technologically *lege artis* and in an environmentally friendly manner.'[76]

## The Schenker affair and the question of supervision

In 1986, as Kuhn started with the levoprotiline trial, the Thurgau healthcare system was shaken by a scandal surrounding the cantonal physician, Hans Schenker, which would take several years to make its way through the courts. Even though there were no direct ties to Kuhn, there were many indirect connections, which is why in 1989 he eventually received an official request for information. In response, Kuhn wrote a detailed declaration on his own behalf, the like of which he had never done before and would never do again.

Hans Schenker, a doctor and psychiatrist from Schaffhausen, directed the former St Katharinental Asylum for the Sick and Elderly near Diessenhofen in Thurgau, which had been renamed as an old-age and nursing home in 1966 and modernised (today it is the Clinic St Katharinental).[77] He had a part-time position there. Until he assumed the office of the Thurgau cantonal physician, he also ran a practice as a family doctor. The highly active man was involved in many fields. Along with being engaged in politics, the military, and some of the region's public associations, he was also the president of the Association of Swiss Cantonal Physicians and produced scientific publications. Indeed, one wonders how anyone could accomplish all this work.

In March 1986, a medical assistant, who worked at the same time as a laboratory technician at the institution, informed the head of the education and medical services department, Arthur Haffter, that clinical trials were being conducted at St Katharinental without the consent of the patients. It took a month before Schenker was summoned to the medical services director and confronted with the accusations. According to the corresponding file note, apart from being reported because of the 'medication trials' themselves, he was primarily accused of not having obtained the patients' consent, conveying partially falsified or contrived investigation results, and exploiting the staff and infrastructure of the cantonal establishment while at the same time obtaining compensation for himself. Schenker was prohibited from continuing the ongoing trials, effective immediately.[78] The review arranged by the cantonal government proceeded extremely discretely, entirely geared towards protecting Schenker. He was not even suspended from office during the proceedings. The medical assistant was never thanked for her courageous act – on the contrary, she was obliged to secrecy.[79] She had only been in the job for half a year when she contacted the government council. For a long time, her predecessor refused to even be questioned, fearful of the influence of the powerful Hans Schenker, who she felt could still harm her professionally. The whistleblower, on the other hand, came from a different canton. Having just moved to the area, she was evidently not yet tied into the regional networks.

Schenker had been conducting trials at St Katharinental for some fifteen years, but they were never thoroughly investigated. Instead, the statute of limitations was applied,[80] and the investigation was limited to the trials of the last five years. Neither was any effort made to question the patients as the parties most affected (supposedly none of them were of sound mind). The guidelines of the Swiss Academy of Medical Sciences (SAMS), which called for safeguarding the 'mental and physical integrity' of patients (albeit without legislative force), were not taken into account.[81] The Great Council was not informed. Not even the supervisory commission of the medical institutions learned anything about the case, which again reveals this commission's modest role, as described earlier.[82] And yet every step of the investigation uncovered new and serious offenses. Schenker had exploited the patients for his own scientific interests, delivered falsified data to the Cilag company in Schaffhausen, defrauded the canton through large-scale tax evasion, and used the staff at Katharinental, which had had to take on a heavy additional workload without ever being informed about the trials.

The disciplinary proceedings ended in September 1986 with a reprimand, the mildest possible measure. Schenker was supposed to stay in office, unless the outcome of the criminal proceedings prevented him from doing so. The public only became aroused once the Social Democratic Party learned about the affair, presumably from the ranks of the personnel of the St Katharinental care home. On 17 November 1986, a Social Democratic member of the Great Council, Thomas Onken, together with sixteen other parliamentarians, submitted an interpellation that posed numerous questions to the cantonal government. Although there was never a great public outcry, the competent medical services director, Arthur Haffter, had to inform the Great Council in detail. In March 1987,

Schenker was pressured into resigning his positions as clinical director and cantonal physician.[83]

One year later, in March 1988, the Diessenhofen District Court sentenced Schenker to an unconditional prison term of twenty-six months and a fine. Schenker challenged the verdict before the Thurgau Court of Appeal, which partially upheld the appeal and reduced the prison term to a conditional fifteen months. In addition, it concluded that the medical services department actually should have known about Schenker's research activities. It noted that Haffter's predecessor, Alfred Abegg, had mentioned the studies in 1979 in the canton administration's journal.[84] Schenker also had regularly sent copies of his published studies to the medical services department. In an interview with the *Bodensee-Zeitung*, the president of the Thurgau medical association (and later cantonal physician), Alfred Muggli, had confirmed as early as November 1986: 'Yes, in principle that was nothing mysterious, for Dr Schenker had published various results of his investigations in specialised journals. Most of the doctors in the canton therefore knew that such medications were being tested at St Katharinental.'[85]

Government Councillor Haffter defended himself, saying he had known nothing about the financial compensation for these studies, which the state's attorney hardly found convincing.

> Even just general life experience speaks against this, and moreover the administration must have been aware of the long-standing practice of the director of the Münsterlingen Psychiatric Clinic, Roland Kuhn, who with the approval of Schenker's predecessor in the office of the cantonal physician likewise received fees from the pharmaceutical industry and kept them for himself.[86]

This brought Kuhn's name into play. To get a better grasp on the Schenker case, in July 1989, two months before the verdict, the Court of Appeal turned to Kuhn with two key questions: 'For your scientific activity, did you receive compensation and reimbursements for expenses from private institutions or enterprises?'; 'With regard to the handling of these compensations and reimbursements for expenses, was there an explicit or tacit agreement with the medical services and education department, or with the cantonal physician?' Detailed questions followed as to how these agreements – if they existed – were worded, or how one had actually proceeded if no such explicit arrangement obtained. Finally: 'Did the medical services and education department or the cantonal physician have knowledge of this operation?'[87]

Kuhn responded within just a few days with a dense five-and-a-half-page text. It is a strange letter. Whereas the inquiry sought to gain an understanding of Schenker's trials, Kuhn responded to numerous questions that were not even asked. The text's exculpatory character and a certain resentment are unmistakeable. Kuhn began by explaining that he needed to 'go further afield than what would be suggested by the simple answer to your question', but then he immediately followed up with a falsehood. 'The circumstances you are asking me about lie decades back. I do not have any files about them and therefore must rely on my memory.'[88] As we know, he possessed large quantities of files – regarding his trials, his contacts in the industry, and his fee payments. At best, one can accept that there were hardly any documents regarding the informing of the cantonal physician and the government about the issue of compensation, which was the focus of the appeals court. According to Kuhn's own statements, only oral arrangements existed, which is not true.[89] He also seemed to assume that an oral agreement with the cantonal physician was equivalent to an approval from the medical services department. As far as concerns the claim that all this occurred 'decades back', it should be recalled that four years earlier he had received the biggest payment yet from Ciba-Geigy, namely, the last contractually agreed share in the revenue from Ludiomil.

Before Kuhn turned to the question of compensation, he extensively justified the major importance of scientific work in psychiatry, pointing out that he had already agreed on this with Director Zolliker when he commenced his duties in 1939. He then explained how the discovery of Tofranil came about, emphasising its worldwide distribution, and underscoring how cautiously and meticulously the trials had been conducted. 'At the beginning of the trial of a new substance, we only administered one quarter of the dosage indicated by the manufacturing company and also immediately undertook an exact clinical observation and investigation of the effects.'[90] He thereby indirectly conceded that such tests also involved risks, but in reality Kuhn by no means proceeded as cautiously as he claimed. He likewise maintained that the chemical industry assumed a 'guarantee for all possible harm resulting from the trials'.[91] However, only for a single trial is there any documentation in which this issue was addressed.[92]

Characterising the substance trials at the clinic, Kuhn wrote, 'In Münsterlingen, scientific work was, of course, always work in free time, both for Director Zolliker and for me.'[93] This was a phrase Kuhn liked to use repeatedly, one with which he underscored his great sacrifice. If one considers the enormous scope of the trials and the associated amount of work, this claim seems absurd, for this 'work in free time' involved the entire clinic. Without the extensive use of the clinic's infrastructure, the trials would not even have been possible. How this could be 'private' and not a unilaterally undertaken expansion of Kuhn's official function remained obscure.[94]

Concerning the consent of the treated patients, Kuhn explained as follows, without being asked.

> The patients were effectively informed that we had a new medication that could perhaps help them better than the previously used remedy. ... Particularly in psychiatry, there are often people whom one cannot first ask whether they are in agreement with a treatment, either because their mental development is insufficient to make a meaningful statement or because their current illness strongly limits their capacity for judgement or even limits awareness. In these cases, it is up to the responsibly minded doctor to decide, or, if a corresponding commission exists, to advocate a treatment request before it.

There was no mention of the patients' relatives or legal representatives. Kuhn appealed entirely to the authority of the physician who acted solely in the patient's interests, which he contrasted with the ignorance of laypeople. But he then moved seamlessly from the good of the individual patient to the good of the general public, which benefited from the development of new, more effective medications. Unfortunately, however, 'for many people [it is] obviously very difficult to assess the importance of medical research and discoveries', he stated. 'Thus even in the Canton of Thurgau, one did not take note of the achievements at the Münsterlingen Psychiatric Clinic.'[95]

With that, Kuhn came to the issue of compensation, where his resentment towards the canton emerged undisguised. 'In Münsterlingen, the senior officials were inadequately paid for decades.' Zolliker had always been forced to take on secondary work just so his family could get by, and he was happy when Kuhn, thanks to his scientific work, was likewise able to increase his income. As Zolliker's successor, he received an allowance of 10,000 francs in addition to his salary back then of 38,000 francs. 'One explained to me, the canton basically does not pay a successor any better than the predecessor.' The cantonal physician at the time, Dr Bütler, had told him he needed to 'increase [his wages] to that of an average general practitioner, which back then would have constituted an amount approximately in the range of three to four times my pay.'[96] Kuhn was heavily exaggerating here, as is illustrated by a note he himself wrote in 1971, which only refers to a doubling of his pay.[97] Besides, the figures were not really comparable, since, as self-employed professionals, general practitioners rendered their accounts in a completely different way. Moreover, the aforementioned figures of 38,000 and, respectively, 48,000 francs were just for Kuhn's basic salary.[98]

Moving on to the question of income from the chemical industry, Kuhn explained that the cantonal physician had told him he had been

> so inadequately paid for decades, that he only considers it right and proper for me to at least get some compensation after the fact. Dr Bütler and later cantonal physician Dr Nufer, whom I informed about my arrangement with his predecessor and who was content with that, were both accurately informed about my financial situation back then. I have also always truthfully declared my secondary income on the tax declaration.[99]

In conclusion, Kuhn stressed that, as a result of the trials, the clinic's medication expenses were reduced 'by five-figure amounts', savings for which the clinic had been explicitly praised.[100] He then summarised:

> I do not know whether and, if applicable, when and how Director Zolliker informed the medical services department about the medications testing. ... For as long as Director Zolliker was in office, there was an agreement between him as my superior and me with regard to the handling of these compensations. To what extent the medical services department was informed by Director Zolliker, I know only in part. I only know that, presumably at the end of the 1950s, the supervisory commission was briefed by Director Zolliker

about the conducting of trials for the chemical industry. Whether back then there was also talk about financial arrangements, I do not know, but this was probably rather unlikely.[101]

What the court of appeals thought of this response is unclear. However, the decision was evidently made not to respond to Kuhn or to investigate his testing practices. Nor do we have any further statements by Kuhn with regard to the court's request for information. There is nothing to be found in his private correspondence either. Consequently, one cannot determine whether, frightened by the first verdict in the Schenker case, he actually felt threatened by a conceivable criticism of his own actions and therefore responded so extensively and apologetically. It is also possible that, out of sheer pride in his accomplishments, he was simply unable to imagine such a turn of events. In that case, the excessive information would be explained merely by his hunger for recognition and by his resentment at not having been – as he saw it – adequately appreciated and thanked in the Canton of Thurgau and beyond.

At the legislative level, however, the Schenker case, which resulted in this remarkable letter by Kuhn, led to the end of the *laissez faire* that had previously prevailed. In June 1987, the new Health Act of 1985 was supplemented with an Ordinance on the Legal Status of Patients in Cantonal Facilities of the Healthcare System.[102] This ordinance included the first introduction of the terms *Heilversuch* (i.e., non-standard therapeutic use) and 'scientific testing', whereby the latter meant the testing of medications for research purposes.[103] Written information and consent were now indispensable. Trials with people lacking mental capacity were prohibited, and clinical trials were explicitly excluded as secondary income. In addition, in 1987, Thurgau became the first Swiss canton to create a 'medical ethics commission', an innovation that elicited a certain pride.[104] The commission had to determine the 'medical and therapeutic value' of every new trial and inform the medical services director about it.[105] In any case, the era of large-scale, wholly unsupervised trials was long gone. During the 1980s and 1990s, only a few isolated clinical trials took place at the Münsterlingen clinic, about which little is known.[106] Roland and Verena Kuhn, on the other hand, were still occupied with the testing of levoprotiline in their private practice at the time. They did not need the approval of the medical ethics commission for this because the commission did not exist when they started the trials in 1986.[107]

### Controversial memories: Kuhn becomes historical

Kuhn's accomplishments related to the discovery of Tofranil's antidepressant effect were recognised by large numbers of experts in the field, albeit with some delay. Public accolades began in the 1970s, remarkably first in the United States, even though his contacts there had always been limited due to his poor English skills.[108] Starting in 1981, he received three honorary doctorates: from Louvain in Belgium (1981), from the prestigious Sorbonne in Paris (1986), and finally also from the medical faculty of the University of Basel (1992), which referred in part to his accomplishments in daseinsanalysis and in part to those in psychopharmacology.[109] He was frequently invited as a contemporary witness to events that dealt with the early development of psychotropic drugs. For Tofranil's fortieth anniversary, the Psychiatric University Hospital Frankfurt organised a symposium where he also spoke.[110] 'I myself am thus slowly becoming a historical person', he wrote to a former colleague in 1998.[111]

In March 1982, the psychiatrists Hans Heimann and Gerhard Langer reached out to Kuhn; they wanted to publish a manual on 'Psychotropic Drugs: Fundamentals and Therapy' and dedicate it to him. 'We would like to honour you as one of the pioneers of clinical psychology', wrote Heimann, who was friends with Kuhn, 'and make the reader aware that essential impulses for the development of this therapy method are thanks to the European and here the German-language region'.[112] In the manual, Kuhn was commended as a 'European clinician and researcher' who managed to combine extensive theoretical knowledge with practical experience in therapy and was able to 'situate the limited problems of psychopharmacological treatment, its fundamentals, and its practice in a comprehensive theoretical horizon of human existence'.[113] Lofty praise indeed. Kuhn responded with delight and, when the manual appeared in early 1984, he immediately offered suggestions for additions. This would certainly be possible in the second edition, Heimann assured him.[114]

Then *The Antidepressant Era* was published in 1997, a book by the British psychiatrist and historian of psychiatry David Healy, which was about the introduction and distribution of antidepressants.[115] Healy had conducted numerous interviews with surviving pioneers in the development of psychopharmaceuticals and also published these discussions in three volumes, which in turn became a foundation for his book on antidepressants.[116] In September 1996, Healy had been accompanying the Canadian historian Edward Shorter on a visit to Scherzingen to also conduct an interview with Kuhn.[117] The latter had gotten an inkling about the book's content as it pertained to him by no later than summer 1999, when Jules Angst wrote him about a lecture David Healy had given in Zurich, which mentioned the name of the former Geigy employee Paul Schmidlin. Angst noted, 'I would be interested in how you assess the role of Paul Schmidlin, who until his death repeatedly stated that, based on the clinical observations made by you and others, he concluded that imipramine [Tofranil] is an antidepressant.'[118] In Zurich as in Basel, according to Angst, Schmidlin had repeatedly put forth this view on things. Kuhn answered in detail, but he did not consult Healy's book.[119] For linguistic reasons alone, he was far removed from the English-language literature. Not until the turn of year 2000/2001 did he catch up on the readings, namely, after someone had told him that Healy's book cast substantial doubt on his central role in the development of Tofranil.[120]

Now Kuhn was very angry; memories came flooding back. When reading other volumes published by Healy and colleagues, he became annoyed all over again as he discovered statements about himself that he found insulting.[121] In August 2001, he protested to David Healy in a long letter.[122] This was not about opinions and interpretations, he complained, but rather about facts. The statements of Paul Schmidlin reproduced in Healy's book gave the impression that he – Roland Kuhn – had appropriated someone else's intellectual property by failing to disclose that the Geigy employee had given him the decisive suggestion to also test the drug later called Tofranil against depression.[123] Healy had actually never spoken with Schmidlin, who had died in 1984. Schmidlin's views had only been fed to him by a third party, without Healy providing clear information about this.[124] With an archaic turn of phrase, Kuhn insisted that this account offended his honour and his family's good name; he demanded a correction.[125]

David Healy apologised because of the obvious personal offence, but referred to his documentation. According to Healy, in his interviews he had deliberately taken a slightly provocative approach to get the discussion going. He conceded that, in connection with Kuhn's role, he had noticed a certain animosity on the part of other parties that he could not explain.[126] With such contradictory opinions, a confrontation of the participating interview partners would have been appropriate, but he failed to organise such an exchange with the opportunity to reply. Since another volume of documentation was already nearing completion, Healy managed to appease Kuhn by giving him space in the new publication to explain his position in detail.[127] The deadline was short and Kuhn set to work in great haste. He started combing through and reorganising his material. Every now and then, he filed a note indicating that these documents were historically significant – a reference for future researchers: 'This folder contains the important files for the history of my contributions to psychopharmacology', he noted, for instance, on a slip of paper.[128]

Whether Kuhn recovered his peace of mind when room was also made for his version of the history of the discovery of Tofranil, however, remains unclear. While he maintained courtesy towards Healy and spoke about 'mistakes' that he wanted corrected, he sounded much harsher in his private correspondence. He obviously saw himself as the victim of 'defamation', thus of deliberate malice.[129] In May 2001, he went so far as to suspect that he was no longer being invited to conferences on the history of antidepressants because Healy's account in *The Antidepressant Era* was being widely believed, although he never explained who his invisible opponents were.[130]

Kuhn was proud of his work, which occupied a central place in his memory. For a long time, he primarily defined it through daseinsanalysis. In old age, however, psychopharmacology also gained ground, for it was here that he could show tangible accomplishments. When this was not appropriately appreciated, he quickly became resentful.

On the occasion of Kuhn's ninetieth birthday in 2002, a symposium was held in his honour at the Münsterlingen clinic. In his own contributions, as well as in those of his well-wishers, he appears as a subtle, philosophically schooled observer and analyst of human sensitivities. Quite a few years later, after Kuhn's death in October 2005, a different picture emerged from our interviews with contemporary witnesses. In the meantime, the incipient public discussion brought forth some key points of criticism and, in particular, problematised the clinical trials; unqualified admiration was no longer in the cards. Nobody doubted that he had been an unbelievably hard and industrious worker. 'The entire life in the clinic [had been] almost monastic', recalled Albert Lingg, an assistant and then senior physician in the 1970s.[131] Kuhn lived entirely for the clinic, and he was strict – in the eyes of many, all too strict. He was criticised for his aloofness, for example, in how he conducted rounds – the way he spoke to patients was mechanical, without any perceptible appreciation of them as people.[132] 'He was not an approachable person', maintains a former clinic employee; he was 'bad at contact', says another.[133] Verena Kuhn at his side had a countervailing effect, far warmer in social relationships, sometimes even affectionate.[134] Primarily important to him was that one followed his advice and orders. Closer encounters were most likely to occur if Kuhn found someone useful or interesting, as when a patient was able to communicate and became a discussion partner. Sometimes he developed longstanding relationships with individual ambulatory patients – those involved have favourable memories of him. An attentive and approachable observer, or an unsociable person concerned primarily about respect for his hierarchical status? Here we can only note this contradiction; it cannot be resolved.

What remained in Kuhn's very advanced age, in the last chapter of his life, was a concern for his posthumous memory, his scientific legacy. As shown by the notes he left behind, even after the dispute with David Healy, he was still preoccupied with sifting through his personal holdings. This sustained interest became immediately apparent when the state archivist of the Canton of Thurgau contacted him in April 2005.[135] The state archives had in the meantime taken over the clinic's files, systematically incorporating them into its holdings, and the archive was interested in adding to them. Kuhn reacted immediately and favourably; a personal meeting and an initial inspection of his private archive took place just a few days later. Kuhn felt that the transfer of his papers to the state archive was a good solution. Death thwarted his intention to carry this out in person; Kuhn died in 2005 at the age of 93. The remarkable holdings did not make their way to the state archive until 2012/ 2013. They constitute a unique place of knowledge, without which this book would have been impossible.

## Notes

1 See, for example, interview with Karl Studer, 3 November 2016; StATG, 9'40, 1.0.2/2.
2 PKM archive, directorate archive Studer, 1.62.04, letters to the *Schweizerische Bodensee-Zeitung*, 14 February 1980.
3 *Ibid.*, *Thurschau, Zeitschrift für Politik und Kultur*, no. 3, March 1980, 1–2, 6–7. (quote 7). Dahinden criticised, among other things, 'the one-sided concentration on the medical, medicamentous treatment of the patients' and brought up the term 'guinea pigs'. 'Patients are filled up with medications, made to be quiet. Much to the delight of the pharmaceutical industry, for whom the Münsterlingen patients occasionally also get to play as guinea pigs'; *ibid.*, 7.
4 See, for example, Assmann, *Der lange Schatten*; Wimmer, *Archivkörper*. On the power of archiving, see also Derrida, *Dem Archiv*; Stoler, *Along the Archival*.
5 On the impact of files, Vismann, *Files*; on textualisation, for instance, Becker and Clark, *Little Tools*.
6 Usually, the first stage of a field's historicisation is made not by historians but by protagonists. The same applies to psychopharmacology – for example, with Healy, *The Psychopharmacologists*.
7 On 'biographical illusion', see Bourdieu, 'L'illusion'.
8 StATG, 9'40, 12/326, Kuhn to Prof Ulrich Honegger, University of Bern, 17 February 2001.
9 See König, 'Besichtigung einer Weltindustrie', 255–264.
10 Kuhn's successor requested the return of the patient medical files; StATG, 9'40, 2.2/0, Karl Studer to Kuhn, 18 March 1985.
11 Various contemporaries mention Kuhn's frequent presence; he also had free access to the medical files.
12 Interview with a former administrative employee of the clinic, 28 November 2016; StATG, 9'40, 5.0.4/2, Kuhn to Ciba-Geigy, 5 March 1980; PKM archive, directorate archive Studer, 1.60.01, medication research, MHPG. The study was about the level of the excretion value of MHPG, a metabolite of adrenaline and noradrenaline. In 1980, the hypothesis was put forward that depression altered the metabolism of noradrenaline.

13 StATG, 9'40, 9.0, lectures at the University of Zurich, 1948–1998.
14 See StATG, 9'40, 12/413, circular letter, 28 May 2003 (with enclosed list of addresses). The manuscripts of Kuhn's lectures have been published since 2013 in the series *Münsterlinger Kolloquien*, 6 vols., Würzburg 2013–2018, StATG, 9'40, 8.0/316.
15 StATG, 9'40, 12/0, handwritten annotation regarding the blue folders, possibly filed for future persons using his private archive. This section of the private archive now fills twenty-two archive boxes.
16 StATG, 9'40, 12/250, Kuhn to Prof. Shota Gamkrelidze, Tbilisi, 26 February 2002: 'Now I am also able to write you by email!'
17 See correspondence 2002–2004 in StATG, 9'40, 12/368.
18 StATG, 9'40, 12/733, Kuhn to Dr Stahl, 22 August 2001.
19 StATG, 9'40, 12/344, filing on the balladeer Hanns In der Gand, notice dated 8 November 2004.
20 StATG, 9'40, 3.1.11/0, Kuhn to Wolfgang Blankenburg, 10 November 1980, 2.
21 StATG, 9'40, 3.2.0/4, Kuhn to Dr Scherer, 14 May 1980.
22 Thirty-five publications appeared between 1980 and 1989, twelve with a psychopharmacological topic; thirty-seven appeared between 1990 and 1999, eight of which were psychopharmacological.
23 StATG, 9'40, 3.1.11/0, Kuhn to Blankenburg, 17 April 1978.
24 StATG, 9'40, 8.4.3/8, Bein to Kuhn, 2 July 1980.
25 StATG, 9'40, 3.1.42/0, Kuhn to Heimann, 8 March 1982.
26 StATG, 9'40, 8.4.0, 8.4.3 and 8.4.4 contain numerous text fragments from this period.
27 StATG, 9'40, 12/295, Kuhn to Heimann, 28 August 2003.
28 See Kuhn, *Psychiatrie mit Zukunft*. The preceding attempts with various publishing houses are documented in StATG, 9'40, 12/329; 9'40, 12/353; 9'40, 12/127. See also StATG, 9'40,12/295, Kuhn to Heimann, 28 August 2003.
29 StATG, 9'40, 12/367, Kuhn to the cantonal physician Alfred Muggli, 29 July 2002.
30 CA Novartis, Ciba-Geigy, PH 2, Division Pharma, siting decision of Ciba-Geigy products 1975/76, 21 October 1976, 2–3.
31 CA Novartis, Ciba-Geigy, PH 4.00.2, Division Pharma, pharma research committee, 21 June 1978.
32 Hess et al., *Testen*, 70, note 17 states that the drug was first intended for cardiac arrhythmia; that must be an error because the research committee was already talking about an antidepressant in 1978.
33 The following information according to Hess, *Testen*, 71–80; see also Steger and Jeskow, *Das Antidepressivum* with further information on the relocation to the German Democratic Republic.

34 Hess et al., *Testen*, 73. In the district hospital of Ansbach, unapproved substances or drugs taken off the market were tested on psychiatric patients without their consent.
35 *Ibid.*, 81–87.
36 Interview with Alexandra Delini-Stula, 19 June 2017.
37 See Chapter 5, 183–184.
38 StATG, 9'40, 5.0.4/1, Kuhn to Director Max Wilhelm, 1 August 1986; the substance to be tested is not named, but it must have been CGP 12013.
39 *Ibid.*
40 Novartis clinical archive, doc 205 (A), arch no: M-850, confidential, CGP 12103 A, levoprotiline, trial protocol EN/P 01, Ciba-Geigy, Basel, research and development, undated, 2.
41 StATG, 9'40, 5.0.4/20.1, Delini-Stula, Ciba-Geigy, to a doctor from Porrentruy, 8 September 1987.
42 Novartis clinical archive, box 112, binder 3/12, acc. no. 23646, meeting on the clinical study EN/PO 1 (levoprotiline), Basel, 13 November 1989.
43 StATG, 9'40, 5.0.4/20.1, Bein to Delini-Stula, Ciba-Geigy, 30 October 1988; trial protocol CGP 12103 A, September 1987, 9.
44 StATG, 9'40, 5.0.4/20.1, Delini-Stula to Kuhn, 10 November 1986.
45 *Ibid.*, Kuhn to Delini-Stula, 17 July 1987, 3.
46 Possibly also in connection with the drug scandal in West Germany. See above, note 34.
47 StATG, 9'40 5.0.4/20.2, consent declarations of seventeen patients for a trial with CGP 12103, 1987–1989.
48 StATG, 9'40, 5.0.4/20.1, trial protocol CGP 12103 A (levoprotiline), September 1987 (first draft), 11.
49 Novartis clinical archive, box 112, binder 3/12, acc. no. 23646, Dr Rosselet, meeting on clinical study EN/PO 1 (levoprotiline), Basel, 13 November 1989.
50 StATG, 9'40, 8.2/152, Vorläufige Mitteilung über erste Erfahrungen mit Levoprotilin Ciba-Geigy, Basel, 12 November 1987.
51 *Ibid.*, 6; such information is not available for all of the patients involved.
52 *Ibid.*, 2.
53 *Ibid.*
54 *Ibid.*, 8.
55 StATG, 9'40, 5.0.4/20.1, Kuhn to Max Wilhelm, 28 December 1987.
56 *Ibid.*, Max Wilhelm to Kuhn, 28 January 1988.
57 *Ibid.*, Delini-Stula to Kuhn, 10 August 1989.

58 Novartis clinical archive, box 112, binder 3/12, acc. no. 23646, Dr Rosselet, discussion about clinical study EN/PO 1 (levoprotiline), Basel, 13 November 1989 (also in StATG, 9'40, 5.0.4/20.1).
59 *Ibid.*, Rosselet and Wilhelm to Kuhn, 26 November 1990.
60 Novartis research archives, clear folder levoprotiline, Maître to Wilhelm, 25 October 1991, report on AGNP meeting; Wendt, 'Exkurs', 396–397.
61 For the discontinuation of the ketimipramine trial series, see Chapter 4, pp 138–139.
62 StATG, 9'40, 5.0.4/20.1, Kuhn to Max Wilhelm, 7 November 1991.
63 *Ibid.*
64 *Ibid.*, Kuhn to Wilhelm, 9 January 1992, 2.
65 *Ibid.*, Kuhn to Wilhelm, 8 December 1990.
66 *Ibid.*
67 Ibid.; see also StATG, 9'40, 5.0.4/22, Kuhn to Gelzer, Ciba-Geigy, 12 May 1992.
68 StATG, 9'40, 5.0.4/20.1, Kuhn to Wilhelm, 8 December 1990, 3.
69 Ibid.
70 Interview with Alexandra Delini-Stula, 19 June 2017.
71 StATG, 9'40, 12/458, Maître to Kuhn, 6 August 2001. More detailed company documents on this matter have thus far not been made available.
72 Alexandra Delini-Stula, interview with David Healy, November 1994, in Healy, *The Psychopharmacologists*, vol. 1, 434.
73 *Ibid.*, 435.
74 There was one more attempt to revive levoprotiline with the Swedish company Astra; Kuhn tried very hard, but in 1993 the Swedes withdrew as well, referring to the existing placebo studies. See StATG, 9'40, 5.0.4/23, contacts with Astra, Sweden, 1993.
75 StATG, 9'40, 12/458, Kuhn to Maître, 21 February 1996.
76 *Ibid.*, Maître to Kuhn, 25 June 1996.
77 This account follows the detailed treatment by Müller, 'Das Disziplinarverfahren'.
78 *Ibid.*, 4.
79 This was impermissible, for the circumstances reported by the employee had nothing to do with medical confidentiality.
80 Müller, 'Das Disziplinarverfahren', 12. This was permissible only within the framework of the disciplinary proceedings; in criminal proceedings conducted at the same time, the (longer) limitation periods under criminal law would have applied.
81 Quoted in *ibid.*, 11.

82 See Chapter 1, 26.
83 The criminal investigation only started after the conclusion of the disciplinary proceedings. The Thurgau government council concluded the disciplinary proceedings against Schenker in summer 1986 and then directed various potential criminal offences to the criminal court.
84 Müller, 'Das Disziplinarverfahren', 23.
85 *Bodensee-Zeitung*, 21 November 1986, 21, quoted in Müller, 'Das Disziplinarverfahren', 25, note 125.
86 Müller, 'Das Disziplinarverfahren', 23–24.
87 StATG, 9'40, 1.05/5, vice president of the court of appeals, Thomas Zweidler, to Kuhn, 10 July 1989.
88 *Ibid.*, Kuhn to Zweidler, 17 July 1989.
89 See Chapter 5, 188.
90 StATG, 9'40, 1.05/5, Kuhn to Zweidler, 17 July 1989, 2.
91 *Ibid.*, 4.
92 See the trial of Ciba 24160 in 1959; StATG, 9'40, 5.0.2/2, Kaufmann to Kuhn, 1 December 1959.
93 StATG, 9'40, 1.05/5, Kuhn to Zweidler, 17 July 1989, 2.
94 See Chapter 5, 185.
95 StATG, 9'40, 1.05/5, Kuhn to Zweidler, 17 July 1989, 2–3.
96 *Ibid.*, 4.
97 See StATG, 9'10, 1.2.8/6, meeting with Cantonal Physician Julius Bütler, file note Kuhn, 26 June 1971, 1.
98 See Chapter 5, 186. In Switzerland in 1971, male white-collar service-sector employees with a degree or completed apprenticeship earned an average of just under 30,200 Swiss francs per year. Ritzmann, *Historische Statistik*, 470.
99 StATG, 9'40, 1.05/5, Kuhn to Zweidler, 17 July 1989, 4. See Chapter 5, 181–182, 185, 188.
100 StATG, 9'40, 1.05/5, Kuhn to Zweidler, 17 July 1989, 5.
101 *Ibid.*, 5–6; the minutes of the supervisory commission suggest that the trials were in fact discussed in June 1960; see StATG, 4'840'33, minutes of the supervisory commission, 29 June 1960.
102 Müller, 'Das Disziplinarverfahren', 31–35.
103 This made the SAMS's distinction in 1970 between the 'research studies in the interests of the persons to be studied' and 'those that serve general medical research' (see Chapter 6, 205) legally binding.
104 On the history of the ethics commissions in Switzerland, see Jenni, *Forschungskontrolle*.
105 Quoted in Müller, 'Das Disziplinarverfahren', 33.
106 A few references are found in the files of Studer's directorate archive; see PKM archive, 1.60.01, medication research: Sandoz NB 106–689, 1984/1985; risperidone for schizophrenics, 1993/1994.

107 Information from Rainer Andenmatten, former cantonal pharmacist and president of the cantonal ethics commission from 1996 to 2016; email to Marietta Meier, 6 January 2019.
108 He himself emphasised the early accolades from the United States; see Kuhn, 'Roland Kuhn', 224.
109 See StATG, 9'40, 13.0, 13.1, 13.3. In Paris, he was honoured for his work in daseinsanalysis, in Basel for imipramine, and in Louvain for both. Many of his texts on daseinsanalysis were translated into French.
110 StATG, 9'40, 12/73, correspondence with Prof. H.-G. Baumgarten, Berlin.
111 StATG, 9'40, 12/429, Kuhn to Angst, 8 May 1998.
112 StATG, 9'40, 3.42/0, Hans Heimann to Kuhn, 2 March 1982.
113 Langer and Heimann, *Psychopharmaka*, dedication.
114 StATG, 9'40, 3.42/0, Heimann to Kuhn, 1 March 1984 (answer to Kuhn's response to the book, which has not survived).
115 See Healy, *The Antidepressant Era*. Healy continued to publish in the field (Healy, *The Creation*). In the meantime, he strongly campaigned against the hasty prescription of antidepressants, particularly to young people (suicide risk), and appeared as an expert witness in trials against large corporations; see his ample website: https://davidhealy.org/ (accessed 8 April 2024).
116 See Healy, *The Psychopharmacologists*.
117 Published in Healy, *The Psychopharmacologists*, vol. 2, 93–118.
118 StATG, 9'40, 12/31, Angst to Kuhn, 28 June 1999.
119 *Ibid.*, Kuhn to Angst, 5 July 1999.
120 Who informed Kuhn remains unclear. The first documented response to the readings is found in StATG, 9'40, 12/144, Kuhn to Arvid Carlsson, Göteborg, 23 January 2001.
121 Ban et al., *The Rise*.
122 Printed in Ban et al., *From Psychopharmacology*, 286–288.
123 See Chapter 2, 61–62.
124 In early 2001, Kuhn contacted one of these sources by mail, namely, the Basel psychiatrist Raymond Battegay, a student of Kielholz; their correspondence remained quite reserved. See StATG, 9'40, 12/71.
125 Kuhn to Healy, in Ban et al., *From Psychopharmacology*, 288.
126 Healy to Kuhn, 23 August 2001, in *ibid.*, 289–290.
127 Ban et al., *From Psychopharmacology*. The volume contains an 'imipramine dossier', which includes correspondence with David Healy, Pierre Simon, and Edward Shorter, a response by Kuhn to statements in Healy's *The Antidepressant Era* of 1997, as well as a series of documents from Kuhn's private archive, among other things.
128 StATG, 9'40, 5.1.0/0.2.

## The 1980s

129 See StATG, 9'40, 12. These holdings contain various letters by Kuhn from this period in which the term defamation appears; thus 9'40, 12/144, to Carlsson, 23 January 2001; 9'40, 12/71, to Battegay, 30 January 2001; 9'40, 12/593, to Pollmächler, Max Planck Institute Munich, 14 April 2001; 9'40, 12/458, to Maître, 22 August 2001.
130 StATG, 9'40, 12/140, Kuhn to Charles Kahn, Montreal, 14 May 2001.
131 Interview with Albert Lingg, 7 September 2016.
132 Telephone interview with a former nurse who worked at the Münsterlingen Psychiatric Clinic in the 1970s, 11 November 2016.
133 Interview with a former administrative employee, 28 November 2016; interview with Jürg Grundlehner, who from 1971 to 1974 completed an apprenticeship at the Münsterlingen Psychiatric Clinic, 23 August 2017.
134 This from various statements from contemporary witnesses: interview with a former administrative employee, 28 November 2016; interview with Karl Studer, Kuhn's successor, 3 November 2016; interview with a former assistant physician, 6 March 2018.
135 StATG, 9'99, 04.20.19, holding 9'40, state archive's letter to Kuhn, 28 April 2005.

# Conclusion

The results of our research cannot be summarised in just a few lines. *On trial* not only describes the progression and scope of the Münsterlingen trials but also categorises them and charts the changing circumstances and framework conditions. The chronological structure with thematic components depicts this entangled history. Starting in the 1950s, psychiatric clinics underwent radical change. Fences disappeared, the range of therapeutic services expanded, and the number of outpatient treatments grew. Many of these innovations were also related to the psychopharmacological revolution; in 1953, Largactil ushered in the era of modern psychotropic drugs and the pharmaceutical industry underwent a veritable boom. The first neuroleptics were soon joined by antidepressants and tranquillisers, and the drug market continuously expanded. Whereas in the 1950s clinical trials still took an exploratory and open approach, by 1962, the first regulations regarding drug approvals, risks, side-effects, and testing methods began taking hold. Step by step, the trials were now supposed to be standardised and brought in line with statistical, quantitative criteria. The impulse for this change came not just from the authorities but also from the pharmaceutical industry itself. With the Declaration of Helsinki in 1964 and the guidelines for research studies on humans issued by the Swiss Academy of Medical Sciences in 1970, new ethical principles were finally introduced.

The trials at Münsterlingen must therefore be viewed against a background which was itself evolving. In this respect, one can describe some important shifts. In the 1960s, Roland Kuhn developed more and more into an anachronistic investigator who rejected innovations that elsewhere prevailed. This raises the central question about the categorisation of his clinical trials: did the investigations at Münsterlingen deviate from contemporary testing practices? Was the clinic part of an entire line of trial centres engaged in similar practices? Were Kuhn's trials more problematic than others? Or were these simply darker times, when there was still less concern about the wellbeing of patients, less awareness of ethical issues, and when a strong faith in pharmacological progress still reigned?

From a categorisation of the Münsterlingen trials, one quickly arrives at their evaluation. A historical perspective can bring to light findings that are important and helpful to both, for underlying the questions outlined above is the idea of a linear forward motion: that things are better today, that our society, medicine, and psychiatry has made progress and established clear norms, and that we, looking back from our present heights, can measure the past according to today's standards. From this perspective, the above questions can then also be easily – but ahistorically – answered: nowadays one would do things differently; one would not be allowed to do things that way today. But the social values for what is considered permissible in the fields of medicine and psychiatry changed as well throughout the entire period. Ethical norms, too, have a history.[1]

For our study, this means that the standards against which we assess Kuhn's trials are not stable either. Thus one must first ask: when did which norms apply? How did the awareness of the risks, dangers, and side-effects of psychoactive substances evolve? Did the testing procedures at Münsterlingen fall outside the parameters of what was permissible or common practice? Along with this categorising perspective, we decided on a strategy of close observation. For example, did Kuhn continue testing even though he knew that a substance was dangerous? Did he intentionally expose certain patient groups to greater risks? Were others more likely to be spared? *On trial* has examined how exactly the Münsterlingen trial site functioned and changed, and how it should be situated in the landscape of clinical trials. To do so, first the perspective was reversed; we put ourselves in Roland Kuhn's shoes, so to speak, and went through the times and his private archive step by step. Having undertaken this march, we realised that Kuhn as an individual could be situated and understood in relation to the broader historical trend.

The troublesome elements, we feel, lie above all in fine discrepancies, in the quotidian transgressions of boundaries. When out of scientific fervour and pressed for time, he dispensed with preliminary investigations that were actually already commonplace. When, as a precaution, Kuhn stopped giving one patient a dangerous test substance but at the same time accepted new patients into the same trial series. When a trial was aborted by the company but was still informally continued at Münsterlingen. When there was too little attention and not enough supervision to notice in time that rapid physical deteriorations were taking place that might otherwise have been stopped. When substances with an unpredictable effect were first given to hopeless, so-called serious cases to obtain an initial picture, and afterwards one switched to patients with more favourable prognoses. When test substances were administered to patient groups whose diagnoses did not match the sought-for effect. When non-registered substances were given in disguise or patients were increasingly pressured to take substances. When patients were included in trials without being informed and without their consent, even though this was already called for by existing guidelines. When, not least for financial reasons, Kuhn pursued the strategy of treating large numbers of patients with test substances rather than with approved medications.

### On the scope of the trials

What distinguishes the Münsterlingen trial site from the experimental landscape of its times is the exceptional documentation, which for the first time has made it possible to track clinical trials so closely. Apart from that, it is the sheer scope of the experiments. This applies to the number of substances, the long duration of many of the trials, and the number of patients involved. In 1946, Kuhn carried out the first trial with Parpanit; the last trial, with levoprotiline, ended in 1990 in his private practice. With one exception, they all took place under his control; Clinical Director Zolliker started testing a drug for Huntington's disease in the 1960s, but Kuhn then took over the trial.

For the Geigy company, Kuhn tested at least thirty-two substances, and he tested eleven for Ciba. After the merger, he conducted clinical trials with eight Ciba-Geigy preparations. Five test substances from the Hoffmann-La Roche company made their way to Münsterlingen; from Wander there were four; and trials with six substances are documented for Sandoz. Kuhn also conducted a trial for the American company Wyeth. In total, we recorded 117 substances in our database. For many, there is no sound evidence that Kuhn actually tested them after the company's inquiry, but for sixty-seven substances there is clear evidence of a trial.[2] This minimum number does not include trials in which substances were revisited; nor did we count substances for which only deliveries are documented. The forms of the documented trials varied strongly – along with rapid tests performed on just a few individuals, there were large-scale trials involving more than 1,000 cases.

Our database includes the names of 1,112 people who were administered at least one test substance. This number, too, is a minimum value, for not all of the names could be deciphered or attributed to a person. Random samples from the medical files also revealed that none of the source holdings are really reliable; in some medical files, we found references to test substances without the relevant person showing up in the trial documentation. Conversely, the administration of test substances was not systematically recorded in the medical files, even for patients who were mentioned by name in the trial documentation. Thus there are gaps everywhere – on the one hand, more than 1,000 identifiable test patients; on the other, an unknown number that must make the total significantly higher. All told, Kuhn's test reports and records make mention of 2,789 cases. This number, too, is conservative since Kuhn did not always count all of the cases, nor did he indicate for every substance how many persons were involved. Moreover, some test reports are missing, and the number of cases does not correspond to the number of patients because some patients were involved more than once.

The most reliable gauge for the dimensions of the trials is probably the volume of substances. Throughout the entire period, at least 3 million individual doses of test substances found their way to Münsterlingen. The discrepancy between these immense delivered quantities and the number of patients known by name is huge; Kuhn's statements in his reports to the pharmaceutical industry also suggest that the number of affected persons was much higher, even when one considers that the case and patient numbers are not the same. This also applies to the number of substances that were administered to the individual patients. For more than one third of the patients known by name, only one test substance is documented. On the other end of the spectrum, there are twenty-nine patients who received at least six test substances. One female schizophrenic patient was in fact given at least thirteen test substances over a period of twenty years. An estimate of how many patients were involved in trials and how many test substances they received on average would require a systematic sampling from the medical files. But this result, too, would only be a minimum value.

Both sexes were pretty much equally represented in the trials.[3] Kuhn admittedly found it more difficult to evaluate a substance's effect in the case of women because of their menstrual cycle, but this evidently did not impact testing practices. Until the end of the 1950s, test substances were primarily administered to patients with organic and schizophrenic disorders; they were joined as of 1957 by persons with affective disorders. In the 1960s, the number of the latter grew until it caught up with and finally surpassed that of patients with organic disorders. The number of schizophrenic patients who were involved in trials, on the other hand, remained more or less constant until the late 1970s, when, with Kuhn's transition to private practice, tests were chiefly carried out with depressive patients.

To enable a categorisation, these trial dimensions must be compared to those of other clinics. However, little is currently known about clinical trials in Switzerland. Nevertheless, it is clear that trials were conducted in many places.[4] The holdings we consulted mention a broad spectrum of additional trial sites, both domestic and foreign, ranging from clinics through to children's homes and private practices. Particularly in the case of non-university clinics, such as Münsterlingen, financial aspects and the availability of new drugs must have been a decisive factor. In smaller clinics, experiments were not necessarily utilised for publications. Since such publications were more likely to emerge from university clinics, their trials are more visible upon first glance. Even though clinical trials have hardly been researched, one can now already say that the pharmaceutical companies provided test substances to many domestic and foreign clinics, which in exchange reported on their experiences. Thus even if Switzerland may not have had a second 'Kuhn', recently there have been more and more indications that Münsterlingen is not an exception, and that elsewhere there are comparable practices to review.

## Beyond the biographical perspective

Roland Kuhn was polarising. This book has cited various voices that have presented Kuhn in completely contradictory ways. What mainly stuck in people's minds were concise verbal images. According to one nurse, Kuhn was called 'Daddy-Long-Legs';[5] another felt that, despite his primness, he clearly had a certain power of persuasion. Described as having little charisma, the psychiatrist in 'Jesus sandals' could evidently obtain respect among his immediate colleagues at Münsterlingen through the clinic's hierarchy, his seriousness, and his enthusiasm for work.[6] His discussion evenings, secretly called 'peppermint parties', are characteristic for this perception of Kuhn.[7] The peppermint tea served on these occasions is virtually emblematic of his key qualities: an invariably teetotaling, ascetic severity, mixed with a seemingly Protestant zeal for work (to the point of hyperactivity), an iron discipline with himself and the employees, and a broad sober-mindedness that only seemed to recede when he scaled philosophical heights. According to a former assistant physician, Kuhn only opened up with employees when someone mentioned the key word 'daseinsanalysis', while, in contrast, he treated those uninterested in the topic as 'second-class citizens'.[8]

His private archive conveys the impression of a doctor who, with advancing age, felt misunderstood, a man who believed he had been destined for higher things but always found himself on the margins and made numerous efforts to belong. He painstakingly collected everything he could find about himself and worried about 'properly' going down in the annals of history. He perceived errors in media reporting as defamation and his unsuccessful university appointments as rejections and exclusions by his colleagues. In the course of his life, he found various forums for his quest for recognition, first in research on Rorschach tests, later on daseinsanalysis, both of which gave him entry to an intellectual community. Particularly dear to him was his exchange with Ludwig

Binswanger in the neighbouring clinic of Bellevue, who on account of his age was more of a teacher than colleague. The partnership and collaboration with actors from the pharmaceutical industry also constituted an important forum. His correspondence with partners in the industry shows that he by no means just delivered minimalistic results but rather was searching for something more; he wrote up his thoughts, created hypotheses, and searched for and found interaction, attention, and recognition. His relationships with Geigy and later also Ciba went well beyond mere transactions of knowledge, substances, and remunerations. There were shared interests on many levels. Ultimately, his research achievements were also honoured in the scientific community; Kuhn received three honorary doctorates and made his way into the major psychiatric reference books of his times as the discoverer of antidepressants.

His second important partnership was private in nature: with 'Vreni', Verena Kuhn-Gebhart, his wife. Even at ninety years of age, he wrote in a letter, 'I discuss my cases regularly with Vreni, and she discusses her cases with me'.[9] Compared to her husband, who meticulously kept notes and collected things, Verena Kuhn is far more difficult to get to know. Whereas Roland Kuhn haunts these pages and his private archive as an ambivalent and somewhat enigmatic figure, Verena Kuhn is practically impossible to get a grip on from the files. She disappears behind her husband (and probably also did so during their lifetimes), who engaged in correspondence, held lectures, published texts, and conducted psychopharmaceutical research in both their names. She was a 'quiet, withdrawn woman', recalls a nurse. 'She smiled. She gave ... one the feeling that she was concerning herself with you. But very reticently.' In contrast to the secretary, who walked as if she was in somebody else's shoes, Verena Kuhn was herself, even in the way she moved. Quite different than Mathilde, the senior nurse, who strutted around with her royal poodle. The staff also enjoyed making jokes about how the couple told each other their dreams each morning.[10] Other contemporaries described Verena Kuhn less sympathetically as a 'grey mouse'.[11] But in the practice, especially in the outpatient department, she played a central role. There she supervised numerous patients, specialised in children and youth, and also administered test substances; typical for her is the sentence she frequently used when starting to administer a test substance: 'we want to try it once with this remedy'.

We know little about the relationship of the Kuhns as a couple. But their interactions must have been close and strongly dominated by professional matters and clinic practicalities. The sources we examined show no evidence of conflicts or differences of opinion; Roland and Verena Kuhn functioned very much as a team. With respect to pharmacological substances, they both seem similarly open-minded; they generally believed in the efficacy of psychopharmacological therapies. The trials of psychotropic drugs were also in the service of this idea; they were necessary to obtain even better drugs, to advance pharmacological progress, which, almost incidentally, also reaped certain benefits for the clinic. That the couple could rub people the wrong way is shown not least by the numerous internal conflicts, for the staff incessantly struggled with excessive workloads. Roland and Verena Kuhn both used their psychotherapeutic meetings with female nurses to plumb them for information about quarrels in the wards and thus deal with conflicts indirectly. The mood towards the Kuhns among the assistant physicians was not always positive either.

The biographical perspective that is suggested by a personal archive brings many things to light, but it also conceals a lot. The historian runs the risk of being taken in by her informants, of assigning them too much weight, disregarding other actors and perpetuating her informants' self-representations. Correspondence is given more weight than the Kuhns' daily conversations; written documents outweigh practical everyday matters. Above all, however, there is the risk of losing sight of other actors and structural aspects: the large-scale changes in the pharmaceutical market, the transformation of psychiatric clinics and government supervision and regulation, the hierarchically structured but complex fabric of work and life in the microcosm of the Münsterlingen clinic and its connections to the outside world. Patients, nurses, assistant physicians, relatives, a landlady, referring general practitioners, letter correspondents, pharmacists, chemists, pharmacologists, forms, questionnaires, EEG devices, and not least the substances themselves were all actors in this far-reaching network of the Münsterlingen trial site. Inputs and outputs – not only of patients, but also of information, knowledge, money, and substances – were at least as important here as the inner life of the clinic itself. Thus one can imagine the subject of our investigation as a node in this network: with one branch extending to the cantonal authorities in Thurgau; a second to the companies in Basel; another to the world of science with its publications and lectures; and many smaller ones to medical practices and to the homes of ambulatory patients.

## Partnerships between Basel and Münsterlingen

Roland Kuhn was polarising as a person, but initially not so much because of his trials. It was only after his death that the focus fell on the testing of psychotropic drugs, pushed in that direction by media reports and the statements of affected persons. During his lifetime, criticism was practically inaudible, with isolated voices mainly criticising his methodology and analyses as being impressionistic and largely unscientific.

Disputes with the pharmaceutical companies arose primarily when Kuhn's assessment of a new substance did not concur with company resolutions or the evaluations of other investigators – most prominently with regard to Keto and levoprotiline. But there are no documented conflicts regarding his procedures. Instead, it seems that the pharmaceutical companies were dependent on their investigators and went to great lengths to ensure that they were not put off. Not only the companies but also Kuhn acted strategically at times in this partnership. If he believed in a substance, he could disregard all hierarchical levels and, in a tactical coup, play various contact persons off against each other.

If one scrutinises the practice of their collaboration, however, one can clearly make out a change; Kuhn's role as investigator shifted over time, provoked by changes in the drug approval process and in testing methods. He developed an actual testing philosophy, which for him was validated by the 'discovery' of Tofranil, and which he then vehemently adhered to for the rest of his life. In sum, it consisted – and in this respect actually more as a philosophy than as a methodology – of the following elements: his observing gaze as a lead investigator; an exploratory approach that did not test for predetermined indications but rather searched openly for substance effects, often across several diagnostic categories; a long trial period; the variation of dosages; as well as the rejection of placebos, statistical analyses, and the use of control substances. In the process, Kuhn claimed to have a holistic view, one that did not reduce the patients to numbers, curves, and statistics, but rather took in the entire human being. But ever since the changes in the pharmaceutical industry started taking place in the mid-1960s, such a philosophy was no longer in keeping with the times. This could have meant the end of the Münsterlingen trial site, yet the opposite was the case; Kuhn filled an important niche in the roundelay of testing. The companies used him as a rapid investigator for so-called pilot tests, that is, at the very beginning of the clinical testing phase of a new substance, or they gave his enthusiasm free rein in long-term trials.

Measured against the standards that since 1962 had arisen within and outside the pharmaceutical industry, Kuhn's testing practices deviated from the norm in the following three respects.

*First*, some of the substances that came to Münsterlingen for testing had not yet gone through the already common preliminary tests. This occurred particularly in the case of Geigy, when Kuhn made suggestions for substance modifications. Some substances were given to Kuhn for testing 'out of scientific interest', as the company put it. The trial phases commonly used today for testing substances were first defined in the 1960s. Accordingly, a new substance in the preclinical phase was first supposed to be tested for toxicity, followed by tolerability tests on healthy volunteers. Only afterwards did the clinical phase begin with testing on patients. In some cases, however, the toxicology tests on animals were not yet completed when Kuhn started with the clinical trial, and sometimes not all of the usual tests were carried out. Several statements are documented in which Kuhn says he wants first to test the toxicity of a new substance on a chronic case. A number of test substances thus made their way to Münsterlingen without ever going through all of the already common stages of preliminary testing, especially if the point was to test Kuhn's proposals for sidechains and his pharmacological hypotheses.

*Second*, Kuhn did not follow the new methodological requirements. True, for a long time they were not legally binding, but they were necessary for approval applications in the United States and, as of the 1970s, also in Switzerland. Consequently, his results took on an admittedly important but informal status. Moreover, Kuhn did not adhere to the starts and endings of trials stipulated by the companies but instead continued using certain substances after the trials had been discontinued. Finally, he also distributed substances even when a trial had already come to an end. It seems unlikely that he sent remainders back to Basel, as requested by some firms.[12] He blatantly ignored trial protocols that started being set up in many places in the late 1960s. Such a trial protocol would have required, for example, a predetermined number of patients, clear diagnoses, and prescribed dosages, no combining of substances, and clearly defined questions.

*Third*, the Nuremberg Code of 1947 and the Declaration of Helsinki of 1964 had established guidelines for testing on humans, which required that patients be informed and give their consent. And the Swiss Academy of Medical Sciences also published guidelines for research on humans in 1970.[13] By then at the latest, there was a growing awareness of ethical issues in clinical trials on humans and, concomitantly, of the associated risks and dangers. But there are also indications that Kuhn was far from the only doctor who hardly paid attention to them at first. Moreover, many psychiatrists initially considered the use of placebos to be unethical because it meant one was knowingly giving patients ineffective substances. At Münsterlingen, the boundaries between therapeutic research and scientific experimentation – thus between treatment efforts and experiments without therapeutic intent – were repeatedly blurred. Although common today, this distinction was not introduced until the Declaration of Helsinki in 1964; prior to that, there was no common practice of distinguishing between the two. In Switzerland, the innovations for clinical trials that took hold in 1960s were introduced above all by the pharmaceutical companies, who were pressured to do so by approval authorities in the English-speaking world. On the other hand, however, it must be noted that the pharmaceutical companies virtually never intervened when Kuhn did not follow their standards. They only went as far as isolated, friendly reminders, but without further insistence – after all, the companies were dependent on this important trial partner, who could give them first impressions of a new substance.

## Consent, information, and deception

Despite the emerging ethical awareness since Helsinki and new research guidelines, for a long time the gap between testing norms and Kuhn's practices remained surmountable. Admittedly, there had been various tense moments over the years when Kuhn suddenly faced criticism – but not with regard to his testing.

One example is the Schenker case, where Kuhn reported at length about his trials and evidently managed to assuage the authorities. Another occurred in the wake of the ever more vociferous critique of psychiatry in the 1970s, which scrutinised and publicly debated the conditions in the clinics. In the Canton of Thurgau, there was an interpellation, which turned above all on staff conflicts, the desolate conditions of the premises, and 'custodial psychiatry'. As elsewhere, the discussion concentrated first and foremost on the clinic regimen and the stigma associated with mental illness; when psychotropic drugs were mentioned, the focus was on their routine use a 'chemical club'.

The tide did not turn until the late 1980s; the first written patient consent forms found among Kuhn's records are for the levoprotiline trial in 1987. Two years later, Kuhn received a letter from a budding historian of medicine. He was asking about the 'attendant circumstances' in the discovery of Tofranil and at the same time posed new questions: about ethical guidelines, patient consent, and Kuhn's approach.[14] The latter responded by return mail. In doing so, he left the question about self-experiments unanswered, but provided all the more candid information on other aspects. Back then, there were 'no requirements whatsoever, let alone legal regulations'. During the trials, blood pressure, pulse, and blood count were always checked, and through his close observation of the patients he always personally made sure 'to identify possible harms early on and to abort the trials immediately'. In fact, however, there was no consistent, close monitoring; incidents, some with a fatal outcome, could not always be avoided.

Especially illuminating, however, is the question about consent. Kuhn wrote about it frankly.

> We never asked patients for their consent to taking a test preparation. We always started with patients who suffered severely from their illnesses and whom we could not improve with the remedies

at our disposal. We then told them, we have a new medication that perhaps might help after all, and so we actually had no difficulties, neither with the patients nor with their relatives nor with the nursing staff or even with the assistants.[15]

For Kuhn, the vocal demands since the 1970s for the informed consent of patients seemed rather to be an obstacle because, in his opinion, they too strongly influenced the selection of probands. To give consent declarations, patients needed to understand what was being proposed. Moreover, the consent process distorted the results of a trial because it created expectations, hopes, and fears.[16] However, Kuhn never reflected on his own expectations as a lead investigator and observer. In the medical files of the Münsterlingen Psychiatric Clinic, we found no references to patient consents for clinical trials. Instead, our source work gave the impression that Kuhn relied on linguistically vague phrases: we have a new remedy that might help. It was a formulation that never disclosed that he was referring to a test substance and not to an approved drug.

In contrast, for electroshocks or lobotomies, the consent of patients or their relatives was being obtained throughout Switzerland. They were major interventions in the patient's physical integrity and thus had a different status than chemical substances. By comparison, a pill, capsule, or injection could be seen as a lower-threshold intervention with less severe physical consequences. Moreover, contrary to the aforementioned somatic therapies, these consequences seemed reversible, since medications could be discontinued and it was believed that their undesired effects would then disappear as well. The striking contrast between these consent policies might therefore be traced back to the difference between physical and mental treatments. On the other hand, it could also be related to the severity of the intervention, for in the case of somatic therapies doctors wanted to make sure to protect themselves in the event of any incidents.

Kuhn's statements, however, suggest that the test status itself justified dissimulation when administering test substances; it was the patients' lack of knowledge that allowed him to freely select patients in the first place, and it ensured that expectations did not distort the results. The clearest evidence that Kuhn deliberately kept his patients in the dark comes from the substances themselves.

## Conclusion 293

He repeatedly requested that the materiality of a test substance match that of a known substance so the test substance could be dispensed in disguise. In 1960, he suggested that Geigy make a new preparation exactly the same colour as Tofranil so that the patients did not notice they were receiving a different preparation. As late as 1976, he asked Ciba-Geigy to produce a test substance that looked like a different medication that was already approved. Whether the companies accommodated these requests is unknown.

Fully voluntary patient participation in clinical testing was rare at Münsterlingen. With the advent of psychoactive pills, dragees, and injections, the spectrum between coercion and voluntariness had become more diverse; there was now more latitude for camouflage, persuasion, and pressure. Inpatients who did not want to take a drug were sometimes given test substances mixed in their coffee or soup. How long these practices persisted is unclear. For later periods, there is evidence that trials were stopped if patients successfully resisted. There were variously subtle strategies of both resistance and countermeasures. Along with the frequent practice of persuasion and convincing, there were also cases of coercive administration, such as using injections, as well as strategies for increasing pressure. The latter included, above all, threatening to isolate someone or to transfer them to a different ward.

In some instances, especially in the case of outpatients or patients with psychiatric training, Kuhn provided more precise information, but sometimes only after being asked. Thus several nurses asked whether they had to pay for the substances they were being given as part of psychotherapy. Only then did Kuhn tell them that some of the substances were free. Others, on the other hand, were relatively comprehensively informed about test substances, especially 'favourite patients' with a positive attitude towards medications. When it came to ambulatory patients, Kuhn was more dependent on their cooperation because they had to take the substances on their own and report how they did with them. This also influenced information practices.

Compared to elsewhere at the time, the consent policy at Münsterlingen no doubt hardly deviated from the ordinary. Presumably, for a long time trials were also carried out at other institutions without informed patient consent. When this changed is a question for further research. For the Psychiatric University

Hospital Zurich, the first isolated but clear references to written consents and education appear in the period after 1978.[17] For Kuhn, such verifiable references do not appear until slightly less than a decade later. In clinical practice, it was long common to withhold information; thus patients did not always know what drugs they were taking, and whether these were test substances or approved medications.

## Many things are not what they seem

What Kuhn wrote was not always consistent with what he did. The number of cases that he named in his test reports, for instance, usually did not correspond to the number of patients actually involved. In his evaluations for the pharmaceutical industry, he left patients out, albeit not necessarily cases that were particularly problematic. Rather, he seems to have excluded the so-called preliminary tests from the evaluations because he saw them as an initial reconnaissance to become familiar with a substance. At this point, the testing was not yet about finding the effect in the proper sense of the term. But scepticism is called for at other levels, too, for his testing philosophy could simply not be consistently implemented in practice. So what did Kuhn's testing practices look like if one mistrusts his descriptions? Can recurring patterns be discerned? Were certain patient groups particularly affected?

Kuhn's testing philosophy conformed to his practices insofar as he proceeded exploratively and justified this with daseinsanalytical deliberations. His rejection of systems, numbers, data, statistics, and other methods that would have relativised his observer position can also be ascertained in the daily routine of testing. It is implausible, however, that this resistance was linked with the close observation and supervision of the test patients. Constantly struggling with an excessive workload, the clinic staff at all levels simply lacked the time to closely supervise the probands, meticulously record everything in reports, and always carry out all of the desired supporting examinations. The idea that Kuhn alone observed the most important effects and side-effects of new substances is likewise unrealistic. Even at the written level, one can trace how Kuhn made use of nursing reports and substantially enriched 'his' observations.

Furthermore, there is evidence of group discussions on substances, in which assistant physicians reported on their patients. Kuhn's discovering gaze actually consisted of many observing gazes that were hierarchically subordinated to him.[18]

Whether the tests followed a pattern is difficult to answer. The process often seems arbitrary; whenever we believed we could make out a pattern, it fell apart again upon closer inspection. Nonetheless, there are a few cornerstones. Kuhn preferred a long testing period, especially for substances that he assessed positively. But, on the other hand, in the case of 'uninteresting' substances, the tests could indeed be brief and small-scale, sometimes with only a single proband. No rules and arrangements were stipulated in advance; the process always remained open and intuitive. Kuhn constantly expanded trials; thus he did not begin with a predefined number or group of patients. The same applied to diagnoses, for the greatest possible flexibility prevailed here as well. Kuhn brought patients with other diagnoses into a trial series at his discretion if an effect in this direction seemed possible. If he found that a substance did indeed have an antidepressant effect, but that it also had other active components, he immediately brought patients with the corresponding diagnoses into the trial without consulting with the pharmaceutical company. These diagnostic expansions were often tied to pharmacological-theoretical deliberations.

However, this pattern too must be qualified. Around half of all the test substances that made their way to Münsterlingen were intended as antidepressants. The clinic's population, however, did not consist of that many depressed patients. In practice, this meant that the substances beings tested as potential antidepressants were increasing being tested on ambulatory patients. When it came to inpatients, the trials included many subjects with other diagnoses, for example, psychotic disorders. Even more bewildering is the fact that Kuhn sometimes included patients with diagnoses such as reduced intelligence or organic lesions in antidepressant trials. It is extremely doubtful that such diagnoses and the sought-for effect of the substance somehow matched in these cases; therefore, other criteria must have been a factor. Schizophrenias and depressions, as well as the associated substance groups, neuroleptics and antidepressants, were admittedly more closely linked for Kuhn than for others; for some schizophrenias, Kuhn suspected depressive components, and for a few potential antidepressants he suspected neuroleptic effects. However, discerning a connection between the sought-for effect and the diagnosis is by no means always possible.

The exact temporal sequence of a test brings another pattern into view, which also explains why diagnosis groups like reduced intelligence were included in trials. Kuhn often first tested a new substance on chronic patients – the so-called severe cases with little hope of recovery. The goal here was always 'to learn something' about the unknown substance and to determine its tolerability and the appropriate dosage. However, he felt these patients were unsuitable for more precise testing because they often only showed a weak response, expressed themselves poorly compared to other patients, and suffered from many different physical ailments. Therefore, the next step for Kuhn was to switch to a second patient group that responded more strongly and allowed for more observations of the effect. For the trials, Kuhn therefore had a clear patient hierarchy in the back of his mind. But this did not mean that certain patient groups were categorically excluded from trials. Even his 'favourite patients' were given test substances, albeit usually substances that already had shown positive effects.

Roland and Verena Kuhn did not generally treat children and youth any differently than adults, except the dosages were smaller, and they tried more often to confirm already known effects or to use them therapeutically. Therefore, one can only stress the diversity of the range of test subjects. All types of people were given test substances. Categories such as legal guardianship, social origin, or gender seem not to have played any role in the selection of patients. In his pharmacological optimism, Kuhn evidently proceeded democratically – with the exception of those chronic, serious cases that he had given up on and used to familiarise himself with new substances.

This is what makes the involvement of severely and chronically ill patients especially troublesome from today's perspective.[19] Their clinical picture often did not match at all with the intended effect of a test substance; another factor was often the patients' poor general physical condition. A few were quite well adjusted to a standard medication, which was then discontinued because of a test. Therefore, it is not true that Kuhn only selected patients for whom all other therapies had failed.

Another pattern pertains to the combining of substances. Kuhn freely combined test substances with approved medications or with other test substances. A patient's treatment with existing medications was not systematically discontinued before the patient was included in a trial. Kuhn was convinced that combinations could lead to improved results; in his eyes, they helped to clarify the effects and to alleviate side-effects. In his opinion, test substances therefore could work to each other's strengths. He was certain he could discern the effect of an individual test substance even from drug cocktails. This approach contradicted systematic, scientific testing programmes, but the pharmaceutical companies nonetheless let him have his way. Scepticism was rarely expressed.

In Kuhn's eyes, side-effects and risks by no means meant that substances were unsuitable or ineffective. Quite the contrary; from his perspective, complicated substances could be highly effective. If problems arose, to him this meant that the dosage had to be adjusted, or other patients were needed to better discern the effect. This had consequences for his handling of risk. For Kuhn, large risks did not automatically mean that a trial had to be aborted. There is evidence that Kuhn halted trials for four substances. These were substances that seemed too problematic for him or led to complications. Much more often, however, trials were stopped by the company, whether due to market considerations, patent-related reasons, or because the substance's effect seemed too marginal.

### Motives and regulatory oversight

Kuhn repeatedly invoked financial reasons for his testing activities. Münsterlingen did not have enough money for Largactil, he noted, which was why he continued the trials for Geigy. Modern psychopharmaceuticals, which emerged in 1953 with Largactil, were in fact expensive. Kuhn also argued that clinical testing considerably reduced the pressure on the clinic's medication budget. Thus one killed two birds with one stone, gaining access to the newest substances while saving money for the clinic and the canton.

The experiments were repeatedly discussed with the higher authorities. They therefore knew the score, but they never looked too closely. Their surviving exchanges with the clinic refer almost exclusively to individual patients or to financial, building-related, or staffing issues. The clinical trials were never monitored. Kuhn was not asked to give an account of them, and as far as we know the trial documentation was never inspected. The higher authorities took it for granted that research was being conducted, which moreover reduced the spending on medications, and they were content with that. Research on humans was not legally regulated in Thurgau until the 1980s, when the first cantonal ethics commission was set up in Switzerland. This was in part a reaction to the Schenker scandal, through which the authorities gained an initial awareness of the problem.

Clinical research made Roland Kuhn a wealthy man. All told, his research income amounted to around 8 million francs (as per 2015 prices). Practically all of the compensation went to him personally. Kuhn always emphasised that he carried out the clinical trials in his free time. But he made no mention of the fact that he relied on the clinic's personnel and infrastructure, as well as – not least – on its patients.

The question as to Kuhn's personal motives cannot be definitively answered; in his case, research interests and financial motives can hardly be separated. His lifestyle was hard-working and middle-class; he was variously described as a frugal man. Money per se did not seem that important to him, nor was it important for supporting an upscale lifestyle or as a sign of social advancement. For him it was more of a confirmation of success and form of recognition.

Clinical research gave Kuhn a chance to gain prestige. He was known as the 'father' of Tofranil and, ever since its success, the 'discovery' of new medications was for him a preordained path that could lead to fame and honour. Kuhn was not satisfied with a contemplative existence; he wanted to interact with the intellectual giants of his time and find acceptance among his colleagues. The exchange of expertise with pharmaceutical experts must also have been quite important to him. Only this explains why he ventured so far from his home territory of psychiatry and engaged in speculations about the laws of chemistry and pharmacology. Questions are raised in particular by his stubborn commitment to substances such as ketimipramine or levoprotiline. For him, was this perhaps all about 'discovering', by hook or by crook, a new

Tofranil, which had brought such financial success and recognition? In any event, financial success and professional recognition could both be had through clinical testing.

Apart from research interests and a strong need for affirmation, Kuhn was also characterised by a great pharmacological optimism. He advocated the use of medications for a wide range of complaints and believed in the efficacy of chemical substances. Other therapeutic approaches meant little to him – here, one can mention psychoanalysis or social-psychiatric approaches, which were critical of a purely pharmacological therapy. Instead, Kuhn struck a balancing act, trying to link his clinical trials with daseinsanalysis and combining psychopharmacological and psychotherapeutic approaches. Remarkably often, Kuhn assessed substances more positively than other investigators; only rarely did he find substances uninteresting or ineffective. This optimism seems strange at times, and it was tied to an occasionally risky approach when administering test substances. Moreover, Kuhn would continue his trial series for an extraordinarily long time. Admittedly, the long duration was for him an epistemological alternative to placebos, through which he wanted to eliminate suggestive effects. However, the transition from testing to purely therapeutic applications appears to have been seamless.

### The end of the beginning

*On trial* must leave certain key questions unanswered. The systematic, comprehensive sampling of medical files allowed us to supplement Kuhn's private archive with another central source base. This was all the more important since we had previously been unable to calculate more accurate figures. How many patients received test substances without their names being listed in Kuhn's private archive? How many serious incidents and fatalities took place? Were there other patient groups who received test substances? And were there groups who never received any test substances whatsoever?

Even if Kuhn was in many respects an extraordinary and especially eager investigator, it should be pointed out that clinical tests with psychoactive substances took place not only in Münsterlingen but also in numerous other institutions. A deeper understanding and more contextualised evaluation of the Münsterlingen trial site would require comparisons with other clinics. Only then could one answer questions about the nature of the national and international testing landscape, about the degree to which testing practices elsewhere differed from those of Kuhn, and about changes to the practice of educating patients about trials and obtaining their consent. But what especially distinguishes the Münsterlingen case is the source material itself. Roland and Verena Kuhn's private archive constitutes a remarkably abundant body of sources, which can be profitably linked with the archive of the Münsterlingen Psychiatric Clinic. In the medical files of the latter, Kuhn rarely appears; showing up here instead are countless individual fates, entire lives with their vicissitudes, which taken as whole would enable not only a sociological study of the Canton of Thurgau, but also a large-scale picture of the postwar society.

## Notes

1 This history starts no later than with the Nuremberg Code of 1947, when the experiments on humans in the Nazi concentration camps were condemned and ethical norms were formulated, including the voluntary consent of test subjects and the eschewing of arbitrary, superfluous testing and unnecessary suffering.
2 These are those drugs for which we could find testing records or that were referred to in medical files. The trials took place at the Münsterlingen Psychiatric Clinic or in Kuhn's private practice.
3 The database includes 537 women and 523 men; the sex of 52 persons is unclear.
4 For an overview of studies from the German-speaking word, see Germann, 'Medikamentenversuche'.
5 Photo album of former nurse Marlies Verhofnik, interview of 12 September 2016.
6 Interview with former trainee nurse, 18 April 2018.
7 Interview with René Bloch; interview with former administrative employee, 28 November 2016.
8 Interview with René Bloch, 14 March 2018.
9 StATG, 9'40, 12/367, Kuhn to cantonal physician Alfred Muggli, 29 July 2002. At this time, Kuhn still had one or two consultations a week with private patients.

10 Interview with a former trainee nurse, 18 April 2018.
11 Interview with Alexandra Delini-Stula, 19 June 2017.
12 After the dissolution of the clinic pharmacy at the end of 1986, twelve metal boxes remained, which each contained between 5,000 and 25,000 capsules or dragees. File note, Rainer Andenmatten, former cantonal pharmacist, for the attention of the Thurgau State Archives, 2 October 2014.
13 These were norms, not laws. To what extent these testing practices already violated the constitutional right to physical and mental integrity is a legal question that we cannot address here.
14 StATG, 9'40, 5.1.2/2, Udo Benzenhöfer to Kuhn, 21 June 1989.
15 StATG, 9'40, 5.1.2/2, Kuhn to Benzenhöfer, 29 June 1989.
16 Kuhn, 'Clinique', 160.
17 Rietmann et al., 'Medikamentenversuche', 245.
18 StATG, 9'40, 5.0.3/11, notice of a discussion with doctors about Yellow II, 4 April 1961.
19 Unfortunately, we cannot answer the question of whether Kuhn's practice with chronic and severely ill patients differed significantly from contemporary practice, but rather only point to the discrepancies with existing guidelines and norms.

# Chronology

| | |
|---|---|
| 1839/1840 | Founding of the Münsterlingen Mental Hospital, consisting of a psychiatric ward and an infirmary |
| 1850 | Thurgau Medical Services Act (remains in force until 1985) |
| 1871 | The two old former monastic building complexes of the Münsterlingen Mental Hospital are separated from each other by a railway line |
| 1895 | Definitive separation of the Münsterlingen 'Mental Asylum' and 'Hospital' |
| 1900 | Agreement between five cantons, which is gradually joined by additional cantons: creation of the Intercantonal Office for the Control of Medicines (IKS), which reviews and registers new drugs |
| 4 March 1912 | Roland Kuhn is born in Biel |
| 1912 | Hermann Wille becomes director of the Münsterlingen Psychiatric Clinic (MPC) |
| 3 August 1921 | Verena Gebhart is born in Kreuzlingen |
| 1929/1930 | Change of name from *Irrenanstalt* (insane asylum) to *Irrenheilanstalt* (mental sanatorium) |
| 1937 | Roland Kuhn: state exams in Bern, position as assistant physician at Waldau under Jakob Klaesi |
| 1938/1939 | Roland Kuhn's first publications on the Rorschach test and on daseinsanalysis
Establishment of an outpatient clinic at the MPC |
| 1939 | Roland Kuhn becomes senior physician at the MPC, Adolf Zolliker becomes director, and Agathe Christ becomes secretary |

# Chronology

| | |
|---|---|
| 1940 | Change of name from the 'Thurgauische Irrenheilanstalt Münsterlingen' (Thurgau Insane Asylum Münsterlingen) to 'Thurgauische Heil- und Pflegeanstalt Münsterlingen' (Thurgau Sanatorium and Care Facility Münsterlingen) |
| 1942 | Establishment of a laboratory at the MPC |
| | Revision of the IKS agreement: now each new medicine must be evaluated and registered before the cantons can approve it |
| 1946 | Start of the collaboration with Geigy: Kuhn sends his first reports to Basel |
| 1947 | Verena Gebhart becomes the fourth assistant physician at the MPC |
| 1949 | At Geigy, the chemist Walter Schindler synthesises the substance G 22355, the later Tofranil |
| 1950 | The first test quantity of G 22150 is tested at MPC |
| 1952 | Verena Gebhart becomes a senior physician at the MPC |
| 1953 | Largactil (chlorpromazine), the first neuroleptic, is introduced at the MPC |
| 1954 | The number of patients at the MPC reaches its highest level with more than 700 people |
| | G 22150 undergoes a large-scale trial at the MPC |
| | Largactil is officially approved in Switzerland |
| | The cantons fully transfer the review and assessment of medicines to the IKS |
| 1954/1955 | G 22355 (Tofranil) arrives and is initially tested for its effect on schizophrenia |
| 1956 | Roland Kuhn's first report to Geigy on the antidepressant effect of G 22355 |
| | Married staff of the MPC may now stay overnight outside of the clinic; work time is reduced to sixty hours per week |
| 1957 | Roland Kuhn completes his postdoctoral qualification (*Habilitation*) at the University of Zurich |
| | The MPC's fencing along the lakeshore is removed |
| | Roland Kuhn's first publication on G 22355 |
| | Paul Schmidlin recommends the commercial launch of G 22355 to his superiors at Geigy |
| 1958 | Marriage of Roland Kuhn and Verena Gebhart |
| | Approval of G 22355 imipramine as Tofranil in Switzerland |

|      |   |
|------|---|
| | Roland and Verena Kuhn, together with Paul Schmidlin, travel to the United States to promote Tofranil |
| 1959 | Approval of Tofranil in the United States |
| | Roland Kuhn receives his first annual Tofranil bonus |
| 1960 | Roche makes contact with Roland Kuhn |
| 1961 | New construction of a medical centre at the MPC; the Kuhn family moves into the new senior physician's apartment |
| | Roche launches its own antidepressant called Elavil (amitriptyline) |
| | Geigy launches Insidon |
| | Thalidomide scandal |
| 1962 | Geigy launches Pertofran |
| | Kefauver–Harris Amendment, which tightens the FDA requirements in the United States |
| | Testing of FR 33 at the MPC (until 1964) |
| 1963 | IKS expands the documentation obligation, thereby requiring clinical proof of effectiveness for new preparations |
| | Testing of Ketotofranil (until approximately 1970) |
| 1964 | Declaration of Helsinki ethical research guidelines for clinical trials |
| | Triumphant success of the Roche substances Librium and Valium |
| | Kuhn henceforth receives an annual Tofranil bonus of 60,000 Swiss francs (until 1976) |
| 1965 | Swiss Academy of Medical Sciences (SAMS): reporting obligation for incidents and fatalities that could be related to the administering of test substances or approved medications |
| 1966 | Roland Kuhn becomes honorary professor at the University of Zurich |
| | Testing of Ciba 34276 (Ludiomil) at the MPC (until 1972) |
| | Geigy launches Anafranil |
| | Change of name from 'Thurgauische Heil- und Pflegeanstalt Münsterlingen' (Thurgau Sanatorium and Care Facility Münsterlingen) to 'Psychiatrische Klinik Münsterlingen' (Münsterlingen Psychiatric Clinic) |
| 1967 | Merger of Sandoz and Wander |
| 1970 | Merger of Ciba and Geigy as Ciba-Geigy |

# Chronology

| | |
|---|---|
| 1970 | Opening of the nursing school and staff building at the MPC |
| | SAMS: Guidelines for 'research studies on humans' |
| 1971 | Roland Kuhn takes over the directorate of the MPC |
| | A pool for secondary income is established at the MPC |
| | IKS assumes responsibility for monitoring the manufacturing of new medications |
| 1972 | Approval of Ludiomil |
| | Roland Kuhn receives his first revenue share for Ludiomil (until 1985) |
| | Verena Kuhn becomes a leading physician at the MPC |
| 1972/1973 | Public criticism of Kuhn and the conditions at the MPC; interpellation in the canton parliament |
| 1973 | The director and leading physicians are now officially allowed to provide consultations and expert evaluations for their own account |
| 1975 | Agathe Christ retires |
| 1976 | Roland Kuhn for the first time receives an annual revenue share of more than 100,000 Swiss francs (until 1984) |
| 1977 | Roland and Verena Kuhn move from their apartment on the clinic grounds into a single-family home in Scherzingen |
| | IKS: revision of the registration guidelines of 1963, clinical studies on humans are basically supposed to be conducted as controlled clinical trials |
| 1978 | Gender desegregation of two wards in the MPC |
| 1980 | Roland Kuhn retires and opens a private practice |
| | Karl Studer becomes clinic director |
| 1981 | Roland Kuhn receives an honorary doctorate from Louvain University in Belgium |
| 1983 | Retirement of Verena Kuhn-Gebhart |
| 1986 | Roland Kuhn receives an honorary doctorate from Sorbonne University in Paris |
| | Schenker affair: disciplinary and criminal proceedings against the cantonal physician Hans Schenker (until 1989) |
| 1987 | Establishment of a medical ethics commission in the Canton of Thurgau |
| | The Thurgau Health Act is supplemented with an Ordinance on the Legal Status of Patients in Cantonal Facilities of the Healthcare System, which includes provisions on clinical trials |

| | |
|---|---|
| 1992 | Roland Kuhn receives an honorary doctorate from the University of Basel |
| 1995 | IKS: regulations on medications in clinical trials enter into force |
| 1996 | Merger of Sandoz with Ciba-Geigy as Novartis |
| 1998 | Roland Kuhn's teaching activity at the University of Zurich ends |
| 2002 | Therapeutic Products Act enacted at the federal level |
| 10 October 2005 | Death of Roland Kuhn |
| 2012 | The Thurgau State Archives obtain the private archive of Roland Kuhn and Verena Kuhn-Gebhart through donation by the Kuhns' joint heirs |
| 20 April 2015 | Death of Verena Kuhn-Gebhart |

## List of test substances

| Test number | Internal company name | Substance name | Trade name | Manufacturer | Request | Trial | Approval |
|---|---|---|---|---|---|---|---|
| 38904 Ba (Alival) | | Nomifensine hydrogenmaleinicum | Alival | Ciba-Geigy Farbwerke Hoechst | 09/1973 | 07/1976–08/1976 | 16/03/1977 |
| AMPT | | Alpha-methyl-p-tyronsine | | Astra Läkemedel | | 07/1976–11/1976 | |
| AW 143076 | | | | Wander | 03/09/1978 | 03/1969–04/1969 | |
| AW 151129 | | | | Wander | 06/07/1967 | 07/1967–09/1968 | |
| Ba-49802 B | | Oxaprotiline | | Ciba-Geigy | 05/11/1976 | | |
| BY 54 | | | | Sandoz | 08/10/1958 | 10/1958–01/1960 | |
| BY 107 | | Ciclopramine | | Byk Gulden | 25/02/1975 | | |
| C 7245 | | | | Cilag-Chemie | 01/1964–06/1964 | | |
| CGP 12103 | | Levoprotiline | | Ciba-Geigy | 07/1986 | 11/1986–11/1990 | |
| CGP 14175 | | Citatepine mesylate | Tetral | Ciba-Geigy | 31/03/1988 | 05/1988–1988 | |
| Ciba 10870 | | | | Ciba | 15/09/1954 | 10/1954–1955 | |

*(continued)*

List of test substances (Cont.)

| Test number | Internal company name | Substance name | Trade name | Manufacturer | Request | Trial | Approval |
|---|---|---|---|---|---|---|---|
| Ciba 10870 | | | | Ciba | 02/12/1957 | | |
| Ciba 17040 | | | | Ciba | 07/1956 | 07/1956–1960 | |
| Ciba 20068 | | | | Ciba | 02/1967 | | |
| Ciba 20068 | | | | Ciba-Geigy | 01/1972 | 03/1972 | |
| Ciba 21024 | | | | Ciba-Geigy | 01/1972 | 03/1972–07/1973 | |
| Ciba 21401 | | Tribenoside | Glyvenol | Ciba | 11/1968 | | 06/04/1967 |
| Ciba 24160 | | | | Ciba | 11/1959 | 12/1959–01/1960 | |
| Ciba 27937 | | | | Ciba | 05/1962 | 06/1962–11/1964 | |
| Ciba 30803 | | Benzoctamine | Tacitin | Ciba | 29/05/1962 | 1963–1967 | 03/04/1970 |
| Ciba 30803 | | Benzoctamine | Tacitin | Ciba | 17/11/1964 | | 03/04/1970 |
| Ciba 30803 | | Benzoctamine | Tacitin | Ciba | 15/03/1967 | | 03/04/1970 |
| Ciba 32143 | | | | Ciba | 1962 | 06/1964–10/1965 | |
| Ciba 34276 | Ciba remedy | Maprotiline | Ludiomil | Ciba | 10/1965 | 01/1966–10/1972 | 10/11/1972 |
| Ciba 34647 | | Baclofen | Lioresal | Ciba | 15/03/1967 | 03/1967–1969 | 18/12/1970 |

List of test substances (Cont.)

| Test number | Internal company name | Substance name | Trade name | Manufacturer | Request | Trial | Approval |
|---|---|---|---|---|---|---|---|
| Ciba 34647 | | Baclofen | Lioresal | Ciba-Geigy | 01/1975 | 01/1975–1976 | 18/12/1970 |
| Ciba 34799 | | | | Ciba | 1962/1963 | 06/1964–11/1964 | |
| Ciba 39089 | | Oxprenolol | Trasicor | Ciba | | 06/1974–1980 | 21/05/1968 |
| Ciba 42694 | | Beta-melanotropin, beta-MSH | | Ciba-Geigy | 06/1973 | 06/1973–1975 | |
| EMD 25004 | | | | Merck | 01/1976 | | |
| FR 33 | | Butyrophenone | | Sandoz | 08/1962 | 08/1962–09/1964 | |
| G 2747 | | Parpanit | Parpanit | Geigy | 03/1946 | 04/1946–12/1946 | 30/12/1946 |
| G 14133 | | | | Geigy | 04/1950 | 04/1950 | |
| G 14134 | | Parpanit tartrate | | Geigy | 10/1946 | 11/1946 | |
| G 21302 | | | | Geigy | 1962 | | |
| G 22150 | Geigy White | | | Geigy | 10/1950 | 10/1950–12/1951 | |
| G 22150 | Geigy White | | | Geigy | 03/1954 | 04/1954–12/1956 | |
| G 22355 | Geigy Red | Imipramine | Tofranil | Geigy | 08/1954 | 11/1954–03/1958 | 13/03/1958 |

(*continued*)

List of test substances (Cont.)

| Test number | Internal company name | Substance name | Trade name | Manufacturer | Request | Trial | Approval |
|---|---|---|---|---|---|---|---|
| G 22355 R 1683/1 and other extended release formulations | | Tofranil fumarate, imipramine fumarate | | Geigy | 1958 | 09/1958–03/1959 | |
| G 23746 | Geigy Yellow | | | Geigy | 07/1956 | 07/1956–03/1957 | |
| G 24075 | | | | Geigy | 02/1951 | | |
| G 24415 | Geigy Blue | | | Geigy | 07/1956 | 08/1956–08/1957 | |
| G 24575 | | | | Geigy | 03/08/1951 | | |
| G 27032 | | | | Geigy | 09/1958 | 09/1958–12/1959 | |
| G 28342 | Geigy Brown | | | Geigy | 10/1956 | 07/1957–08/1958 | |
| G 28364 | Geigy Black | Dichlorimipramine | | Geigy | 10/1956 | 03/1957–11/1957 | |
| G 28568 | Geigy Green | | | Geigy | 10/1955 | 11/1955–10/1956 | |
| G 31002 | Geigy White (II) | | | Geigy | 06/1956–07/1956 | 07/1956–1960 | |

List of test substances (Cont.)

| Test number | Internal company name | Substance name | Trade name | Manufacturer | Request | Trial | Approval |
|---|---|---|---|---|---|---|---|
| G 31220 | Geigy Green (II), Geigy Orange | | | Geigy | 15/08/1956 | 08/1956–11/1956 | |
| G 31220 | Greigy Green (II), Geigy Orange | | | Geigy | | 09/1959–01/1960 | |
| G 31406 | Geigy Pink, Stilben Tofranil | | | Geigy | 12/07/1957 | 08/1957–12/1960 | |
| G 31531 | | | | Geigy | 07/1965 | | |
| G 31531 | | | | Geigy | 15/06/1966 | 06/1966–07/1966 | |
| G 32883 | | Carbamazepine | Tegretol | Geigy | 06/1962 | 07/1962–12/1963 | 05/06/1963 |
| G 32883 | | | Tegretol | Ciba-Geigy | 07/1974 | 1974–1975 | 05/06/1963 |
| G 33006 | Geigy Blue (II) | | | Geigy | 10/12/1958 | 06/1959–03/1961 | |
| G 33040 | Geigy (II), Geigy Violet | Opipramol | Insidon | Geigy | 09/1958 | 01/1959–11/1960 | |
| G 33040 | Geigy (II), Geigy Violet | Opipramol | Insidon | Geigy | | 01/1961–1961 | 12/10/1961 |

(*continued*)

List of test substances  (Cont.)

| Test number | Internal company name | Substance name | Trade name | Manufacturer | Request | Trial | Approval |
|---|---|---|---|---|---|---|---|
| G 33679 | Geigy Violet, Metabolite I | | | Geigy | 09/06/1958 | 06/1958–12/1958 | |
| G 33679 | Geigy Violet, Metabolite I | | | Geigy | 17/11/1961 | 12/1961–12/1962 | |
| G 34586 | Chloride Tofranil, Monochloride Tofranil | Clomipramine | Anafranil | Geigy | 10/03/1960 | 04/1960–1961 | 25/10/1966 |
| G 35020 | Metabolite III | Desipramine, desmethylimipramine | Pertofran | Geigy | | 09/1961–06/1962 | 06/06/1962 |
| G 35259 | Keto | Ketotofranil, ketimipramine | | Geigy | 08/1963 | 10/1963–12/1970 | |
| G 35570 | Geigy Green (III) | | | Geigy | 19/06/1959 | 1960–1976 | |
| G 35754 (R 1875) | | | | Geigy | 11/1959 | | |
| G 35878 | | | | Geigy | 16/09/1960 | | |
| G 36526 | Metabolite VI | | | Geigy | 1964 | 1964–1966 | |
| G 36526 | Metabolite VI | | | Geigy | 15/06/1966 | | |

List of test substances (Cont.)

| Test number | Internal company name | Substance name | Trade name | Manufacturer | Request | Trial | Approval |
|---|---|---|---|---|---|---|---|
| G 37329 | | | | Geigy | 22/11/1961 | 11/1961–03/1963 | |
| G 37329 | | | | Geigy | | 01/1964–12/1964 | |
| G 37815 | | | | Geigy | 11/1961 | | |
| G 37816 | | | | Geigy | 11/1961 | | |
| G 38038 | | | | Geigy | 09/01/1963 | 01/1963–12/1964 | |
| G 38462 | | | | Geigy | 31/10/1963 | 11/1963–04/1967 | |
| G 38462 | | | | Geigy | 15/06/1966 | | |
| GP 41369 | | | | Geigy | 01/1967 | 02/1967–02/1968 | |
| GP 43011 | | | | Ciba-Geigy | 01/1972 | | |
| GP 44964 | | | | Ciba-Geigy | 01/1972 | 02/1972–02/1972 | |
| GP 47680 | Keto Tegretol, Tegretol successor | Keto carbamazepine, oxcarbazepine | Trileptal | Ciba-Geigy | 09/1977 | 10/1977–1978 | 23/12/1994 |
| GP 49203 | | | | Ciba-Geigy | 01/1972 | 02/1972–05/1972 | |
| H 102/09 | | Zimelidine | Normud | Astra Läkemedel | 11/1976 | | 19/05/1982 |

(*continued*)

List of test substances (Cont.)

| Test number | Internal company name | Substance name | Trade name | Manufacturer | Request | Trial | Approval |
|---|---|---|---|---|---|---|---|
| HF 1854 | | Clozapine | Leponex | Wander | 06/07/1967 | 07/1968–05/1969 | 02/11/1972 |
| HF 1854 | | Clozapine | Leponex | Wander | | 09/1972–11/1972 | 02/11/1972 |
| HH 222 | | | | Hommel | 03/1969 | | |
| I.C.I 58834 | | Viloxazine | Vivalan | Imperial Chemical Industries | 08/06/1973 | | 11/01/1977 |
| IB 503 | | | | Sandoz | 02/1965 | 02/1965–12/1965 | |
| IB 503 | | | | Sandoz | 05/1967 | 05/1967–07/1967 | |
| IB 503 | | | | Sandoz | 18/09/1967 | 10/1967–1969 | |
| IBD 78 | | | | Sandoz | 08/1965 | | |
| (Irgapyrin) | | | Irgapyrin | Geigy | 28/06/1950 | 07/1950–08/1950 | 01/04/1950 |
| IS 884 | | | | Sandoz | 18/12/1968 | | |
| (Largactil) | | | Largactil | Specia | | 09/1953–02/1954 | 11/02/1954 |
| NR 286 | | Flutizenol, thienobenzodiazepine | | Sandoz | 05/1970 | 06/1970–1971 | |
| PSP 900 | | | | Sandoz | 07/1965 | 08/1965–06/1966 | |

List of test substances (Cont.)

| Test number | Internal company name | Substance name | Trade name | Manufacturer | Request | Trial | Approval |
|---|---|---|---|---|---|---|---|
| PSP 900 | | | | Sandoz | | 06/1966–05/1967 | |
| R 1899/1 | | | | Geigy | 06/1959 | 08/1959–02/1960 | |
| R 5147 | | Spiroperidol | | Cilag-Chemie | 06/1964 | | |
| Ro 4-9661 | | | | Hoffmann-La Roche | 04/05/1966 | 06/1966–11/1966 | |
| Ro 6-2728 | | | | Hoffmann-La Roche | 01/12/1966 | 12/1966–07/1967 | |
| Ro 6-5136 | | | | Hoffmann-La Roche | 1967 | 08/1967–11/1967 | |
| Ro 6-5670 | | | | Hoffmann-La Roche | 1968 | 1968–10/1969 | |
| (Serpasil) | | Reserpine | Serpasil | Ciba | 05/1954–06/1954 | 06/1954–05/1955 | 23/09/1953 |
| (Serpasil and Ritalin) | | | | Ciba | 05/1954–06/1954 | 06/1954–11/1954 | |
| (Solcoderm) | | | Solcoderm | Solco | 29/06/1978 | 1978–1979 | 12/03/1984 |

(*continued*)

List of test substances (Cont.)

| Test number | Internal company name | Substance name | Trade name | Manufacturer | Request | Trial | Approval |
|---|---|---|---|---|---|---|---|
| (Solcoseryl) | | | Solcoseryl | Solco | | | 03/01/1957 |
| SUM 3170 | | Loxapine | | Wander | 08/1969 | 08/1977 | |
| Wy 3263 | American drug | Iprindole | Galatur | Wyeth | 03/11/1961 | 10/1969–01/1971 | |
| YF 181 | | Indenopyridine | | Sandoz | 1970 | 11/1961–08/1962 | |
| | | | | | | 12/1970–03/1971 | |

*Notes*: Substances in brackets in the 'test number' column are only referred to by their substance or trade name in the book.
Some of the information in the 'request' and 'trial' columns is approximate, particularly if larger time periods are indicated.
Approval: first approval of the active substance. The approval information comes from Swissmedic or was reviewed by Swissmedic.

# Bibliography

## Sources

### Archival sources

*Archive of the Psychiatric Museum Bern*
Akten Ernst Grünthal (1894–1972), Waldau

*Archive of the Münsterlingen Psychiatric Clinic, Münsterlingen*
1.53.01 Regierungsrat und Departement: Korrespondenz (1978–1992)
  Departement ab Januar 1987
  Regierungsrat und Departement: Korrespondenz
1.54.03 Labor: Akten und Korrespondenz
1.60.01 Medikamentenforschung
1.62.04 Pressetexte und Dokumentationen (1980–1994)
Personnel file of Verena Kuhn-Gebhart

*Archive of Swissmedic, Bern*
Clinical documentation and copies from approval dossiers related to Anafranil, Glyvenol, Insidon, Leponex, Lioresal, Ludiomil, Melleril, Pertofran, Serpasil, Tacitin, Tegretol, Tofranil, Trasicor

*Novartis AG, Basel*
**Company archive (CA Novartis)**

Ciba
FO 5.03, Forschung. Zweckforschung, chemische Protokolle, Pharma-Forschungsausschuss, Nr. 1/63–16/70 (1.6.1963–23.9.1970)
PE 4.01 (Hugo Bein, CIBA)
Vf 1, Pharma-Informations-Comité, Protokolle, 1953–1963
  Verkauf. Pharma-Protokolle, Pharma-Planungsausschuss, 1966–1970

Verkaufs- und Werbeausschuss, Pharma-Protokolle, 1967–1970
Vg 1.101 Verwaltung, Geschäftsleitung, Pharma-Protokolle, 1964–1970

Ciba-Geigy
RE 14.02 ZF Recht, Freie Mitarbeiter, Aufstellung der Zahlungen, 1982–1986
PH 8.01.01 Division Pharma, Pharma Schweiz, Pharmazeutischer Spezialitäten-Umsatz, Ciba-Linie 1970–1983
VR 1, 1973/1974
Z 9.01 Zentralsekretariat, Darstellungsservice, Organigramme Stammhaus, 1970
PH 1, Divison Pharma, Protokolle der Divisionsleitung, Index für die Jahre 1976–1981
PH 2, Division Pharma, Berichte, Psycho-Neuropharmaka, Standortbestimmung der Ciba-Geigy Produkte 1975/1976, 21.10.1976
PH 4.00.2, Division Pharma, Forschung, Protokolle, Pharma-Forschungs-Ausschuss, 1970–1978
PH 4.02, Division Pharma, Forschung Konzern, Research Conference Basle/USA 1975
PH 7.01, Marketing-Medizinisch-pharmazeutische Information, Psyche + Soma 1975–1980
PH 7.04, Division Pharma, Präparate und Information, diverse
PH 8.06, Pharma-International, PHI-Protokolle 1983–1984

Geigy
FB 1, Material zu Dr med. Paul E. Schmidlin (1917–1984)
FB 4/3, Firmengeschichte, Biographisches, Dr Robert Boehringer (1884–1974), Berichte und Beobachtungen, Pharma.
FB 4/4 Firmengeschichte, Biographisches, Dr Robert Boehringer (1884–1974), Korrespondenz mit Carl Koechlin-Vischer, 1948–1957
G_JU/V, ZF Recht, Abgelaufene Verträge, Nr. 2081–2219; Geigy-Verträge, Nr. 2183–2250
GB 26, Technische Jahresberichte 1956–1959
GL 10–11, Geschäftsleitender Ausschuss, Protokolle 1955–1958
PP 1a, Produktion Pharma, Geigy-Pharmaka, Jahresberichte, 1947, 1950, 1962–1966, 1. Quartal 1967
PP 1b: Produktion Pharma, Jahresberichte, Diverses
PP 3, Produktion Pharma, Pharmazeutische Abteilung, Gründung, Forschung & Entwicklung
PP 9/2, Produktion Pharma, Pharma Fassionierungsbetrieb, Sammlung Dr K. Reber, Quartals- und Jahresberichte 1954–1958
PP 12/1–3, Produktion Pharma, Pharma-Gremium, Protokolle, 1952–1957, 1960–1967
PP 12/4, Produktion Pharma, Pharma-Gremium, Protokolle: Geigy Pharmaka/Pharma-Planung, Forschungs- und Vertriebssitzung, Piraten-Komitee, Pharma Engagement, 1953–1956

PP 12/5, Produktion Pharma, Medizinische Abteilung, Sachgebietsprotokolle
PP 22/6-7, Produktion Pharma, Psychopharmaka, Tofranil
PP 36, Produktion Pharma, Forschung, Quartalsberichte 1965–1970, Sammlung Dr E. Girod
PP 42, Produktion Pharma, Medizinische Abteilung, Jahresberichte 1964–1967
PP 50, Produktion Pharma, Pharmakologische Abteilung, Klinik-Präparate, Entwicklungspräparate, Statistische Jahresberichte 1955–1966
PP 52, Produktion Pharma, Medizinische Abteilung, Planung, Organisation, Prüfungsprogramme, Entwicklungspräparate 1969–1971
PP 130, Produktion Pharma, Jahresberichte der Pharmazeutischen Abteilung, 1947–1959

Sandoz
C 304.001, 1957–1969
C 307.000, 1967–1969
H 101.002/003
H 205.003/205.004
H 205.006, 1959–1960
H 209.005, 1956–1966
H 209.006–209.008, Protokolle der Sitzungen der Klinischen Forschungsabteilung
H 121.000, Pharmazeutisches Departement, Protokoll der Geschäftsführung

Wander
Companies 1968/1969
Annual reports of subsidiaries 1968, 1969, 1970
Subsidiaries 1968–1971

**Novartis AG clinical archive and research archive**

Individual documents

*Roche AG, Basel*
**Roche historical archive**

Interne Mitteilung Dr H. Bruderer, VI/Chem., H.W. Roth, VI/ZS, Present State and Prospects in the Field of Antidepressants, 23.5.1975
Rapport Nr. B-53'543, Interner Forschungsbericht. Ein Bericht über Neuroleptika, Dr E. Kyburz, 29.9.1975
Rapport Nr. 54'333, Dr L. Havas, Bactrim Injektionslösung Ro 06–2580/022. Ergebnisse über Therapie und Verträglichkeit. 25.4.1972
Rapport Nr. 70'563. Abschlussbericht von Dr G. J. Foglar, Abt. VI/Klin., Präparat Ro 6-5670, 24.3.1970
Rapport Nr. 71'499, Dr J. E. Blum, Vergleichende Beurteilung von Benzodiazepinen in verschiedenen pharmakologischen Tests, 4.1.1968

## Bibliography

*Fribourg State Archives*

**Cantonal Psychiatric Hospital, Marsens**

HPC 49, Traitement du personnel, 1953–1954
HPC 202, Pensionnaires, 1956–1968
HPC 305, Correspondances, 1954–1961
HPC 446, Commission administrative, sous-commission médicale, Rapports, séances, 1959–1963

*Thurgau State Archives (StATG)*

**Finance department**

4'30 Finanzdepartement allgemein (1803–)
4'34 Finanzverwaltung: Staatsanstalten III (1804–1990)

**Health office**

9'14, 5.2.6 Psychiatrische Klinik Münsterlingen (1962–1996)

**Great council**

2'30'331-A, 54/9-1, Allgemeine Akten Grosser Rat, Botschaft des Regierungsrats zum Gesetz über das Gesundheitswesen, 8.9.1981

**Münsterlingen Psychiatric Clinic**

9'10. 0 Rechtliche Grundlagen (1840–1978)
9'10, 1 Direktion und Verwaltung (1840–1995)
9'10, 2 Rechnungswesen (1851–1992)
9'10, 3 Bauwesen (1843–1980)
9'10, 4 Personalwesen (1850–1994)
9'10, 5 Patienten und Patientinnen stationär (1839–1959)
9'10, 6 Patienten und Patientinnen ambulant (1916–1980)
9'10, 8 Testverfahren, Diagnostik (1926–1994)
9'10, 9 Forschung, Therapie (1844–1994)
9'10, 10 Pflege (1909–1980)

**Private archive of Roland Kuhn/Verena Kuhn-Gebhart**

9'40, 1 Roland Kuhn: Oberarzt und Klinikdirektor (1935–1993)
9'40, 2 Roland Kuhn: Der Schreibtisch des Jahres 2005 (1934–2006)
9'40, 3 Roland Kuhn: Korrespondenz (1912–2014)
9'40, 4 Roland Kuhn: Dokumentationen (1862–2005)
9'40, 5 Roland Kuhn: Psychopharmakologie (1946–2002)
9'40, 8 Roland Kuhn: Publikationen und Vorträge (1940–2014)
9'40, 9 Roland Kuhn: Der Universitätslehrer (1942–2000)
9'40, 11 Roland Kuhn: Krankengeschichten (1878–2014)
9'40, 12 Roland Kuhn: Blaue Ordner (ca. 1800–2008)

# Bibliography

9'40, 13 Roland Kuhn: Ehrungen (1980–2004)
9'40, 14 Roland Kuhn: Privatpraxis ab 1980 (1980–1992)
9'40, 15 Roland Kuhn: Kleinobjekte (ca. 1920–ca. 2000)
9'40, 21 Verena Kuhn-Gebhart: Berufliche Tätigkeit (1952–2006)
9'40, 22 Verena Kuhn-Gebhart: Krankengeschichten (1950–2008)
9'40, 23 Verena Kuhn-Gebhart: Kleinobjekte (ca. 1960–ca. 2000)

## Health services department

4'800 Manuale (1970–1990)
4'802 Allgemeine Akten (1803–1990)
4'803 Allgemeines, Personelles, Gesetzgebung (1869–1987)
4'840'33, Protokolle Aufsichtskommission (1935–1970)

## Criminal courts

6'10'50 Obergericht Criminale: Protokoll (5.1.1989–15.12.1989)
6'11'** 1989 Obergericht Criminale: Akten, S 48

## St Iddazell Association and Children's Home, Fischingen

8'943, 6 Kinderdossiers
8'943, 11 Nachlieferungen ab 1. März 2014 (1969–1985)

## Transitional archive

Files of the tax administration
Inpatient medical files of the Münsterlingen Psychiatric Clinic
Outpatient medical files of the Münsterlingen Psychiatric Clinic

## Oral history sources

### Interviews with contemporary witnesses

#### Non-anonymised persons

Jules Angst, Dr med., 1969–1994 professor for clinical psychiatry and director of the Research Department of Psychiatric University Hospital Zurich, 9 May 2016
René Bloch, Dr med., 1970–1972 assistant physician, 1973–1974 deputy senior physician at the Münsterlingen Psychiatric Clinic, 14 March 2018
Alexandra Delini-Stula, Dr med., 1966–1970 researcher at Geigy, 1971–1989 at Ciba-Geigy, 19 June 2017
Colette Grosspietsch, 1973–1977 apprenticeship as psychiatric nurse, since then psychiatric nurse at the Münsterlingen Psychiatric Clinic, 13 September 2016
Jürg Grundlehner, 1970–1974 apprenticeship as psychiatric nurse at the Münsterlingen Psychiatric Clinic, 23 August 2017

Albert Lingg, Dr med., 1975–1977 assistant physician, 1977–1978 deputy senior physician, 1978–1979 senior physician at the Münsterlingen Psychiatric Clinic, 7 September 2016

Doris Meli-Nyffenegger, 1971–1974 apprenticeship as psychiatric nurse, then until 2015 psychiatric nurse at the Münsterlingen Psychiatric Clinic, 13 September 2016

Uwe Moor, primary school teacher and historian from the Canton of Thurgau, 15 November 2016

Ernst Müller, 1970/1971 as young adult treated twice as an inpatient at Münsterlingen Psychiatric Clinic, 29 November 2016

Ingrid Ruoss, 1960 at age 28 initially treated as an outpatient, then for three and a half weeks as an inpatient at the Münsterlingen Psychiatric Clinic, 14 November 2016

Marianne Sax, as a child examined as an outpatient in the Münsterlingen Psychiatric Clinic, 30 November 2016

Karl Studer, Dr med., 1980–2006 head physician at the Münsterlingen Psychiatric Clinic, 3 November 2016

Marlies Verhofnik, 1958–1961 apprenticeship as psychiatric nurse, 1963–1978 night shift nurse, 1986–1991 psychiatric nurse at the Münsterlingen Psychiatric Clinic, 12 September 2016

Heinz Wiederkehr, as a child examined and treated as an outpatient at the Münsterlingen Psychiatric Clinic in the early 1960s, 16 December 2016

Kaspar Winterhalter, Dr med., 1970–1974 member of the Friedrich Miescher Institute (a foundation established in 1970 on the initiative of Ciba and Geigy that conducts basic medical research) and consultant for the Solco company, 1977–2005 professor for biochemistry at the ETH Zurich, 11 December 2017

Ernst Wyrsch, 1966–1973 deputy head nurse, 1973–2003 head nurse at the Münsterlingen Psychiatric Clinic, 19 August 2016

**Anonymised persons**

Man treated by Roland Kuhn as an outpatient from 1963 to 1981, 21 July 2016

Doctor employed as an assistant physician at the Münsterlingen Psychiatric Clinic from 1984 to 1986, 28 July 2016

Two sisters whose mother was treated as an outpatient at the Münsterlingen Psychiatric Clinic for several years in the early 1960s, 23 November 2016

Woman employed as an administrator at the Münsterlingen Psychiatric Clinic in the 1980s, 28 November 2016

Man treated as an inpatient at the Münsterlingen Psychiatric Clinic several times in the 1970s and 1980s

Man employed as an assistant physician at the Münsterlingen Psychiatric Clinic in 1959/1960 and then in the pharmaceutical industry from 1964 to 1970, 6 June 2018

Woman who completed an apprenticeship as a psychiatric nurse at the Münsterlingen Psychiatric Clinic in 1957–1960 and was treated as an outpatient by Verena Kuhn from 1958 to 1960, 18 April 2018

Man who as a youth was treated as an outpatient by Verena Kuhn in 1965/1966, 12 January 2018

*Telephone interviews with twenty-nine contemporary witnesses*

Telephone interviews were conducted with thirty former inpatients and outpatients of the Münsterlingen Psychiatric Clinic (8 November 2016–3 March 2017), nine relatives and acquaintances of former patients of the Münsterlingen Psychiatric Clinic (9 November 2016–7 February 2017), five former employees of the Münsterlingen Psychiatric Clinic (9 November 2016, 11 November 2016, 5 December 2016, 13 February 2017, 17 January 2018), one former government agency employee (10 November 2016), and one additional person (10 November 2016).

*Printed sources*

Angst, J. (1969) 'Leerpräparate in Therapie und Forschung', *Praktische Psychiatrie* 47(1), pp. 2–12.

Angst, J. (1973) 'Doppelblindversuch', in Müller C. (ed.) *Lexikon der Psychiatrie*. Berlin, Heidelberg, and New York: Springer, p. 140.

Angst, J. and Pöldinger, W. (1963) 'Klinische Erfahrungen mit dem Butyrophenonderivat Methylperidol (Luvatren). Vergleichender Beitrag zur Methodik pharmakopsychiatrischer Untersuchungen', *Schweizerische Rundschau für Medizin* 52(44), pp. 1348–1354.

Angst, J. et al. (1967) 'Über das gemeinsame Vorgehen einer deutschen und schweizerischen Arbeitsgruppe auf dem Gebiet der Psychiatrischen Dokumentation', *Schweizer Archiv für Neurologie, Neurochirurgie und Psychiatrie* 100, pp. 207–211.

Angst, J. et al. (1969) 'Das Dokumentations-System der Arbeitsgemeinschaft für Methodik und Dokumentation in der Psychiatrie', *Arzneimittel-Forschung* 19, pp. 399–405.

Angst, J. and Theobald, W. (1970) *Tofranil (Imipramin)*. Bern: Stämpfli.

Bein, H.J. (1974), 'Psychopharmakologie: Quo vadis', *Schweizer Archiv für Neurologie, Neurochirurgie und Psychiatrie* 115, pp. 17–25.

Bein, H.J. (1977) 'Prejudices in Pharmacology and Pharmacotherapy: The So-Called Anticholinergic Effect of Antidepressants', *Agents and Actions* 7, pp. 313–315.

Birkmayer, W. (ed.) (1976) *Anfall – Verhalten – Schmerz. Internationales Symposium St. Moritz, 6.–7. Januar 1975*. Bern, Stuttgart, and Vienna: Huber.

Brodie, B. et al. (1961) 'Preliminary Pharmacological and Clinical Results with Desmethylimipramine (DMI) G 35020 a Metabolite of Imipramine', *Psychopharmacologia* 2, pp. 467–474.

Ciba Aktiengesellschaft (ed.) (1970) *Entspannung – neue therapeutische Aspekte. Internationales Symposium St. Moritz, 16. Januar 1970.* Basel.

Ciba Aktiengesellschaft (ed.) (1971) *Entspannungstherapie psychosomatischer Störungen. Internationales Symposium St. Moritz, 11.–13. Januar 1971.* Basel.

Gebhart, V. (1952) 'Zum Problem der intellektuellen Entwicklung im Rorschachschen Formdeutversuch', *Monatsschrift für Psychiatrie und Neurologie* 124, pp. 91–125.

Grünthal, E. (1946) 'Über Parpanit, einen neuen, extrapyramidalmotorische Störungen beeinflussenden Stoff', *Schweizerische Medizinische Wochenschrift* 50, pp. 1286–1289.

Interkantonale Kontrollstelle für Heilmittel (1972) *Interkantonale Vereinbarung über die Kontrolle der Heilmittel (vom 3. Juni 1971).* Bern.

Interkantonale Kontrollstelle für Heilmittel (1977) *Richtlinien der IKS betreffend Anforderungen an die Dokumentation für die Registrierung von Arzneimitteln der Humanmedizin (Registrierung-Richtlinien),* 16.12.1977 Bern.

Jungi, W.F. et al. (1977) 'Gehäufte durch Clozapin (Leponex) induzierte Agranulozytosen in der Ostschweiz?' *Schweizerische Medizinische Wochenschrift* 107(49), pp. 1861–1864.

Kielholz, P. (ed.) (1972) *Depressive Zustände: Erkennung, Bewertung, Behandlung. Internationales Symposium St. Moritz, 10.–11. Januar 1972.* Bern, Stuttgart, and Vienna: Huber.

Kielholz, P. (ed.) (1973) *Die larvierte Depression. Internationales Symposium St. Moritz, 8.–10. Januar 1973.* Bern, Stuttgart, and Vienna: Huber.

Kielholz, P. (ed.) (1978) *Betablocker und Zentralnervensystem. Internationales Symposium St. Moritz, 5.–6. Januar 1976.* Bern, Stuttgart, and Vienna: Huber.

Kielholz, P. and Battegay, R. (1958) 'Behandlung depressiver Zustandsbilder. Unter spezieller Berücksichtigung von Tofranil, einem neuen Antidepressivum', *Schweizerische Medizinische Wochenschrift* 88(3), pp. 763–767.

Kuhn, R. (1954) *Maskendeutungen im Rorschachschen Versuch*, 2nd revised and expanded edition. Basel: Karger.

Kuhn, R. (1957) 'Über die Behandlung depressiver Zustände mit einem Iminodibenzylderivat (G 22,355)', *Schweizerische Medizinische Wochenschrift* 87(35–36), pp. 1135–1140.

Kuhn, R. (1959) 'Probleme der klinischen und poliklinischen Anwendung psychopharmakologischer Substanzen', *Schweizer Archiv für Neurologie, Neurochirurgie und Psychiatrie* 84(1–2), pp. 319–329.

Kuhn, R. (1961), 'Medikamentöse Behandlung der Depression und der Nervosität', *Zeitschrift für ärztliche Fortbildung* 50(7), pp. 518–528.

Kuhn, R. (1963) 'Daseinsanalyse und Psychiatrie', in Gruhle, H.W. et al. (eds) *Psychiatrie der Gegenwart*, Volume 1. Berlin: Springer, pp. 853–902.

Kuhn, R. (1970) 'Beobachtungen und Erfahrungen an einem psychiatrischen Ambulatorium während 30 Jahren', *Schweizer Archiv für Neurologie, Neurochirurgie und Psychiatrie* 106(2), pp. 345–353.

Kuhn, R. (1970) 'Vorwort', in Angst, J. and Theobald, W. (eds), *Tofranil (Imipramin)*. Bern: Stämpfli, p. vi.

Kuhn, R. (1972) 'Klinische Erfahrungen mit einem neuen Antidepressivum', in Kielholz, P. (ed.), *Depressive Zustände: Erkennung, Bewertung, Behandlung. Internationales Symposium St. Moritz, 10.–11. Januar 1972*. Bern, Stuttgart, and Vienna: Huber, pp. 195–202.

Kuhn, R. (1974) 'Ambulante Depression', in Kielholz, P. (ed.), *Die Depression in der täglichen Praxis. Internationales Symposium St. Moritz, 7.–8. Januar 1974*. Bern, Stuttgart, and Vienna: Huber, pp. 98–101.

Kuhn, R. (1976) 'Die psychotrope Wirkung von Carbamazepin bei nicht-epileptischen Erwachsenen', in Birkmayer, W. (ed.), *Anfall – Verhalten – Schmerz. Internationales Symposium St. Moritz, 6.–7. Januar 1975*. Bern, Stuttgart, and Vienna: Huber, pp. 267–270.

Kuhn, R. (1976) 'Über die neuroleptische Wirkung von Baclofen bei chronisch Schizophrenen', *Arzneimittel-Forschung* 26, p. 1187.

Kuhn, R. (1978) 'Erkennung thymoleptischer Wirkungen im klinischen Bereich', in Kielholz, P. (ed.), *Ergebnisse der Anwendung von Antidepressiva, vorgetragen anlässlich des von den Troponwerken Köln am 6. Mai 1977 veranstalteten Symposions*. Cologne: Tropon Arzneimittel, pp. 7–12.

Kuhn, R. (1994) 'Beitrag zur Daseinsstruktur von Suchtverhalten', in Nissen, G. (ed.), *Abhängigkeit und Sucht: Prävention und Therapie*. Bern: Huber, pp. 54–61.

Kuhn, R. (2007 [1986]) 'Clinique et expérimentation en psychopharmacologie', in Marceau, J. (ed.), *Ecrits sur l'analyse existentielle*. Paris: Harmattan, pp. 149–165.

Kuhn, R., Taeschler, M., and Schoch, J. (1966) 'Pharmakologische und klinische Eigenschaften eines neuen Butyrophenon-Derivates (FR 33)', *Psychopharmacologia* 9, pp. 351–362.

Kuhn-Gebhart, V. (1976) 'Die psychotrope Wirkung von Carbamazepin bei nicht-epileptischen Kindern', in Birkmayer, W. (ed.), *Anfall – Verhalten – Schmerz. Internationales Symposium St. Moritz, 6.–7. Januar 1975*. Bern, Stuttgart, and Vienna: Huber, pp. 263–266.

Mayer-Gross, W. (1959) 'The Idea of a Psychiatric Vocabulary', in Stoll, W.A. (ed.), *2nd International Congress for Psychiatry, Zürich, 1.–7.9.1957*. Zurich: Orell Füssli, vol. IV, pp. 269–271.

Oberholzer, R.J.H. (1964) *Die klinische Prüfung neuer Arzneimittel*. Edited by Informationsstelle der forschenden pharmazeutischen Industrie. Biel: Informationsstelle der forschenden pharmazeutischen Industrie [also in Pharmaceutica Acta Helvetiae 39/465 (1964)].

Osmond, H. (1958) 'Chemical Concepts of Psychosis (Historical Contributions)', in Rinkel, M. (ed.), *Chemical Concepts of Psychosis:*

Proceedings of the Symposium on Chemical Concepts of Psychosis held at the 2nd International Congress of Psychiatry in Zurich, Sept. 1–7, 1957. New York: McDowell, pp. 3–26.

Randow, T. (1963) 'Keine Heilung ohne Risiko: Neue Arzneimittelgesetze in Deutschland und USA', *Die Zeit*, 16 April.

Rinkel, M. (1958) 'Foreword', in Rinkel, M. (ed.), *Chemical Concepts of Psychosis: Proceedings of the Symposium on Chemical Concepts of Psychosis held at the 2nd International Congress of Psychiatry in Zurich, Sept. 1–7, 1957*. New York: McDowell, pp. vii–ix.

Robson, J.M. and Sullivan F.M. (1963) 'The Production of Foetal Abnormalities in Rabbits by Imipramine', *The Lancet* 281 (7282), pp. 638–639.

Schindler, W. and Häfliger, F. (1954) 'Über Derivate des Iminodibenzyls', *Helvetia Chimica Acta* 37 (2), pp. 472–483.

Schwab, R.S. and Leigh, D. (1949) 'Parpanit in the Treatment of Parkinson's Disease', *Journal of the American Medical Association*, 5 March, pp. 629–634.

Schweizerische Akademie der Medizinischen Wissenschaften (SAMS) (1970) *Richtlinien für Forschungsuntersuchungen am Menschen*. Basel: Huber.

Senn, H. et al. (1977) 'Clozapine and Agranulocytosis', *The Lancet* 5, p. 547.

Theobald, W. et al. (1966) 'Zur Pharmakologie von Metaboliten des Imipramins', *Medicina et Pharmacologia Experimentalis* 15, pp. 187–197.

Wille, H. (1944) *Hundert Jahre Heil- und Pflegeanstalt Münsterlingen 1840–1940*. Frauenfeld: Huber.

Woggon, B. and Angst, J. (1978) 'Grundlagen und Richtlinien für erste klinische Psychopharmaka-Prüfungen (Phase I, II) aus der Sicht des klinischen Prüfers', *Arzneimittelforschung* 28, pp. 1257–1259.

World Medical Organization (1996) 'Declaration of Helsinki 1964', *British Medical Journal* 313, pp. 1448–1449.

## Research literature

Akermann, M. et al. (2015) *Kinder im Klosterheim: Die Anstalt St. Iddazell Fischingen 1879–1978*. Frauenfeld: Verlag des Historischen Vereins des Kantons Thurgau.

Ammann, J. and Studer, K. (eds) (1990) *150 Jahre Münsterlingen: Das Thurgauische Kantonsspital und die Psychiatrische Klinik 1840–1990*. Weinfelden: Thurgauisches Kantonsspital, Psychiatrische Klinik.

Ankele, M. and Majerus, B. (eds) (2020) *Material Cultures of Psychiatry*. Bielefeld: Transcript.

Appadurai, A. (1986) 'Introduction: Commodities and the Politics of Value', in Appadurai, A. (ed.), *The Social Life of Things: Commodities*

*in Cultural Perspective*. Cambridge: Cambridge University Press, pp. 3–63.
Assmann, A. (2006) *Der lange Schatten der Vergangenheit: Erinnerungskultur und Geschichtspolitik*. Munich: Beck.
Bacopoulos-Viau, A. and Fauvel, A. (2016) 'The Patient's Turn: Roy Porter and Psychiatry's Tales, Thirty Years on', *Medical History* 60, pp. 1–18.
Balz, V. (2010) *Zwischen Wirkung und Erfahrung: eine Geschichte der Psychopharmaka. Neuroleptika in der Bundesrepublik Deutschland, 1950–1980*. Bielefeld: Transcript.
Ban, T.A., Healy, D., and Shorter, E. (eds) (1998) *The Rise of Psychopharmacology and the Story of CINP*. Budapest: Animula.
Ban, T.A., Healy, D. and Shorter, E. (eds) (2000) *The Triumph of Psychopharmacology and the Story of CINP*. Budapest: Animula.
Ban, T.A., Healy, D., and Shorter, E. (eds) (2002) *From Psychopharmacology to Neuropsychopharmacology in the 1980s and the Story of CINP*. Budapest: Animula.
Ban, T.A., Healy, D. and Shorter, E. (2004) *Reflections on Twentieth-Century Psychopharmacology*. Budapest: Animula.
Becker, P. and Clark, W. (eds) (2001) *Little Tools of Knowledge: Historical Essays on Academic and Bureaucratic Practices*. Ann Arbor: University of Michigan Press.
Bersot, H. (1936) *Die Fürsorge für die Gemüts- und Geisteskranken in der Schweiz*. Bern: Huber.
Bersot, H. (1939) *Das Pflegepersonal der öffentlichen und privaten psychiatrischen Anstalten der Schweiz*. Bern: Huber.
Beyer, C. et al. (2021) *Wissenschaftliche Untersuchung der Praxis der Medikamentenversuche in schleswig-holsteinischen Einrichtungen der Behindertenhilfe sowie in den Erwachsenen-, Kinder- und Jugendpsychiatrien in den Jahren 1949 bis 1975*. Lübeck.
Bonah, C. et al. (eds) (2009) *Harmonizing Drugs: Standards in 20th-Century Pharmaceutical History*. Paris: Editions Glyphe.
Borch-Jacobsen, M. (2002) 'Psychotropicana', *London Review of Books* 24(13), pp. 17–18.
Bourdieu, P. (1986) 'L'illusion biographique', *Actes de la recherche en sciences sociales* 62–63, pp. 69–72.
Brandenberger, K. (2012) 'Psychiatrie und Psychopharmaka: Therapien und klinische Forschung mit Psychopharmaka in zwei psychiatrischen Kliniken der Schweiz, 1950–1980'. PhD thesis, University of Zurich.
Braunschweig, S. (2013) *Zwischen Aufsicht und Betreuung: Berufsbildung und Arbeitsalltag der Psychiatriepflege am Beispiel der Basler Heil- und Pflegeanstalt Friedmatt, 1886–1960*. Zurich: Chronos.
Burke, P. (2016) *What Is the History of Knowledge?* Cambridge: Polity Press.
Callon, M. (1986) 'Some Elements of a Sociology of Translation: Domestication of the Scallops and the Fishermen of St Brieuc Bay', in Law, J. (ed.), *Power, Action and Belief: A New Sociology of Knowledge?* London: Routledge, pp. 196–223.

Campbell, N.D. and Stark, L. (2015) 'Making up "Vulnerable" People: Human Subjects and the Subjective Experience of Medical Experiment', *Social History of Medicine* 28, pp. 825–848.

Cantor, D. (1992) 'Cortisone and the Politics of Drama, 1949–1955', in Pickstone, J.V. (ed.), *Medical Innovations in Historical Perspective*. London: Macmillan, pp. 165–184.

Condrau, F. (2007) 'The Patient's View Meets the Clinical Gaze', *Social History of Medicine* 20(3), pp. 525–540.

Croissant, J.L. (2014) 'Agnotology: Ignorance and Absence or Towards a Sociology of Things That Aren't There', *Social Epistemology: A Journal of Knowledge, Culture and Policy* 28(1), pp. 4–25.

Daemmrich, A. (2002) 'A Tale of Two Experts: Thalidomide and Political Engagement in the United States and West Germany', *Social History of Medicine* 15(1), pp. 137–158.

Daemmrich, A. (2004) *Pharmacopolitics: Drug Regulation in the United States and Germany*. Chapel Hill: University of North Carolina Press.

Dammann, G. (2015) 'Zur Einführung: Phänomenologische Psychiatrie heute und ihr geschichtlicher Bezug zur Klinik Münsterlingen', in Damman, G. (ed.), *Phänomenologie und psychotherapeutische Psychiatrie*. Stuttgart: Kohlhammer, pp. 11–19.

Daston, L. (2017) 'The History of Science and the History of Knowledge', *KNOW: A Journal on the Formation of Knowledge* 1(1), pp. 131–154.

Daston, L. and Galison, P. (2010) *Objectivity*. New York: Zone Books.

Derrida, J. (1997) *Dem Archiv verschrieben: Eine Freudsche Impression*. Berlin: Brinkmann und Bose.

Doering-Manteuffel, A. and Raphael, L. (2008) *Nach dem Boom: Perspektiven auf die Zeitgeschichte seit 1970*. Göttingen: Vandenhoeck & Ruprecht.

Dommann, M. (2011) 'Handling, Flowcharts, Logistik: Zur Wissensgeschichte und Materialkultur von Warenflüssen', *Nach Feierabend: Zürcher Jahrbuch für Wissensgeschichte* 7, pp. 75–103.

Dornes, M. (2016) *Macht der Kapitalismus depressiv? Über seelische Gesundheit und Krankheit in modernen Gesellschaften*. Frankfurt am Main: Fischer.

Dumit, J. (2012) *Drugs for Life: How Pharmaceutical Companies Define Our Health*. Durham, NC: Duke University Press.

Dyck, E. and Delille, E. (2022) 'Human Experimentation and Clinical Trials in Psychiatry', in McCallum, D. (ed.), *The Palgrave Handbook of the History of Human Sciences*. Singapore: Palgrave Macmillan, pp. 1357–1378. https://doi.org/10.1007/978-981-15-4106-3_93-1

Ehlers, S. (2019) *Europa und die Schlafkrankheit: Koloniale Seuchenbekämpfung, europäische Identitäten und moderne Medizin 1890–1950*. Göttingen: Vandenhoeck & Ruprecht.

Ehrenberg, A. (2010) *The Weariness of the Self: Diagnosing the History of Depression in the Contemporary Age*. Montreal: McGill-Queen's University Press.

Ehrenbold, T. (2017) *Samuel Koechlin und die Ciba-Geigy: Eine Biografie*. Zurich.

# Bibliography

Erni, P. (1979) *Die Basler Heirat: Geschichte der Fusion Ciba-Geigy*. Zurich: Neue Zürcher Zeitung.

Fischer, P. (1975) 'Werdegang, Aufgaben und Organisation der Interkantonalen Kontrollstelle für Heilmittel', in Interkantonale Kontrollstelle für Heilmittel (ed.), *75 Jahre interkantonale Heilmittelkontrolle (1900–1975)*. Bern: Interkantonale Kontrollstelle für Heilmittel, pp. 33–51.

Fleck, L. (1979) *Genesis and Development of a Scientific Fact*. Chicago, IL: University of Chicago Press.

Galison, P. and Jones, C.A. (1999) 'Factory, Laboratory, Studio: Dispersing Sites of Production', in Galison, P. and Thompson, E. (eds), *The Architecture of Science*. Cambridge, MA: The MIT Press.

Gaudillière, J. and Hess, V. (2013) 'General Introduction', in Gaudillière, J. and Hess, V. (eds), *Ways of Regulating Drugs in the 19th and 20th Centuries*. Basingstoke and New York: Palgrave Macmillan, pp. 1–16.

Gaudillière, J. and Thoms, U. (eds) (2015) *The Development of Scientific Marketing in the Twentieth Century: Research for Sales in the Pharmaceutical Industry*. London: Pickering & Chatto.

Gerber, L. (2015) 'Marketing Loops: Clinical Research, Consumption of Antidepressants and the Reorganization of Promotion at Geigy in the 1960s and 1970s', in Gaudillière, J. and Thoms, U. (eds), *The Development of Scientific Marketing in the Twentieth Century: Research for Sales in the Pharmaceutical Industry*. London: Pickering & Chatto, pp. 167–189.

Gerber, L. and Gaudillière, J. (2016) 'Marketing Masked Depression: Physicians, Pharmaceutical Firms, and the Redefinition of Mood Disorders in the 1960s and 1970s', *Bulletin of the History of Medicine* 90, pp. 455–490.

Germann, U. (2017) *Medikamentenprüfungen an der Psychiatrischen Universitätsklinik Basel, 1953–1980. Pilotstudie mit Vorschlägen für das weitere Vorgehen*. Bern: Universität Bern. www.img.unibe.ch/forschung/medikamentenversuche/index_ger.html

Germann, U. (2022) 'Medikamentenversuche in der Deutschschweizer Psychiatrie 1950–1990: Zum aktuellen Stand der Forschung', *Schweizerische Zeitschrift für Geschichte* 1, pp. 75–91.

Goliszek, A. (2003) *In the Name of Science: A History of Secret Programs, Medical Research, and Human Experimentation*. New York: St Martin's Press.

Goltermann, S. (2022) *Victims: Perceptions of Suffering and Violence in Modern Europe*. Oxford: Oxford University Press.

Gomart, E. (2002) 'Methadone: Six Effects in Search of a Substance', *Social Studies of Science* 32(1), pp. 93–135.

Gooday, G. (2008) 'Placing or Replacing the Laboratory in the History of Science?', *Isis* 99(4), pp. 783–795.

Greene, J. (2007) *Prescribing by Numbers: Drugs and the Definition of Disease*. Baltimore, MD: Johns Hopkins University Press.

Greene, J. (2014) *Generic: The Unbranding of Modern Medicine.* Baltimore, MD: Johns Hopkins University Press.

Greene, J. and Podolsky, S. (20212) 'Reform, Regulation, and Pharmaceuticals: The Kefauver-Harris Amendments at 50', *New England Journal of Medicine* 367(16), pp. 1481–1483.

Greene, J., Condrau, F., and Siegel Watkins, E. (eds) (2016) *Therapeutic Revolutions: Pharmaceuticals and Social Change in the Twentieth Century.* Chicago, IL: University of Chicago Press, pp. 65–96.

Hacking, I. (1986) 'Making up People', in Heller, T., Morton S., and Wellbery, D. (eds), *Reconstructing Individualism: Autonomy, Individuality, and the Self in Western Thought.* Stanford, CA: Stanford University Press, pp. 222–236.

Hacking, I. (1995) 'The Looping Effects of Human Kinds', in Sperber D., Premack, D., and Premack, A.J. (eds), *Causal Cognition: A Multidisciplinary Debate.* Oxford: Clarendon Press, pp. 351–383.

Hägele, R.H.W. (2004) *Arzneimittelprüfung am Menschen: Ein strafrechtlicher Vergleich aus deutscher, österreichischer, schweizerischer und internationaler Sicht.* Baden-Baden: Nomos.

Hähner-Rombach, S. and Hartig, C. (2019) *Medikamentenversuche an Kindern und Jugendlichen im Rahmen der Heimerziehung in Niedersachsen zwischen 1945 und 1978.* Hannover: Niedersächsisches Ministerium für Soziales, Gesundheit und Gleichstellung. www.ms.niedersachsen.de/themen/gesundheit/psychiatrie_und_psychologische_hilfen/versorgung-psychisch-kranker-menschen-in-niedersachsen-14025.html

Haller, L. (2012) *Cortison: Geschichte eines Hormons, 1900–1955.* Zurich: Chronos.

Hanley, A. and Meyer, J. (eds) (2021) *Patient Voices in Britain, 1840–1948.* Manchester: Manchester University Press.

Healy, D. (1996, 1998, 2001) *The Psychopharmacologists: Interviews,* 3 vols. London: Arnold.

Healy, D. (1997) *The Antidepressant Era.* Cambridge, MA: Harvard University Press.

Healy, D. (2002) *The Creation of Psychopharmacology.* Cambridge, MA: Harvard University Press.

Henckes, N. (2016) 'Magic Bullet in the Head? Psychiatric Revolutions and their Aftermath', in Greene, J., Condrau, F., and Siegel Watkins, E. (eds), *Therapeutic Revolutions: Pharmaceuticals and Social Change in the Twentieth Century.* Chicago, IL and London: University of Chicago Press, pp. 65–96.

Herzberg, D. (2009) *Happy Pills in America: From Miltown to Prozac.* Baltimore, MD: Johns Hopkins University Press.

Hess, V., Hottenrott, L., and Steinkamp, P. (2016) *Testen im Osten: DDR-Arzneimittelstudien im Auftrag westlicher Pharmaindustrie.* Berlin: be.bra Wissenschaft.

Hirshbein, L.D. (2006) 'Science, Gender, and the Emergence of Depression in American Psychiatry, 1952–1980', *Journal of the History of Medicine and Allied Sciences* 61, pp. 187–216.

*Historische Statistik der Schweiz*, Zurich: Chronos. https://hsso.ch/

*Historisches Lexikon der Schweiz*. http://hls-dhs-dss.ch/

Hornblum, A., Newman, J.L., and Dober, G.J. (2013) *Against their Will: The Secret History of Medical Experimentation on Children in Cold War America*. New York: Palgrave Macmillan.

Horwitz, A.V. (2021) *DSM: A History of Psychiatry's Bible*. Baltimore, MD: Johns Hopkins University Press.

Itzen, P. and Müller, S. (2016) 'Risk as a Category of Analysis for a Social History of the Twentieth Century: An Introduction', *Historical Social Research* 41(1), pp. 7–29.

Jasanoff, S. (2004) 'The Idiom of Co-Production', in Jasanoff, S. (ed.), *States of Knowledge: The Co-Production of Science and Social Order*. London and New York: Routledge, pp. 1–12.

Jenni, C. (2010) *Forschungskontrolle durch Ethikkommissionen aus verwaltungsrechtlicher Sicht: Geschichte, Aufgaben, Verfahren*. Zurich: Dike.

Kaminsky, U. and Klöcker, K. (2020) *Medikamente und Heimerziehung am Beispiel des Franz Sales Hauses: Historische Klärungen – Ethische Perspektiven*, Münster: Aschendorff.

Klauser, U. (in preparation) ' "Schwierige" Kinder: Abklärung, Therapie und Forschung in der ambulanten Kinder- und Jugendpsychiatrie, 1950–1980'. PhD thesis, Department of History, University of Zurich.

König, M. (2016) *Besichtigung einer Weltindustrie – 1859 bis 2016*, vol. 1 of *Chemie und Pharma in Basel*, edited by Kreis, G. and von Wartburg, B. Basel: Christoph Merian.

König, M., Siegrist, H., and Vetterli, R. (1985) *Warten und Aufrücken: Die Angestellten in der Schweiz 1870–1950*. Zurich: Chronos.

Kuhn, R. (1977) 'Roland Kuhn', in Pongratz, L. (ed.), *Psychiatrie in Selbstdarstellungen*. Bern: Huber, pp. 213–257.

Kuhn, R. (1990) 'Geschichte und Entwicklung der psychiatrischen Klinik', in Ammann, J. and Studer, K. (eds), *150 Jahre Münsterlingen: Das Thurgauische Kantonsspital und die Psychiatrische Klinik 1840–1990*. Weinfelden: Thurgauisches Kantonsspital, Psychiatrische Klinik, pp. 99–125.

Kuhn, R. (2004) *Psychiatrie mit Zukunft: Beiträge zu Geschichte, Gegenwart, Zukunft der wissenschaftlichen und praktischen Seelenheilkunde*. Basel: Schwabe.

Lakoff, A. (2007) 'The Right Patients for the Drug: Managing the Placebo Effect in Antidepressant Trials', *BioSocieties* 2, pp. 57–73.

Landecker, H. (2007) *Culturing Life: How Cells Became Technologies*. Cambridge, MA and London: Harvard University Press.

Langer, G. and Heimann, H. (eds) (1983) *Psychopharmaka: Grundlagen und Therapie*. Vienna: Springer.

Lässig, S. (2016) 'The History of Knowledge and the Expansion of the Historical Research Agenda', *Bulletin of the German Historical Institute* 59, pp. 29–58.

Latour, B. and Woolgar, S. (1979) *Laboratory Life: The Social Construction of Scientific Facts*. Beverly Hills, CA: Sage Publications.

Lemov, R. (2011) 'X-Rays of Inner Worlds: The Mid-Twentieth-Century American Projective Test Movement', *Journal of the History of Behavioral Sciences* 47(3), pp. 251–278.

Lemov, R. (2015) *Database of Dreams: The Lost Quest to Catalog Humanity*. New Haven, CT and London: Yale University Press.

Lenhard-Schramm, N., Dietz R., and Maike, R. (2022) *Göttliche Krankheit, kirchliche Anstalt, weltliche Mittel: Arzneimittelprüfungen an Minderjährigen im Langzeitbereich der Stiftung Bethel in den Jahren 1949 bis 1975*. Bielefeld: Verlag für Regionalgeschichte.

Lienhard, M. and Condrau, F. (2019) *Psychopharmakologische Versuche in der Psychiatrie Baselland zwischen 1950 und 1980: Bericht zuhanden der Psychiatrie Baselland*. Liestal and Zurich. www.pbl.ch/medikamententests

Lopez-Muñoz, F. and Alamo, C. (2009) 'Monoaminergic Neurotransmission: The History of the Discovery of Antidepressants from 1950s Until Today', *Current Pharmaceutical Design* 15, pp. 1563–1586.

Lüönd, K. (2009) *Rohstoff Wissen: Geschichte und Gegenwart der Schweizer Pharmaindustrie im Zeitraffer*. Zurich: Neue Zürcher Zeitung.

Majerus, B. (2016) 'Making Sense of the "Chemical Revolution": Patient's Voices on the Introduction of Neuroleptics in the 1950s', *Medical History* 60, pp. 54–66.

Marks, H.M. (1997) *The Progress of Experiment: Science and Therapeutic Reform in the United States, 1900–1990*. Cambridge: Cambridge University Press.

Marks, H.M. (2009) 'What Does Evidence Do? Histories of Therapeutic Research', in Bonah, C. et al. (eds), *Harmonizing Drugs: Standards in Twentieth-Century Pharmaceutical History*. Paris: Editions Glyphe, pp. 81–100.

Martin, E. (1994) *Flexible Bodies: The Role of Immunity in American Culture from the Days of Polio to the Age of AIDS*. Boston, MA: Beacon Press.

Meier, M. (2015) *Spannungsherde: Psychochirurgie nach dem Zweiten Weltkrieg*. Göttingen: Wallstein.

Meier, T., Jenzer, S., and Keller, W. (2017) *Eingeschlossen: Alltag und Aufbruch in der psychiatrischen Klinik Burghölzli zur Zeit der Brandkatastrophe von 1971*. Zurich: Chronos.

Meyers, T. (2013) 'Pharmacy and its Discontents', *BioSocieties* 8(4), pp. 507–511.

Mohun, A.P. (2016) 'Constructing the History of Risk: Foundations, Tools, and Reasons Why', *Historical Social Research* 41(1), pp. 30–47.

Moncrieff, J. (2008) *The Myth of the Chemical Cure: A Critique of Psychiatric Drug Treatment*. Basingstoke: Palgrave Macmillan.

Müller, N. (2018) 'Das Disziplinarverfahren gegen den Thurgauer Kantonsarzt Hans Schenker im Jahr 1986 und seine Folgen'. BA thesis, University of Zurich.

Petryna, A. (2005) 'Ethical Variability: Drug Development and the Globalization of Clinical Trials', *American Ethnologist* 32(2), pp. 183–197.

Petryna, A., Lakoff, A., and Kleinman, A. (eds) (2006) *Global Pharmaceuticals: Ethics, Markets, Practices*. Durham, NC: Duke University Press.

Pidoux, V. (2010) 'Expérimentation et clinique électroencéphalographiques entre physiologie, neurologie et psychiatrie (Suisse, 1935–1965)', *Revue d'histoire des sciences* 63, pp. 439–472.

Pignarre, P. (2001) *Comment la dépression est devenue une épidémie*. Paris: La Découverte.

Pignarre, P. (2006) *Psychotrope Kräfte: Patienten, Macht, Psychopharmaka*. Zurich: Diaphanes.

Polanyi, M. (1966) *The Tacit Dimension*. Chicago, IL: University of Chicago Press.

Porter, R. (1985) 'The Patient's View: Doing Medical History from Below', *Theory and Society* 14, pp. 175–198.

Proctor, R.N. and Schiebinger, L. (eds) (2008) *Agnotology: The Making and Unmaking of Ignorance*. Stanford, CA: Stanford University Press.

Radin, J. (2017) *Life on Ice: A History of New Uses for Cold Blood*. Chicago, IL: University of Chicago Press.

Ratmoko, C. (2010) *Damit die Chemie stimmt: Die Anfänge der industriellen Herstellung von weiblichen und männlichen Sexualhormonen 1914–1938*. Zurich: Chronos.

Rees, W.L. and Healy D. (1997) 'The Place of Clinical Trials in the Development of Psychopharmacology', *History of Psychiatry* 8, pp. 1–20.

Reubi, D. (2012) 'The Human Capacity to Reflect and Decide: Bioethics and the Reconfiguration of the Research Subject in the British Biomedical Sciences', *Social Studies of Science* 42(3), pp. 348–368.

Reubi, D. (2013) 'Re-Moralising Medicine: The Bioethical Thought Collective and the Regulation of the Body in British Medical Research', *Social Theory and Health* 11(2), pp. 215–235.

Rheinberger, H. (2001) *Experimentalsysteme und epistemische Dinge: Eine Geschichte der Proteinsynthese im Reagenzglas*. Göttingen: Wallstein Verlag.

Richli, P. (2018) *Bericht über den Umgang mit Arzneimittelversuchen in der Luzerner Psychiatrie in den Jahren 1950–1980 aus rechtlicher Sicht*. Lucerne: Im Auftrag des Gesundheits- und Sozialdepartementes des Kantons Luzern. www.lu.ch/-/media/Kanton/Dokumente/GSD/Publikationen/2018_11_23_Bericht_1_Arzneimittelversuche_A4.pdf?la=de-CH

Rietmann, T., Germann, U., and Condrau, F. (2018) ' "Wenn Ihr Medikament eine Nummer statt eines Markennamens trägt": Medikamentenversuche in der Zürcher Psychiatrie 1950–1980', in Gnädinger, B. and Rothenbühler V. (eds), *Menschen korrigieren: Fürsorgerische Zwangsmassnahmen und Fremdplatzierungen im Kanton Zürich bis 1981*. Zurich: Chronos, pp. 201–254.

Rigal, C.S. (2008) 'Neo-Clinicians, Clinical Trials, and the Reorganization of Medical Research in Paris Hospitals after the Second World War: The Trajectory of Jean Bernard', *Medical History* 52(4), pp. 511–534.

Ritzmann, H. (ed.) (1996) *Historische Statistik der Schweiz*. Zurich: Chronos.

Rodgers, D.T. (2011) *Age of Fracture*. Cambridge, MA: Belknap Press of Harvard University Press.

Roelcke, V. and Maio, G. (eds) (2004) *Twentieth Century Ethics of Human Subjects Research: Historical Perspectives on Values, Practices, and Regulations*. Stuttgart: Franz Steiner.

Rose, N. (2007) 'Psychopharmaceuticals in Europe', in Knapp, M., Roelcke, V., and Maio, G. (eds), *Mental Health Policy and Practice across Europe*. Maidenhead: McGraw-Hill, pp. 146–187.

Rosenberg, C.E. (1977) 'The Therapeutic Revolution: Medicine, Meaning and Social Change in Nineteenth-Century America', *Perspectives in Biology and Medicine* 20(4), pp. 485–506.

Sadowsky, J. (2021) *The Empire of Depression: A New History*. Cambridge, MA: Polity Press.

Scheidegger, T. (2011) 'Der Lauf der Dinge: Materiale Zirkulation zwischen amateurhafter und professioneller Naturgeschichte in der Schweiz um 1900', *Nach Feierabend: Zürcher Jahrbuch für Wissensgeschichte* 7, pp. 53–73.

Schillings, P. and van Wickeren, A. (2015) 'Towards a Material and Spatial History of Knowledge Production: An Introduction', *Historical Social Research* 40(1), no. 151, pp. 203–218.

Schläpfer, L. (2016) *Probandenschutz, Qualität und Transparenz in der klinischen Arzneimittelforschung: Die Rolle des Sponsors*. Basel: Helbing Lichtenhahn Verlag.

Schlich, T. and Troehler, U. (eds) (2006) *The Risks of Medical Innovation: Risk Perception and Assessment in Historical Context*. London and New York: Routledge.

Schmidt, U. and Frewer, A. (eds) (2007) *History and Theory of Human Experimentation: The Declaration of Helsinki and Modern Medical Ethics*. Stuttgart: Franz Steiner.

Schmuhl, H. and Roelcke, V. (eds) (2013) *'Heroische Therapien': Die deutsche Psychiatrie im internationalen Vergleich, 1918–1945*. Göttingen: Wallstein.

Schoefert, A.K. (2015) 'The View from the Psychiatric Laboratory: The Research of Ernst Grünthal and his Mid-Twentieth-Century Peers'. PhD thesis, Cambridge University.

Schwerin, A. (1961) 'Die Contergan-Bombe: Der Arzneimittelskandal und die neue risikoepistemische Ordnung der Massenkonsumgesellschaft', in Eschenbruch, N. and Volker, H.-W. (eds) (2013) *Arzneimittelgeschichte des 20. Jahrhunderts: Historische Skizzen von Lebertran bis Contergan*. Bielefeld: Transcript, pp. 255–282.

Shorter, E. (1997) *A History of Psychiatry: From the Era of the Asylum to the Age of Prozac*. New York: Wiley.

Shorter, E. (2009) *Before Prozac: The Troubled History of Mood Disorders in Psychiatry*. Oxford and New York: Oxford University Press.

Shorter, E. (2011) 'Brief History of Placebos and Clinical Trials in Psychiatry', *Canadian Journal of Psychiatry* 56(4), pp. 193–197.

Shorter, E. (2013) *How Everyone Became Depressed: The Rise and Fall of the Nervous Breakdown*. Oxford and New York: Oxford University Press.

Snelders, S., Kaplan, C., and Pieters, T. (2006) 'On Cannabis, Chloral Hydrate, and Career Cycles of Psychotropic Drugs in Medicine', *Bulletin of the History of Medicine* 80(1), pp. 95–114.

Sparing, F. (2020) *Medikamentenvergabe und Medikamentenerprobung an Kindern und Jugendlichen: Eine Untersuchung zu kinder- und jugendpsychiatrischen Einrichtungen des Landschaftsverbandes Rheinland 1953 bis 1975*. Berlin: Metropol.

Spiegel, R. (1995) *Einführung in die Psychopharmakologie: Für Ärzte, Psychologen, Sozialarbeiter, Juristen und Pflegepersonal*, revised and expanded 2nd edition. Bern: Huber.

Sprumont, D. (1993) *La Protection des Sujets de Recherche*. Bern: Stämpfli.

Steger, F. and Jeskow, J. (2018) *Das Antidepressivum Levoprotilin in Jena: Arzneimittelstudien westlicher Pharmaunternehmen in der DDR, 1987–1990*. Leipzig: Leipziger Universitätsverlag.

Stephens, T. and Brynner, R. (2001) *Dark Medicine: The Impact of Thalidomide and Its Revival as a Vital Medicine*. Cambridge, MA: Perseus.

Stewart, L. and Dyck, E. (eds) (2017) *The Uses of Humans in Experiment: Perspectives from the 17th Century to the 20th Century*. Leiden and Boston, MA: Brill Rodopi.

Stoler, A.L. (2008) *Along the Archival Grain: Epistemic Anxieties and Colonial Common Sense*. Princeton, NJ: Princeton University Press.

Stupnicki, R. (1953) *Die soziale Stellung des Arztes in der Schweiz*. Bern: P. Haupt.

Tobbell, D. (2009) '"Who's Winning the Human Race?" Cold War as Pharmaceutical Political Strategy', *Journal of the History of Medicine and Allied Sciences* 64(4), pp. 429–473.

Tornay, M. (2015) 'La gentille dame Largactil, la méchante dame Geigy: La clinique psychiatrique de Münsterlingen vers 1954', in Bert, J. and Basso, E. (eds), *Foucault à Münsterlingen: A l'origine de l'Histoire de la folie*. Paris: Editions EHESS, pp. 57–68.

Tornay, M. (2016) *Zugriffe auf das Ich: Psychoaktive Stoffe und Personenkonzepte in der Schweiz, 1945 bis 1980*. Tübingen: Mohr Siebeck.

Tornay, M. (2020) *Träumende Schwestern: Eine Randgeschichte der Psychoanalyse*. Vienna: Turia & Kant.

Tröhler, U. (2007) 'Doctors' Ethos and Statute Law concerning Human Research in Europe', in Schmidt U. and Frewer A. (eds), *History and Theory of Human Experimentation: The Declaration of Helsinki and Modern Medical Ethics*. Stuttgart: Franz Steiner, pp. 27–54.

Undritz, N. (ed.) (1992) *Rechtshandbuch für das Gesundheitswesen mit besonderer Berücksichtigung des Krankenhauswesens*, 3rd edition. Aarau: VESKA.

Valier, H. and Timmermann, C. (2008) 'Clinical Trials and the Reorganization of Medical Research in post-Second World War Britain', *Medical History* 52, pp. 493–510.

Van der Geest, S., Reynolds Whyte, S., and Hardon, A. (1996) 'The Anthropology of Pharmaceuticals: A Biographical Approach', *Annual Review of Anthropology* 25, pp. 153–178.

Vismann, C. (2008) *Files: Law and Media Technology*. Stanford, CA: Sanford University Press.

Wagner, S. (2019) 'Ein unterdrücktes und verdrängtes Kapitel der Heimgeschichte: Arzneimittelstudien an Heimkindern', *Sozial. Geschichte Online* 19, pp. 61–113. http://sozialgeschichteonline.wordpress.com

Wagner, S. (2020) *Arzneimittelversuche an Heimkindern zwischen 1949 und 1975*. Frankfurt am Main: Mabuse Verlag.

Weindling, P. (2001) 'The Origins of Informed Consent: The International Scientific Commission on Medical War Crimes, and the Nuremberg Code', *Bulletin of the History of Medicine* 75, pp. 37–71.

Weindling, P. (2004) *Nazi Medicine and the Nuremberg Trials from Medical War Crimes to Informed Consent*. Basingstoke: Palgrave Macmillan.

Wendt, G. (1993) 'Exkurs: Levoprotilin', in Peter R., Laux, G., and Pöldinger, W. (eds), *Antidepressiva und Phasenprophylaktika*, vol. 3 of *Neuro-Psychopharmaka: Ein Therapie-Handbuch*. Vienna: Springer, pp. 396–399.

Wille, H. (1944) 'Hundert Jahre Heil- und Pflegeanstalt Münsterlingen 1840–1940', in *Thurgauische Beiträge zur vaterländischen Geschichte* 80, 35–142.

Wimmer, M. (2012) *Archivkörper: Eine Geschichte historischer Einbildungskraft*. Konstanz: Konstanz University Press.

Wüst, F. (1969) *Die Interkantonale Vereinbarung über die Kontrolle der Heilmittel vom 16. Juni 1954*. Muri bei Bern: Interkantonale Kontrollstelle für Heilmittel.

Wüst, F. (1970) 'Die Arzneimittelkontrolle in der Schweiz', *Orientierungen* 53, p. 9.

# Index

Note: 'n.' after a page reference indicates the number of a note on that page.

Abegg, Alfred, government councillor (1914–1998) 264
administrative directorate of the Münsterlingen Psychiatric Clinic 25, 178, 188, 210
Ammann, Rudolf (pseudonym) 100, 114n.24
Angst, Jules, Prof. Dr med. (1926–) 79–80, 161n.79, 176, 206, 214, 270
animal testing 38, 120–121, 123–124, 131, 139, 158n.36, 161n.79, 200, 289
antidepressants, development of 3–4, 49, 117–118, 122, 124, 138, 184, 213–215, 254–255, 270–271
antipsychiatry 208, 211, 220, 291
approval see drug approval
approval authorities 5–7, 120–125, 128, 165n.177, 202–206, 223n.33, 237, 243
authorities, cantonal
Great Council (legislature of the Canton of Thurgau) 212, 263
health office 6
medical services department 6, 25–27, 31, 52, 262–268
supervisory commission 6, 24, 26, 179–180, 238, 263, 267

Bachelard, Gaston, philosopher (1884–1962) 152
Bally, Gustav, Prof. Dr med. (1893–1966) 29
Bein, Hugo J., Prof. Dr med. (1919–1994) 139, 198, 253, 257
Bellevue, clinic, Kreuzlingen 95, 286
benzodiazepine 54, 89n.139, 127, 213, 261
Binswanger, Ludwig, Dr med. (1820–1880) 28
Binswanger, Ludwig, Dr med. (1881–1966) 31, 152, 166n.185, 166n.186, 286
Bleuler, Eugen, Prof. Dr med. (1857–1939) 33, 153
Bleuler, Manfred, Prof. Dr med. (1903–1994) 34, 238
Bodmer, Maria (pseudonym) 129
Boehringer Ingelheim 37, 64
Boehringer, Robert, Dr phil. 37, 59, 62–63
Brain Anatomy Institute, Waldau Psychiatric Clinic, Bern 37, 50, 238

# Index

Briner, Otto, Dr med. 27
budget *see* finances
building conditions, infrastructure 3, 18, 20, 23, 26, 31, 168, 180, 208–09, 211, 220, 262, 266, 298
Burghölzli, Psychiatric University Hospital Zurich 27, 33, 36, 79, 115.n41, 116n.55, 184, 214, 238
Bütler, Julius, Dr med., cantonal physician (1908–1982) 267
Byk Gulden 213, 215

Cantonal Hospital Frauenfeld 186, 235
Cantonal Hospital Münsterlingen, 19–20, 24–25, 31, 118, 58, 129, 163n.139, 242, 177, 186, 192, 193, 243–244, 247n.38, 248n.45
Cantonal Hospital St Gallen 201, 238, 244
cantonal physician 26, 178, 180, 186, 191n.48, 253, 262–267
children and youth 24, 34, 96–97, 99–101, 109, 113n.14, 114n.23, 114n.26, 120, 128, 132, 136–140, 169, 201–202, 216, 218, 226n.97, 284, 286, 296
Christ, Agathe 21, 32–33, 66
chronic cases 21, 56, 67–68, 95, 97–101, 128, 131, 142–143, 145, 167n.198, 209, 219, 232–233, 289, 296, 301n.19
Ciba 7, 35–36, 54, 64, 65, 67, 94, 97, 101, 106, 117, 138–139, 155, 173–175, 183–184, 195, 197–202, 207, 231, 251, 254–255, 282, 286
Ciba-Geigy 7, 48–49, 139, 141, 185, 197–199, 202, 214–215, 217–219, 251, 254–255, 257–258, 260–261, 265, 283, 293

Cilag AG 141, 263
clinical director, clinical directorate 6, 11, 13–14, 20–28, 31–32, 38, 45n.74, 52, 66, 82, 97, 143, 178, 180, 185–188, 193n.68, 193n.72, 194n.73, 207–212, 220, 225n.76, 234, 238, 242, 264–267, 282
clinics, psychiatric
  non-university 17n.25, 31, 128, 190n.36, 194n.73, 194n.74
  private 33, 95–96, 286
  university 17n.25, 22, 27–28, 31, 33, 36–37, 51–52, 58, 61, 79, 81–82, 115n.41, 116n.55, 150, 165n.176; 185, 191n.43; 192n.58; 201, 206; 215, 217; 228n.120, 239, 241, 247n.28, 249, 293–294
clinic staff
  nursing staff 8, 18, 20–22, 32, 39, 41, 50, 67, 71, 73, 75–76, 79, 92, 97, 99, 101–104, 107–108, 110–111, 112n.1, 114n.29, 114n.32, 114n.35, 128–130, 135, 142–143, 151, 153–154, 168–169, 171, 176–178, 207–212, 219, 245, 285–287, 292–293
  as patients 101–104, 129–130
  remuneration 30, 182–188, 210, 266–267
  staff shortage 53, 101–102, 208–211, 287, 294
  working conditions 21–22, 208–212, 287, 291, 294
clinical trials
  administration patterns 97–103, 130, 232–234, 295–297
  discontinuation, discontinuation of testing 59, 68–69, 133, 138–141, 145–146, 202, 259–261, 290, 297

## Index

financial remunerations from the pharmaceutical industry 8, 55, 66, 182–188, 286, 298
interests *see* motives
methodology 36, 39, 67, 69, 71, 73, 80, 118–119, 124, 136, 140, 147–156, 205, 213–215, 220, 257, 260, 280, 288–289, 294
motives 12, 131, 147, 212, 286, 297–299
number of trials 282–285
phase models 122, 205, 289
protocols, requirements 41, 61, 124, 138–140, 147–149, 204–205, 257, 290–291, 298
questionnaires 148–149, 213, 244, 287
rapid tests 11, 67, 149, 172, 283, 289
regulation 7, 14, 115n.48, 119–125, 151, 156, 197, 202–207, 222n.31, 254, 260, 280
reports 6, 38–41, 59, 94, 108, 136, 145, 149, 182, 185–186, 199, 230, 235, 284, 295
risks 120–121, 124, 134, 144, 146–147, 156, 177, 205, 229–230, 232, 236, 243–244, 265, 280–281, 290, 297, 299
specialised publications 6, 14, 37, 41, 63, 80–81, 145–146, 152–153, 166n.186, 166n.188, 178, 200, 202, 206–207, 214–215, 217, 222n.31, 245, 251–253, 259, 262, 264, 269–271, 274n.22, 284, 288
standardisation 14, 119, 125, 150–151, 155, 204–205, 214–215, 280, 289–290
test series 58, 66–71, 99, 125, 132, 134, 138, 140–141, 143–145, 170, 260, 282, 295, 299

(voluntary) self-regulation 124–125, 205, 280
coercion 78–79, 107–108, 111, 293
combinations of substances 54, 69, 98, 105, 105, 120, 125, 130, 135–136, 138, 140, 143, 171, 202, 215, 217, 229, 236, 290, 297–299
competition 36, 53, 65, 126, 129, 134, 141, 150, 254
consent to testing 103–106, 115n.48, 125, 205, 257, 262, 266, 268, 275n.34, 282, 290–294, 300, 300n.1
*see also* informed consent
Cornu, Frédéric, Dr med. (1922–2007) 82

daseinsanalysis 28–29, 31, 82, 152–153, 156, 166n.185, 166n.186, 214, 253, 269, 271, 278n.109, 285, 294, 299
database 10, 17n.28, 227n.100, 283, 300, 300n.3
Declaration of Helsinki 125, 205, 257, 280, 290–291
Delini-Stula, Alexandra, Dr med. (1938–2022) 199, 255–256, 258, 261
deliveries of substances 11, 38, 50, 53–55, 69, 84n.29, 118, 125, 133, 141, 168–176, 195, 218, 255, 283
dependence, addiction 35, 54, 74, 127, 166n.186
depression
  definition of 4, 79–83
  endogenous 65, 80, 138, 216, 240
  exogenous (reactive) 115n.47
  vital 80, 256
diagnosis categories 94–96, 98, 113n.13, 148, 150, 155, 288, 290
discontinuation of testing *see* clinical trials

discovery 13–15, 49, 52, 62, 76–77, 84n.26, 104, 126, 197, 207, 211, 214, 219, 250, 265–266, 269, 271, 286, 288, 291, 295, 298
disguise (disguised administration) 107, 115n.46, 282, 293
dispensing of substances despite end of testing 68, 138–140, 146–147, 259
documentation (of the trials) 48–49, 53, 77, 120–121, 125–126, 140, 150, 154, 203–205, 231, 251, 259–260, 282–283, 298
Domenjoz, Robert, Prof. Dr med. (1908–2000) 37, 38, 41, 50, 52–53, 55, 59–63, 66, 69–70
doses, dosage 41, 75, 100, 101, 105, 108, 120, 130, 134, 137, 138, 143–144, 147, 169–172, 176, 189n.9, 201, 229, 232–233, 235, 239–240, 246n.19, 248n.21, 265, 283, 288, 290, 296–297
double-blind studies 36, 119, 135, 151, 153, 156, 202, 213–214, 257
drug approval, drug registration 7–8, 61, 63, 69, 76, 80, 120–121, 128, 130, 137, 149, 172–173, 197–199, 202–205, 213, 226n.98, 242, 254, 260, 280, 288–290

effectiveness
 establishing 1, 8–9, 42, 131, 133, 135–136, 150–151, 232, 233, 260
 witnesses of 38, 41, 71–72, 76–77, 135, 152–154, 219, 256, 294–295
electroencephalogram (EEG) 28, 30, 41, 181–182, 185, 216, 287
Eli Lilly & Co. 149

ethical guidelines 25, 125, 206–207, 257, 280–281, 291
examinations, physical (blood, urine, eyes, etc.) 39, 53, 58, 104, 131, 150, 153, 177, 216, 241–245, 251, 291

fatalities 14–15, 17n.28, 40, 77–79, 94, 140, 143–145, 229–245, 291, 299
finances
 canton budget 26, 30–31, 179–181, 208–209, 263–269
 clinic budget 23, 26, 179–180, 284, 297–298
form of delivery (ampoules, tablets, dragées, etc.) 123, 138, 169–170, 293
Freud, Sigmund, Dr med. (1856–1939) 29
Friedmatt, Psychiatric University Hospital Basel 51–52, 58, 241

galenic form *see* form of delivery
Gebhart, Ernst, Dr med. (1877–1954) 33
Gebhart, Verena, Dr med. *see* Kuhn-Gebhart, Verena (1921–2015)
Geigy, J. R.; Geigy AG 6–7, 13, 18, 23, 35–38, 40–42, 48–50, 52–53, 55–72, 75, 77–79, 81, 99–100, 103, 105, 108, 120–33, 135–139, 148–149, 156, 170–176, 179, 181–185, 188, 197–199, 231, 234–235, 237–238, 240–241, 251, 258, 261, 270, 282, 286, 289, 293, 297
genealogical tables, lineage archive 32, 167n.195
Gerber, Regina (pseudonym) 235
government council (executive of the Canton of Thurgau) 24–26, 179, 187, 191n.48, 209, 211, 263–264

Grünthal, Ernst, Dr med.
  (1894–1972) 28–29,
  37–42, 50–51, 58, 60,
  66–67, 69, 75, 82–83, 131,
  158n.33, 238
  guidelines of the Swiss Academy
  of Medical Sciences (SAMS)
  115n.48, 162n.115,
  206–207, 125, 263, 280, 290

Haffter, Arthur, government
  councillor (1927–2021)
  262–264
Häfliger, Franz, Dr chem.
  37, 42, 50
Healy, David, Dr med. (1954–) 4,
  61, 270–272
Heidegger, Martin, philosopher
  (1889–1976) 28,
  152–153, 156
Heimann, Hans, Dr med.
  (1922–2006) 149, 269
heredity 32–33, 167n.195, 238
Herzog, Heinrich, junior
  (1906–1995) 25
Herzog, Heinrich, senior 25
historicisation 2, 15, 249–250,
  270–274
historiography 3–5, 49, 61–62,
  110–112, 269–273
Hofmann, Albert, Dr chem.
  (1906–2008) 36
Hoffmann-La Roche see Roche
Höppli, Gottlieb, cantonal
  councilman (1916–2009) 26
Huber, Doris (pseudonym)
  102–103
Husserl, Edmund, philosopher
  (1859–1938) 28

incidents (complications) 56, 59,
  94, 121–122, 134, 141–147,
  229–248, 291–292, 299
ineffectiveness 51, 58–59, 136,
  290, 297
informed consent 125, 292

institutionalised and foster children
  100–101, 109, 114n.23,
  114n.26, 137
Intercantonal Office for the
  Control of Medicines (IKS),
  later Swissmedic see approval
  authorities
inventory of substances 55, 67,
  143, 168–176, 278n.107

Janssen Pharmaceutica 141,
  163n.118

Kefauver, Estes (1903–1963) 121
Kefauver-Harris Amendment
  121–122
Kielholz, Paul, Prof. Dr med.
  (1916–1990) 82, 150, 217
Klaesi, Jakob, Prof. Dr med.
  (1883–1930) 27–29,
  31, 37, 81
Klara, nurse (pseudonym) 67,
  168–169, 171
Kline, Nathan S., Dr med.
  (1916–1983) 81
Koechlin, Carl (1889–1969) 63
Koechlin, Hartmann 63
Krebser, Adolf, Dr chem.
  65–66, 126
Kreis, Arthur (1896–1969) 22
Kuhn, Ernst (1874–1969) 27
Kuhn-Gebhart, Verena, Dr med.
  (1921–2015) 6, 8, 13, 22,
  33–35, 52, 56, 97, 100–104,
  109, 118, 128, 137, 176,
  187, 216–218, 253, 255,
  268, 272, 286–287,
  296, 300

laboratory, laboratory staff 22,
  37, 42, 50, 53, 71, 124, 150,
  180, 184–185, 210, 240,
  251, 262
Lang, Deborah (pseudonym)
  239–240
Langer, Gerhard 269

Lausanne, Psychiatric University Hospital 61
law, legal regulations 25, 121, 123–124, 151, 156, 186–187, 197, 203–204, 213, 229, 254, 259, 260, 268, 280, 291, 298
Linder, Sarah (pseudonym) 242
Lingg, Albert, Dr med. (1949–) 272
Littenheid, private clinic 96
lobotomy 24, 56, 292
Löffler, Wilhelm, Prof. Dr med. (1887–1972) 33
Luban-Plozza, Boris, Prof. Dr med. (1923–2002) 256
Lundbeck AG 126

Maître, Laurent, Dr 261
Maldiney, Henri, Prof. Dr med. (1912–2013) 152
marketing 3, 5, 7, 38, 42, 122, 126, 204
Mathilde, head nurse 21, 286
medications, drugs (substances available on the market)
 advertising 55, 64, 87n.87, 120, 252
 distribution 64, 87n.87, 265
 sales 36, 41, 59, 60–61, 63–66, 121, 124, 184, 198, 200, 254
Merck AG 126, 254
mergers, company 7, 138–139, 162n.110, 197–199, 223n.33, 251, 282
Muggli, Alfred, Dr med., Kantonsarzt (1940–) 265
Müller, Jakob, Dr iur., state council member (1895–1967) 27, 31
Münchenbuchsee, Private Clinic 201

narcotics 5, 74, 127
neuroleptics 4, 13, 42, 49, 52, 54, 62–63, 84n.26, 97, 119, 127, 141–147, 174, 232, 241–243, 261, 280, 295–296

non-compliance *see* resistance
Nufer, Kurt, Dr med., cantonal physician (1916–1978) 267
Nuremburg Code 290, 300n.1
nursing staff *see* clinic staff
nutrition, nourishment 40, 144–145, 154

observation, clinical 39, 53, 56, 71, 119, 122, 130, 146, 149, 151–154, 213, 219, 240, 256, 265, 270, 281, 291, 294–296
off-label testing 216, 220
Onken, Thomas, Great Council member (1941–2000) 263
outpatient department (clinic, facility, centre) 24, 30, 32, 53, 95–97, 100, 108, 113n.14, 114n.27, 137, 162n.103, 169–170, 176–177, 178, 187, 191n.47, 194n.73, 209, 243, 286

patents 8, 126–127, 129, 297
patients
 as clinic employees 22, 101–102
 groups 97–98
 hierarchies 17n.28, 76, 97–98, 105, 146, 233–234, 293, 296–297
 numbers (patient population) 53, 94–97
pharmaceutical industry 2–8, 13–15, 19, 35–37, 43n.20, 49, 81, 104, 121–125, 154–156, 178, 180, 182–188, 197–198, 203–204, 207, 214, 220, 222n.31, 230, 232, 234, 236, 241, 250–251, 260, 264, 265, 267–268, 273n.3, 280, 283, 286, 288–289, 294, 297
physician (assistant physician, senior physician, leading physician) 8, 14–15, 20–23, 28–34, 38, 43n.20, 51, 53, 56, 66, 71, 76–77, 79, 81, 97, 124, 154, 178, 182,

185–186, 191n.44, 194n.73,
194n.78, 200–201, 207, 210,
212, 214, 219, 231, 239,
242–243, 266, 272, 285,
287, 295
pilot tests, rapid testing 11, 67,
149, 172, 206, 283, 289
placebo 5, 41, 119, 136, 150–151,
153, 204–205, 257,
259–260, 289–290, 299
practitioner, general (family
physician, family doctor) 33,
40, 96, 118, 129, 138, 156,
175, 176, 177, 218, 235,
253, 262, 267, 287
prioritisation of evaluated
cases 10–11
psychiatrist, privately practicing
15, 33, 96, 110, 106, 176,
201, 251–253, 256–257,
268, 282, 284
psychoanalysis 27–29, 104,
166n.185, 299
psychosis 52–53, 56–57, 59, 61,
81, 141–142, 153, 218,
220, 238
psychotherapy 82, 102, 105,
129–130, 154, 287, 293, 299

Räber, Christine (pseudonym)
238–240
registration *see* drug approval,
drug registration
Reiber, Ernst, medical services
director (1901–1997) 26
Reimann, Hans (pseudonym) 76
relatives, family of patients 14, 18,
33, 40, 41, 77, 96, 104, 106,
108, 138, 154, 174–175,
177, 236–238, 240–241,
266, 287, 292
remunerations from the
pharmaceutical industry *see*
clinical trials
Renz, Bruno (pseudonym) 104–105
Renz, Heinz (pseudonym) 104–105

resistance (non-compliance) 39–40,
107–110, 112, 235, 293
Reutemann, Carl 21
Rickels, Karl, Prof. Dr med.
(1924–) 215
Roche 35–37, 54–55, 126–127,
234, 251, 258, 261, 283
Rorschach test 28–29, 33, 34, 152,
166n.186, 186, 285
Rosegg Psychiatric Clinic in the
Canton of Solothurn 31

Sainte-Anne Psychiatric Hospital in
Paris 51
Sandoz AG 7, 35–36, 54, 58,
65, 97, 110, 141–146, 148,
156, 174, 184, 198, 251,
261, 283
Schenker, Hans, Dr med., cantonal
physician (1926–2000)
262–265, 268, 291, 298
Schindler, Walter, Dr chem.
37, 42, 70
schizophrenia 29, 51–52, 54, 56,
58–59, 62, 69, 72, 76, 78,
96, 98–99, 113n.13,
142–143, 145, 159n.47,
218–219, 227n.114,
227n.116, 231, 234, 237,
243, 277n.106, 284, 295
Schmidlin, Paul, Dr med. 48–49,
60–64, 66–68, 70, 270
self-historicisation vii–viii, 15, 62,
76–77, 152, 249, 252–253,
269, 273
sex, gender 20–21, 72, 201, 209,
284, 296
Shorter, Edward (1941–) 4–5, 270
sidechains 70, 117, 127, 141,
258, 289
side-effects 10, 19, 38, 51, 57–58,
67, 72, 74–75, 89, 98, 110,
119–122, 127–128, 131,
133–134, 146, 148, 150, 170,
201–203, 229, 231–234,
280–281, 294, 297

Staehelin, John E., Prof. Dr med. (1891–1969) 52
standard therapy 138, 140, 143, 150, 201, 205, 296
statistics 71, 73, 79–80, 82, 94, 98, 123–124, 135, 136, 148–153, 155, 202, 205, 213, 259–260, 280, 289, 294
Stenzl, Hans, Dr chem. 37
structures, chemical 58, 68, 70–71, 117–118, 152, 239
Studer, Karl, Dr med. 249
supervision (monitoring) 23, 39, 94, 96–97, 103, 109, 118, 120, 134, 153, 167n.198, 176, 242–243, 282, 286, 291, 294, 298
Suter, Rita (pseudonym) 216–217
Swiss Academy of Medical Sciences (SAMS) 122, 205–206, 237, 263, 280, 290
Swiss Asylum for Epileptics in Zurich 32, 78
Swissmedic *see* Intercantonal Office for the Control of Medicines
symposium, in St Moritz 202, 215, 218

Tanner, Ulrich (pseudonym) 243
Tobler, Silvia (pseudonym) 100–101
tolerability testing 98, 123, 131–133, 148, 158n.27, 158n.33, 160n.71, 200, 232–233, 256, 289, 296
toxicology, toxicology testing 14, 38, 67, 121, 122–124, 131–133, 135, 139, 158n.27, 158n.36, 159n.43, 161n.71, 162n.110, 201, 205, 249n.40, 290
Traber, Franz (pseudonym) 92–97, 108–112

tranquiliser 54, 125, 127, 153, 142, 144, 280
Tuchschmid, Anna (pseudonym) 240
Tuchschmid, Walter, cantonal and national councillor (1893–1963) 26

Vogt, Frieda (pseudonym) 99

Waldau, Psychiatric University Hospital Bern 22, 27–28, 31, 37, 81–82, 201
Wander AG 7, 147, 198, 238–239, 242–244, 251, 283
wards, clinic 23, 55–56, 75, 77–79, 92, 94, 96–97, 99, 108, 115n.47, 116n.55, 129–130, 143, 154, 169, 178, 209, 224n.62, 231–232, 242, 287, 293
Weber, Arnold, Prof. Dr med. (1894–1976) 28
Wenger, Josef (pseudonym) 234–235
Wild, Fräulein (pseudonym) 107
Wilhelm, Max 255, 258
Wille, Hermann, Dr med. (1868–1958) 23–24
Woggon, Brigitte, Prof. Dr med. (1943–2019) 206
Wyeth AG 115n.39, 283
Wyrsch, Jakob, Prof. Dr med. (1963–1982) 28, 81–82

Zihlschlacht, Sanatorium Friedheim, from 1962 Psychiatric Private Clinic Friedheim 33, 96
Zolliker, Adolf, Dr med. (1904–1974) 13, 20, 22–23, 25, 31–33, 38–39, 66, 143, 178–180, 185, 207, 209, 234, 239, 265–267, 282

EU authorised representative for GPSR:
Easy Access System Europe, Mustamäe tee 50,
10621 Tallinn, Estonia
gpsr.requests@easproject.com